COMMON EYE INFECTIONS

Edited by **Imtiaz A. Chaudhry**

Common Eye Infections
http://dx.doi.org/10.5772/45964
Edited by Imtiaz A. Chaudhry

Contributors

Maria C Jimenez-Martínez, Concepcion Santacruz-Valdes, Sergio Estrada-Parra, Mayra Perez-Tapia, Angel Nava, Victor M Bautista-De Lucio, Atzin Robles-Contreras, Oscar Baca-Lozada, Hector Perez-Cano, Alejandro Babayan-Sosa, Virginia Vanzzini, Adnan Haq, Haseebullah Wardak, Narbeh Kraskian, Udo Ubani, Brygida Kwiatkowska, Maria Kazimiera Maślińska, Ana Lilia Perez-Balbuena, Monika Fida, Allma Kocinaj, Xhevdet Krasniqi, Arjeta Grezda, Flora Abazi, Imtiaz A. Chaudhry, Waleed Abduaziz Al-Rashed, Yonca Arat, Osama Al-Shaikh, Hassan Al-Dhibi, Hani Al-Mezaine, Wael Abdelghani

Published by InTech

Janeza Trdine 9, 51000 Rijeka, Croatia

Publishing Process Manager Sandra Bakic
Technical Editor InTech DTP team
Cover InTech Design team

Additional hard copies can be obtained from orders@intechopen.com

Common Eye Infections, Edited by Imtiaz A. Chaudhry
p. cm.
ISBN 978-953-51-0926-6

For EU product safety concerns:
IN TECH d.o.o., Prolaz Marije Krucifikse Kozulić 3, 51000 Rijeka, Croatia,
info@intechopen.com or visit our website at intechopen.com.

Meet the editor

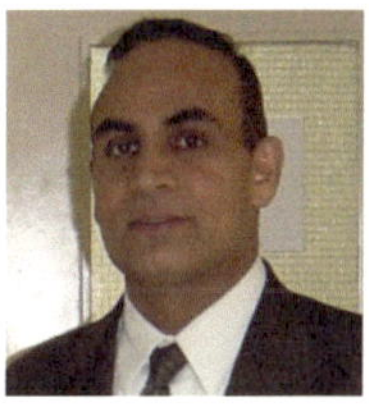

Dr. Imtiaz A. Chaudhry received his MD and PhD degrees from The University of Utah School of Medicine in Salt Lake City. He completed his Internship in Internal Medicine at Yale University School of Medicine and a Residency in Ophthalmology at the prestigious Yale Eye Center, Yale University School of Medicine Department of Ophthalmology and Visual Sciences. Subsequently, he completed his Fellowship in Ophthalmic Plastic and Reconstructive Surgery from Baylor College of Medicine in Houston in 2000. Over the past decade, Dr. Chaudhry has acquired enormous skills in patient care, surgical management of complicated patients, research, teaching and leadership in the field of Ophthalmology. He has enjoyed further expertise in his field by traveling overseas, interacting and teaching other doctors about his advanced techniques of treating many conditions in the field of Ophthalmic Plastic and Reconstructive Surgery. Over these years, his patients have included ambassadors, foreign diplomats and heads of states. During this time, Dr. Chaudhry has helped in training over 50 Ophthalmology residents and 10 Fellows in Oculoplastic Surgery. He has made his presentations in the domestic as well as overseas meetings in the field of Ophthalmic Plastic and Reconstructive Surgery and has taught courses at the American Academy of Ophthalmology and World Ophthalmology Congress. Because of his contribution to the advancement of knowledge in the field of Ophthalmology, American Academy of Ophthalmology honored him with the prestigious "Achievement Award" in 2008. This award honors physicians that exemplify academic success, a high standard of patient care, and surgical expertise.

Contents

Preface

Since ocular infections are one of the most frequent occurrences in ophthalmology, the treatment for these infections must be fast, precise and effective. In order to address this goal, it is important to identify and characterize the culprit microorganisms involved in the pathogenesis of ocular infections. Clinical diagnosis of ocular infections can be confirmed by several techniques based on microbiological test of ocular samples. Some of these techniques include classic microbiological testing in which it is necessary to isolate microorganisms to characterize them by biochemical analysis which require significant resources and timing. Molecular biology techniques on the other hand, such as PCR, real time PCR, microarrays and aptamers (e.g. SOMAmers) can offer the results in a shorter period of time, while keeping a much higher sensitivity and specificity. Recently, mass spectrometry approach has dramatically changed the microbiological field. Some of the advantages of microbiological identification by mass spectrometry include: lack of need for culture and isolation of the microorganisms. Further, fastidious microorganisms can be identified without lengthy wait for their growth. High sensitivity and accuracy for the microorganism identification results in a reduction of sample amount required. And resistance markers and resistance profile can be determined at the same time of identification analysis. In summary, the evolution of microbiological identification methods has improved treatments that impact in the prognosis of ocular infection, reducing complications and avoiding blindness cases, and as a consequence life quality of patients will be better. In the chapter, "Diagnostics Methods in Ocular Infections: From Microorganism Culture to Molecular Methods," Drs. Manuel, Mariana, Antonio, Luz, Carolina, Gustavo, Aurora and Herlinda, discuss current conventional methods for microorganisms identification by the use of cultures, isolation and phenotypic characteristics along-with endpoint PCR, real-time PCR.

Infective conjunctivitis can be acute or chronic and can be caused by several bacterial and viral pathogens. Bacterial conjunctivitis is a relatively common infection and affects all people, although a higher incidence is seen in infants, school children and the elderly. Bacterial conjunctivitis has a higher prevalence in children, and although its incidence is continuing to decrease in developing nations, periodic rises in incidence are seen during the monsoon seasons in many countries such as Bangladesh, and thus, bacterial conjunctivitis is the most common cause of infective conjunctivitis in developing nations. In the developed world, acute infectious conjunctivitis is a common presentation in the primary care setting and many general practitioners may find it difficult to differentiate between bacterial and viral conjunctivitis. The uncertainty of the pathogenic cause of acute conjunctivitis has led to the routine practice of prescribing a broad spectrum antibiotic topically even though the pathogen has not been proved to be bacterial in nature. A diagnosis of conjunctivitis is usually made on the basis of a clinical history and examination by the general practitioner since conjunctivitis is often a self limiting illness and the antibiotics currently used have a good spectrum of pathogen coverage. Swabs and cultures may be indicated in vital situations where a correct diagnosis may be necessary to rule out more serious causes and medical emergencies that would require hospital admission. Such cases may include bacterial keratitis. Hyperacute bacterial conjunctivitis is commonly seen in patients affected with N. Gonorrhoea. The onset is often rapid with an exaggerated form of conjunctival injection, chemosis and copious purulent discharge. Prompt treatment is essential to prevent complications. Chronic bacterial conjunctivitis, ie, red eye with purulent discharge persisting for longer than a few weeks, is generally caused by Chlamydia trachomatis or may be associated with dacryocystitis. Bacterial keratitis is a well known but rare complication of bacterial conjunctivitis. Herpes simplex conjunctivitis is due to a viral pathogens symptoms of which may include a red eye, photophobia, eye pain and mucoid discharge. Herpes zoster ophthalmicus causes shingles of the opthalmic branch of the trigeminal nerve, which innervates the cornea and the tip of the nose. It begins with unilateral neuralgia, followed by a vesicular rash in the distribution of nerve. Once spread to the eye, it may lead to an extremely painful conjunctivitis. Neonatal Conjunctivitis also known as ophthalmia neonatorum is inflammation of the conjunctiva occurring in the first month of life and is caused by a number of different pathogens that may include bacteria, viruses and chemical agents. In recent times prophylaxis has led to decreased morbidity in the developed world. In their chapter, "Infective Conjunctivitis - its Pathogenesis, Management and Complications," Drs. Haq, Wardak and Kraskian describe various causes of infectious conjunctivitis along with its treatment modalities. The authors emphasize that the general practitioners must remain vigilant when diagnosing viral from bacterial conjunctivitis and try to ensure that patient education of the condition is at an optimum level to prevent spread.

Treatment of infectious and allergic conjunctivitis can be challenging because of the diverse infectious agents and immunological mechanisms which can result in the damage of the ocular surface causing significant visual disability. Currently, a wide range of antibiotic and antiallergic topical medications are available and can be confusing due to lack of improvement at the ocular surface in terms of avoiding anatomical changes in severe cases and control of symptoms in the long run. In the chapter, "Treatments in Infectious and Allergic Conjunctivitis: Is Immunomodulation the Future?," Drs. Santacruz, Perez-Tapia, Nava, Estrada-Parra and Jimenez-Martinez, investigate the novel and developing therapies, with special emphasis in immunomodulatory drugs/molecules that could have clinical indication in the treatment of infectious and allergic conjunctivitis in future.

Both the bacterial and fungal keratitis as well as corneal ulceration may be vision threatening ocular condition requiring prompt and accurate diagnosis and early medical intervention to obtain a reasonable outcome. Since keratitis caused by Gram negative bacteria and some fungal pathogens may clinically seem very similar by signs and symptoms, the help which the microbiology service can provide in the differentiation of two entities may be very crucial. Obviously the treatment required by these causative agents require different drugs. Keratitis caused by Gram positive bacteria and yeast like fungus may be too similar in inflammatory signs, however in this cases one smear can make the difference. In Neisseria gonohorroae keratitis, delayed laboratory confirmation of the correct diagnosis may carry a high risk because of the corneal tissue loss since keratitis due to these organisms may not respond well to the commonly applied empirical antibiotics. Other options for detection of yeast or filamentous fungi in corneal samples are PCR techniques especially in cases of previous antibiotics or antifungal therapy and despite having negative cultures. High- resolution melting technique can detect and differentiate yeast and filamentous fungi in keratomycose samples in a more simple, specific and cost- efficient methods. It is very important for the best prognosis in keratitis cases, to confirm the clinical diagnosis by the laboratory work since the first consultation, for to start immediately the specific medical topical treatment. For all those reasons the laboratory support in the clinical diagnosis of keratitis is very important in order to achieve a shorter evaluation time and to avoid any corneal scarring resulting in a reasonable visual prognosis in patients suffering from any infectious keratitis. In their chapter, "Laboratory in the Diagnosis of Bacterial and Fungal Keratitis," Drs. Zago and Perez-Balbuena discuss the role of laboratory in the diagnosis of infectious keratitis.

Microbial keratitis can be a very serious infection that can result in significant visual disability around the world with estimates ranging from 11 cases to almost 800 per 100,000 persons depending on the country and geography. Wide geographical variation exists in the epidemiology of microbial keratitis based on economic and climatic factors. Almost any microorganism can invade the corneal stroma if the normal corneal defense mechanisms are compromised. A wide spectrum of microbial organisms can produce corneal infections and, consequently, the therapeutic strategies adopted for its treatment may be varied. Several potential risk factors such as contact lenses, trauma, aqueous tear deficiencies, neurotrophic keratopathy, eyelid alterations or malposition, decreased immunologic defenses, use of topical corticoid medications and surgery may cause the development of bacterial keratitis. Trauma is a major risk factor for corneal infection in developing countries and the main risk factor for bacterial keratitis in developed countries is the use of contact lenses, particularly extended-wear contact lenses. In the chapter, "Bacterial Keratitis Infection: A Battle between Virulence Factors and the Immune Response,"Drs. Robles-Contreras, Perez-Cano, Babayan-Sosa and Baca-Lozada provide an extensive review of the most common corneal bacterial infections that cause the diseases along with the involvement of the immune system and its regulatory mechanisms which prevent tissue damage. The authors discuss bacterial virulence factors which help the microorganism in evading the host defense mechanisms. There are several clinical features which can be observed in setting of infections due to bacterial keratitis as a result of their unique immunological mechanisms which are evident at the ocular surface when observed carefully. The chapter also focusses on the regulatory defense mechanisms which the host utilizes to minimize the damage caused by the bacterial pathogens.

In the chapter, "Preseptal Cellulitis," Drs. Fida, Kocinaj, Abazi and Grezda, discuss infections of the periorbital area anterior to the septum also called preseptal cellulitis. This is a common infection which tends to be a less severe disease than orbital cellulitis. Preseptal cellulitis can result from the spread of the upper respiratory tract infection, external eye infection or eyelid trauma. Patients with preseptal cellulitis present with acute eyelid erythema and edema along with pain in the absence of any obvious proptosis. The diagnosis is usually made based upon the clinical findings, microbiological and radiological examination. The most common microorganisms causing preseptal cellulitis are Staphylococcus aureus, Staphylococcus epidermidis, Streptococcus species, and anaerobes, known organisms that commonly cause upper respiratory tract infections and external eyelid infections. Cold weather and upper respiratory tract infections are sometimes correlated with increased frequency of sinusitis. Untreated preseptal cellulitis can lead to orbital cellulitis which can be a serious infection especially in children and can result in significant complications including blindness, cavernous sinus thrombosis, meningitis, subdural empyema, and intracranial abscess. The correct treatment of the preseptal cellulitis during the antibiotic era makes these complications less likely but the correct diagnoses and early treatment is important to prevent the life threatening complications. The authors emphasize on the difficulty in distinguishing preseptal cellulitis from orbital cellulitis based just on clinical findings especially in children. In such cases, imaging studies may be helpful in delineating preseptal cellulitis from orbital cellulitis. Antibiotics may be necessary to treat prespetal cellulitis and in certain cases, eyelid abscesses may need to be drained surgically with the incision and drainage while avoiding damage to the critical structures.

Patients with orbital cellulitis may present with swelling of the eyelids, pain, proptosis, conjunctival chemosis, limitation of eye movements and decreased vision. In most patients, the most common predisposing factor for such infection is sinus disease, particularly in the younger age group. Despite advances in diagnosis and in anti-microbial therapy and modern surgical techniques, complications from orbital cellulitis can result. After sinusitis, periocular trauma and history of ocular or periocular surgery are the most common cause of orbital cellulitis. Less common causes of orbital cellulitis include dacryocystitis, dental infection, endophthalmitis and retained orbital foreign bodies. Meningitis and death may be the most feared complication of untreated or undertreated orbital cellulitis. Imaging studies can influence the initial therapeutic plan by demonstrating the size and the location of the abscess. Commonly reported bacteria from the abscesses of the infected orbit may include S. aureus, S. epidermidis, Streptococci, Diphtheroids, H. influenza, E. Coli, multiple species including aerobes and anaerobes. Intravenous antibiotics are usually started once the diagnosis of orbital cellulitis is suspected. Broad-spectrum antibiotics that cover most gram positive and gram negative bacteria are selected initially. In addition to starting intravenous antibiotics, emergent drainage of the orbital abscess has been suggested in patients with compromised vision regardless of patient age. Timely drainage has been recommended for large abscesses, for extensive superior or inferior orbital abscesses, for patients with intracranial complications, for infections of known dental origin in which anaerobes might be expected. In the chapter, "Diagnosis and Management of Orbital Cellulitis," Drs. Chaudhry, Al-Rashed, Al-Sheikh and Arat, emphasize on an individualized therapeutic approach which requires clinician to carefully follow patients with orbital cellulitis and expected abscess. They recommend surgical option when improvement does not occur as expected based on medical treatment. Surgical treatment may be indicated for significant underlying sinus disease, orbital or subperiosteal abscess or both in the younger age group when no improvement occurs as expected. In the adults, sinus surgery remains the most common surgical intervention when there is no improvement with initial systemic antibiotics. The authors mention that the mechanism for loss of vision in orbital cellulitis may involve optic neuritis, ischemia, or compressive effects. Cavernous sinus thrombosis represents the most severe form of postseptal cellulitis which may be suspected clinically by bilateral disease with ophthalmoplegia and loss of vision. Proper management of these patients may include a multidisciplinary team that may include an orbital surgeon, otolaryngologists, neurosurgeon, and infectious disease expert.

Non-Tuberculosis Mycobacteria (NTM), also called "Atypical Mycobacteria" are ubiquitous in soil and water and have been found as normal flora of skin, sputum, and gastric contents. These bacteria are resistant to common disinfectants such as chlorine, formaldehyde and glutaraldehyde. NTM-caused keratitis is rare, having devastating complications along with a diagnostic and therapeutic challenge. Infectious keratitis due to NTM have been reported in several isolated cases as well as in outbreaks. NTM can cause infections of all adnexal and ocular tissues including cornea, iris, lens, retina, choroid and optic nerve. Refractive as well as therapeutic surgical procedures such as LASIK, LASEK, PRK and PKP constitute a risk factor for infection by these organisms. Several factors may contribute to the development of NTM keratitis following corneal procedures. Mycobacterium chelonei, M. abscessus, M. fortuitum, M. szulgai, and M. mucogenicum have been reported usually as the result of improper asepsis. Most NTM infections are caused by M. chelonae and M. fortuitum, belong to the rapid growers group. NTM keratitis can often be mistaken with other bacterial infections that cause non-suppurative keratitis having similar clinical features. In such situations, differential diagnosis include, fungal keratitis, infectious crystalline keratopathy, Nocardia keratitis, herpes simplex virus, and rarely Acanthamoeba keratitis. The principal differential diagnosis must be made between fungal and Nocardia keratitis. Keratitis caused by atypical Mycobacteria is characterized by an indolent course and poor response to antibiotics. The diagnosis requires a high index of suspicion since the early diagnosis of NTM may not be an easy one because the overlying, un-involved corneal stroma may hinder obtaining of sufficient material for culture. Further, such organisms can only be detectable by culture on special media such as Lowenstein-Jensen, and be identified by special stains like Ziehl-Neelsen. In the chapter, "Nontuberculous Mycobacterial Keratitis," Drs. Pérez-Balbuena, Ancona-Lezama and Gutiérrez-Sánchez, focus on keratitis caused by NTM, since a great number of recent clinical reports of NTM ocular infections in the form of keratitis have been reported. The authors describe their 10 years of clinical experience in the diagnosis and treatment of NTM keratitis from México. They substantiate their experience by providing a descriptive retrospective case series of five patients with NTM keratitis treated in their service. Almost all cases of their NTM keratitis had a previous history of surgery, specifically LASIK and PKP. The average age of their patients was of 36.6 years with a range from 12 to 58 years. The average time that took from the onset of symptoms to the establishment of correct diagnosis was over 4 weeks. Antibiotic resistance continues to be an emerging problem in the treatment of NTM keratitis. The authors emphasize the need for vigilance in the follow-up of patients having infectious keratitis. Appropriate adjustment of antimicrobial therapy may be required based on cultures and sensitivity tests when NTM are responsible for keratitis. The authors believe that fourth-generation fluoroquinolones combined with first-line antibiotics constitute the best option to treat NTM keratitis.

Endophthalmitis is one of the most feared ocular infection which may have potential to cause visual, cosmetic and even serious life threatening complications if not diagnosed and treated on a timely basis. Description of epidemiology of endophthalmitis, its diagnosis, management and study of its complications may help in the prognostic evaluation of patients presenting to a clinician. Endophthalmitis is a vital ocular emergency in which most of the patients present with complaints of decreased vision, photophobia, pain or ophthalmoplegia. Any of the clinical features such as decreased visual acuity, chemosis, external ophthalmoplegia, along with radiological evidence of endophthalmitis may require prompt action. Factors responsible for endophthalmitis which may affect the outcome include, demographic such as age, gender, recent and past medical or surgical history and any underlying conditions which might have contributed to the onset of endophthalmitis. In particular, presence of diabetes, cardiac disease, renal disease, organ transplantation, immunodeficiency status and malignancy may enhance chances of having endogenous endophthalmitis. Other risk factors for endophthalmitis include, a recent ocular surgery, trauma, a recent dental procedure, intravenous drug administration, intravenous catheters or indwelling devices. Endophthalmitis is a complex disease and can be caused by a large number of bacterial species, requiring a rapid identification of the causative organism along with the primary infected site. In some cases, the culture of the vitreous samples may not grow any bacteria probably due to the effect of prior antibiotics, nevertheless vitreous biopsy should be considered because a culture of the vitreous sample is more often useful for identifying the responsible bacteria. Visual prognosis of patients with endophthalmitis depends mainly on the underlying microorganisms, which is particularly poor in cases of infection with Gram-positive bacteria or Aspergillus species. There is a trend toward early vitrectomy because of the advancement of vitreous surgery. While the roles of intra-vitreal antibiotics and vitrectomy are evolving and may become more widely accepted as therapeutic modalities in some cases of endogenous endophthalmitis, early antibiotic therapy remains the cornerstone of treatment. In the chapter, "Endophthalmitis: Experience from a Tertiary Eye Care Center," Drs. Chaudhry, Al-Dhibi, Al-Rashed, Al-Mezaine, Arat and Abdelghani, describe their expert opinion of diagnosing and treating endophthalmitis from different causes.

Rheumatoid arthritis is an autoimmune connective tissue disease that manifests itself mostly with symmetrical swelling of the joints characterized by the inflammation of the connective tissue, usually of autoimmunological origin. Although most of the symptoms of the rheumatic diseases concern primarily musculoskeletal system, in many of these disorders pathological changes take also place in various other organs including the eye. Ocular adenxa and the eye may be affected secondary to vascular changes occurring in the course of the primary inflammation or may be the result of complications arising from the therapy of the rheumatic disease. The rheumatoid arthritis and spondyloarthropathies are the most common inflammatory rheumatic diseases. Significantly less frequently juvenile idiopathic arthritis, Sjögren's syndrome, systemic lupus erythematosus and other less frequent connective tissue diseases as scleroderma, dermato-and polymiositis, recurrent inflammation of the cartilage and systemic vasculitis are observed. Patients with different autoimmune disorders may present with conjunctivitis, episcleritis, scleritis, keratitis and uveitis. Impaired secretion of tears occur in all patients with Sjögren's syndrome - either in the initial or more advanced stages of the disease - and constitute one of to the diagnostic criteria. Treatment is based on the use of both symptomatic drugs - moistening eyes and mouth - and of immunosuppressants. Patients with scleroderma may develop secondary Sjorgren's syndrome and symptoms of dry eye. In the course of systemic vasculitis such as polyarteritis nodosa, Churga-Strauss syndrome, Wegener's granulomatosis, Behçet's disease, Takayasu disease, giant cell arteritis and Cogan syndrome there are changes in the eye and ocular adenxa may occur due to vascular changes. The ocular changes in the course of inflammation of the large vessels, such as giant cell arteritis, are mainly associated with ischemia of optic nerve or retina. The treatment of all systemic vasculitis requires aggressive immunosuppressive therapy and high doses of glucocorticoids. Chronic glucocortycoid therapy often leads to cataracts, and glaucoma. In the course of the infection with Chlamydia trachomatis, chronic conjunctivitis may occur in some patients. Clinical symptoms of chlamydial conjunctivitis in reactive arthritis are characterized by moderate redness of an eye, tearing, photophobia and decreased vision. Bacterial keratitis in rheumatic diseases often is a complicated by erosive lesions of the cornea most commonly associated with primary and secondary Sjögren's syndrome. In recent days, many biological drugs have proved effective in the treatment of ocular manifestations of many rheumatic diseases and the exclusion of potential infection is particularly important for the choice of treatment and safety of therapy. In their chapter, "Eye Infection Complications in Rheumatic Diseases," Drs. Kwiatkowska and Maślińska discuss kinds of eye and adnexal complications as a result of various rheumatological disorders.

Trachoma is the leading infectious cause of preventable blindness in the world which is distributed primarily in tropical developing countries including North and sub-Saharan Africa, the Middle East, and the Northern Indian subcontinent. The infection is caused by Chlamydia trachomatis, an obligate intracellular parasite. Children and young women of childbearing age in the low socioeconomic status in areas of poor hygiene are considered to be the primary source of recurrent infections by C. trachomatis. Trachoma has been classified by WHO into 5 classes depending on the severity of the infection. For example in the active stage of the disease (TF), only follicles can be seen in the tarsal conjunctiva, in the trachomatous inflammation (TI), pronounce inflammatory thickening of upper tarsal conjunctiva can be noticed, in the trachomtous scarring (TS), scarring of the tarsal conjunctiva in the form of white band can be noticed, in the trachomatous trichiasis (TT), eye lashes rub the eyeball and in the corneal opacity (CO) stage, one can easily see a visible corneal scar. A presumptive diagnosis of trachoma can be made based on clinical features, especially in an area where trachoma is considered to be present. The World Health Assembly has resolved to eliminate blinding trachoma by the year 2020. To this, the Global Alliance for the Elimination of Blinding Trachoma (GET2020) was formed in 1998. Control activities focus on the implementation of the SAFE strategy, surgery for trichiasis, antibiotics for infection, facial cleanliness (hygiene promotion) and environmental improvements, to reduce transmission of the organism. Each of these components tackles the pathway to blindness at different stages. Antibiotics for treatment of active trachoma may be given locally or systematically, but topical treatment is preferred because: It is cheaper, there is no risk of systemic side-effects, and Local antibiotics are also effective against bacterial conjunctivitis which may be associated with trachoma. Transmission of trachoma is closely associated with personal hygiene and environmental sanitation. In the chapter, "Trachoma and Inclusion Conjunctivitis," the authors nicely outline detailed clinical features, diagnostic strategies with available testing and the effectiveness of the current treatment strategies in the management of trachoma.

Imtiaz A. Chaudhry, MD PhD FACS
Houston Oculoplastics Associates
Memorial Hermann Medical Plaza
Texas Medical Center
Houston, Texas,
United States of America

Chapter 1

Diagnostics Methods in Ocular Infections–From Microorganism Culture to Molecular Methods

Victor Manuel Bautista-de Lucio,
Mariana Ortiz-Casas,
Luis Antonio Bautista-Hernández,
Nadia Luz López-Espinosa, Carolina Gaona-Juárez,
Ángel Gustavo Salas-Lais,
Dulce Aurora Frausto-del Río and
Herlinda Mejía-López

Additional information is available at the end of the chapter

http://dx.doi.org/10.5772/52468

1. Introduction

1.1. Conventional methods of microbiological diagnosis: Culture, isolation and phenotypic identification

Despite advances in the medical field, 4 of the 10 leading causes of death worldwide are due to infectious diseases [1]. At the eye, infections are one of the most common diseases, and bacterias are the first causative agent, followed by fungus and virus. Between these bacterias, *Staphylococcus* genus, *Streptococcus genus, Corinebacterium sp, Chlamydia sp, Pseudomonas aeruginosa, Escherichia coli, Enterococcus sp, Serratia sp*are frequent in keratitis, conjunctivitis, endophthalmitis and cornea ulcer [2]; *Fusarium sp, Aspergillus sp* and *Candida sp,* are the commonly fungus found in keratitis infections [3]; *Adenovirus, HSV-1 (Herpes Simplex Virus-1), HSV-2 (Herpes Simplex Virus-2), VZV (Varicella Zoster Virus), HPV (Human Papilloma Virus)* are important in conjunctivitis and keratitis [4].

In order to reduce complications from ocular infectious diseases is very important to provide appropriate early treatment. To make this possible, is essential microbiological identification of the causative agent of infection in the shortest time possible. However, the microbiological diagnosis by conventional methods considered as gold standards, based on the culture followed by phenotypic identification of the microorganism once isolated, taken between 48 and 72 hours, depending on the requirements of the microorganism, and in the case of fungal infections, identifying and obtaining the antifungal susceptibility profile, come to take over a week. Identification time may be reduced by using automated equipment whose bases are the same as those used for manual identification, through biochemical profile of microorganisms. These tests are based on the ability to ferment, oxidize, degrade or hydrolyze different substrates or to grow on different carbon sources producing changes in pH that may be monitored using compounds that turn color depending on the pH. Automated systems work with cards containing dehydrated culture media with suitable substrates. Culture time elapses while the cards are automatically read and data are collected by a system confronts the data collected with a database through the microorganism is identified. Among the available automated identification systems are the VITEK 2 (bioMérieux, France) and BD Phoenix (USA), these Systems reduce time of identification to 6-12 h.

Although the main disadvantage is the time it takes the identification, cultivation allows the discovery of new or atypical strains, conservation of strains for further characterization and the ability to determine the antimicrobial susceptibility directly [5].

Given the urgency with which requires identification of microorganisms other strategies have been designed which further reduce the periods of time. These include the identification by endpoint PCR, real time PCR, microarrays and mass spectrometry directed to the detection of proteins or nucleic acids.

1.1.1. Endpoint PCR and real time PCR

Although the identification of microorganisms through culture is the gold standard this methodology presents some complications that are resolved using molecular biology techniques such as endpoint PCR and real time PCR, significantly reducing the outcome of days to a couple of hours. The identification of microorganisms using traditional microbiology is limited by slow growing organisms or poorly viable, besides giving false negative results due to treatment of patients with pre antimicrobial sampling [5]. Identification by culturing are required pure colonies, because in mixtures of microorganisms is impossible to identify the components of the mixture. All these constraints are solved by PCR. Using real time PCR is possible the detection of several microorganisms in the same assay [6]. This requires assembling multiple reactions in which the detection of microorganisms is carried out at the end of the amplification when by increasing the temperature gradually build dissociation curve (melt curve). Thus, if we know the temperature to which the DNA strands of amplicons are separated from each microorganism, then microorganisms present in the specimen can be identified [6,7].

Some of the limitations to the identification by PCR are that this reaction requires the use of specific oligonucleotides for each microorganism, then each PCR reaction is performed for one or a particular group of organisms suspected. The design of specific oligonucleotides requires knowledge of the genome of the microorganism as well as genomics variants, sometimes new strains or mutations cause that oligonucleotides designed for the identification might not align correctly. Due to test sensitivity is possible to detect even one copy of the target sequence [6], so that contamination is one of the main problems, one reason for this is the inadequate ways of taking the samples and the presence of microorganisms from normal flora cause false positives [5].

Even with the disadvantages mentioned, there are reasons that justify the use of PCR for diagnosis of ocular infections, due to the importance of receiving prompt treatment to stop the infectious process because otherwise compromises the functionality of the eye. Ocular infections caused by fungi are those with more advantages in the detection by PCR, because fungi growth is very slowly, and detection by molecular means is very quickly, and it allows giving a specific treatment [8].

Sensitivity of culture in cases of endophthalmitis is less than 70% and keratitis is not more than 80% due to the small inoculum [8]. If you have a sample that will uncover the presence fungal crop procedure and identification can take over a week delaying treatment. Therefore, the PCR for fungi provides the sensitivity needed in case of poor sample, even on the day of the sample obtaining [8]. Very few are currently available for clinical diagnostic kits for PCR. Roche provides kits for detection of *Chlamydia trachomatis*, CMV, EBV, Hepatitis A, B and C, HSV 1 and 2, VZV, HIV and *Neisseria gonorrhoeae*, meanwhile Bio-Rad have kits only for *Chlamydia trachomatis* and Mycoplasma. None company offers multiple trials or generic that can detect the presence of fungi and/or bacteria. Generic detection of bacteria is performed using oligonucleotides designed to bind to the conserved region of 16S ribosomal RNA gene, whereas for the detection of fungi, target is the 18S gene. While it is important to know the identity of the organism for appropriate treatment, discrimination between bacteria or fungi as causal agents of infection allows the introduction of generic treatment as early identification of the organism is carried out. The absence of commercial testing kitsallow that diagnostic laboratories use "home" methods at endpoint PCR and real time PCR designed and validated by themselves [8].

1.1.2. Identification by full genome sequencing

Time spent in genome sequencing has decreased. The first genome sequenced in 1995 (*Haemophilus influenzae*) took more than a year [9], whereas today technology is able to sequence hundreds of thousands of times faster. There is currently information around 3,144 complete genome deposited at the GenBank database [10]. All this information makes it possible to implement identification techniques based on sequencing. Through the comparison of sequences obtained from the analysis of clinical samples with the sequences contained in the databases, microbiological identification takes only a few hours with high certainty. These new technologies use PCR to amplify DNA, coupled to a parallel sequencing system using methods such as pyrosequencing, sequencing by ligation and sequencing by synthesis.

Although this technology is available from Roche 454 platforms, SOLID platform from Life Technologies and Illumina platform, plus the costs of technology, interpretation of results is perhaps the greatest barrier to the implementation of the sequencing genome as a routine identification technique in clinical laboratories [10].

In 2005, Yeo *et al.*, reported an outbreak of acute hemorrhagic conjunctivitis in Singapore [11]. Patients were diagnosed clinically with acute hemorrhagic conjunctivitis and it was identified by PCR the presence of an enterovirus and molecular typing confirmed a variant of coxsackievirus A24 (CA24v). Full-length genome sequencing results showed that CA24v virus was responsible for the outbreak and it was evolved from virus emerged 40 years ago.

1.1.3. PCR coupled to mass spectrometry using electrospray ionization (PCR / ESI-MS)

For identification by PCR/ESI-MS using oligonucleotides specific for bacterial groups rather than to a particular species, although variable regions are amplified between species and strains. Additionally, there are species-specific oligonucleotides used as primers that target genes for antibiotic resistance or some pathogenic characteristics [12]. Subsequent to amplification, amplicons are subjected to mass spectrometry and the pattern obtained is compared with those in the databases. The ability to identify an organism without prior knowledge of the Gram, or group of microorganisms is another advantage [12], since the stains are not required or previous isolates that provides fast trial and will always be possible to identify the microorganisms. This technology will be improving the identification of microorganism in ocular infections, it takes some advantages as certainty and specificity, and however the cost is the major disadvantage.

Kaleta *et al.*, designed a study to evaluate the feasibility of the use of PCR/ESI-MS to identify microorganisms directly from blood culture bottles in the clinical microbiology laboratory [12]. The high concordance of the results of this technique with those of standard methods, particularly at the genus level, demonstrates that PCR/ESI-MS technique is capable of rapidly evaluating clinically complex specimens providing information as to the selection and administration of targeted antibiotics.

About eye microorganisms, Pedreira *et al.*,evaluated the efficacy of a prophylactic regimen of daily topical 0.5% moxifloxacin and 5% povidone-iodine in patients with Boston type I. The patients with the prophylactic regimen were sampled and analyzed by standard culture methods and by PCR/ESI-MS [13]. The molecular diagnostic approach using PCR/ESI-MS yielded data comparable with those obtained using standard microbiologic techniques. Because of the high throughput nature and rapid results, the method might be a useful surveillance tool in patients with Boston type I.

2. Microarrays

As we described before, the PCR have several advantages over the culture of to identify microorganisms from infection. However, the disability to work with different genomes at the same time and the obtaining product with the same molecular size, make the PCR not the better method for diagnosis. Therefore, there have been developed new methods of diagnosis that not only reduce the time process; also they have more sensibility and specificity [14].

That is the case of the DNA microarrays, also called biochip, DNA chip, or gene array, which are defined as an orderly arrangement of samples gene for matching known and unknown DNA samples based on base-pairing rules and automating the process of identifying the unknowns and they were created by Brown P.O. y Botstein D. in 1999. An experiment with a single DNA chip can provide to researchers information on thousands of genes simultaneously, a dramatic increase in throughput. Microarray-based technology, with its advantage of highly parallel detection, has been applied to both population profiling and to functional studies of complex microbial communities in the environment [15, 16]. In addition, several studies have reported the use of PCR-amplified genomic fragment sequences as probes.

The gene arrays can be classified as macroarrays or microarrays, depending on the size of the sample spots. Macroarrays contain sample spot sizes of about 300 microns or larger and can be easily imaged by existing gel and blot scanners. The sample spot sizes in microarray are typically less than 200 microns in diameter and these arrays usually contain thousands of spots; microarrays require specialized robotics and imaging equipment.

There are several steps in the design and implementation of a DNA microarray experiment, as is shown in Figure 1.

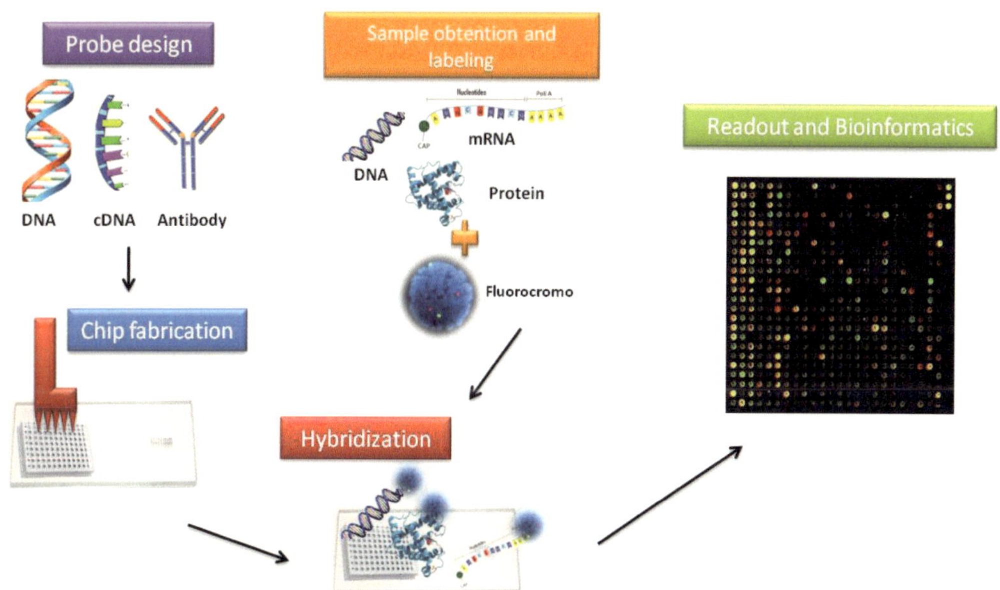

Figure 1. Design and implementation of DNA microarray experiment

It is important to mention that the microarrays made with cDNA are called spotted arrays because the probes are created *in vitro* and the robot put the spots on the microplate. Instead of the microarrays with oligonucleotides which are created *in situ* [17]. Recent studies have used synthesized oligonucleotides as probes because of their flexibility in design and preparation; with intensive specificity evaluation applied to the probe design criteria [18].

Both macroarrays and microarrays can have two application forms for the DNA microarray technology: the identification of sequence (gene/gene mutation) and determination of expression level of genes.

The determination of expression level of genes the microarrays can study the transcriptome or the proteome. For the transcriptome microarrays the probes consist on cDNA that hybridize with the mRNA of the cell. By the other hand, the proteome microarrays can use proteins as probe or the antibody making the antigen-antibody reaction. One example of this microarray is the peptide microarray analysis of *in silico*-predicted epitopes for serological diagnosis of *Toxoplasma gondii* infection in humans [19].

About the identification of gene sequence, microarray should have genomic DNA as probe of a specific chromosome, specifically all the genes that compose the chromosome. Or when a microarray only has a gene with one or more different nucleotides called Single Nucleotide Polymorphism (SNP) can detect a gene mutation [20].

These microarrays are used to determinate the cancer progression; all the changes on these gene are important to establish a clinical forecast [20]. Such microarrays have been used for the detection of specific bacteria [22, 23], species determination [24], and screening of environmental sequences related to a certain function within a community [25, 26].

Chin-I *et al.*, coupled 16S rDNA PCR and DNA hybridization technology to construct a microarray for simultaneous detection and discrimination of eight fish pathogens (*Aeromonas hydrophila, Edwardsiella tarda, Flavobacterium columnare, Lactococcus garvieae, Photobacterium damselae, Pseudomonas anguilliseptica, Streptococcus iniae* and *Vibrio anguillarum*) commonly encountered in aquaculture. The array comprised short oligonucleotide probes complementary to the polymorphic regions of 16S rRNA genes from the target pathogens. The results showed that each probe consistently identified its corresponding target strain with 100% specificity [27].

Yu-Cheng *et al.*, designed the DNA probes and PCR primers for the detection of *Listeria monocytogens, Staphylococcus aureus, Enterobacter sakazakii, Escherichia coli* O157:H7, *Salmonella spp., Vibrio parahaemolyticus, Streptococcus agalactiae*and *Pseudomonas fluorescens* by using two sets of multiplex PCR, followed by a chromogenic macroarray system, these organisms in milk or other food products could be simultaneously detected [28].

An example of microarray designed for infection diagnosis is a microarray developed by Uchida *et al.*, for the direct detection of pathogens in osteoarticular infections by polymerase chain reaction amplification and microarray hybridization [29].

And finally, and the most interesting DNA microarray used for the endophthalmitis diagnosis is the one developed by Tsutomu *et al.* They used 13 samples of vitreous fluid (VF) obtained from 13 patients during vitrectomy. Vitreous fluids from three patients with suspected endophthalmitis and ten controls without infection were subjected to testing for the presence of bacteria and fungi in culture tests, polymerase chain reaction (PCR) analysis, and DNA microarray analysis. The DNA microarray contained the spots for 16S rDNA, variable and conserved areas for bacteria, and the 18S rDNA for fungi. No control sample was positive for bacteria or fungi in the culture test, PCR, or microarray analysis. Specimens from two patients (Cases 1 and 2) with suspected endophthalmitis were positive for bacteria in PCR, and a specimen from one patient (Case 3) was positive for fungi in PCR. *Klebsiella pneumonia* (Case 1), *Streptococcus agalactiae* (Case 2), and *Candida parapsilosis* (Case 3) in the PCR-positive specimens were identified by DNA microarray analysis within 24 hours. Culture results were also positive for *K. pneumonia* in Case 1, *S. agalactiae* in Case 2, and *C. parapsilosis*in Case 3, but required 3 to 4 days to obtain [30].

For infection diagnosis, microarray analysis is complementary to routine cultures for identifying causative microorganisms and is likely to be a useful tool in patients who require rapid diagnosis and early treatment.

3. Aptamers

The term aptamers derives from the Latin *aptus*, it means to adapt [31]. Aptamers are synthetic nucleic acids (DNA or RNA) that bind specifically to a wide variety of molecules including metal ions K^{2+}, Hg^{2+}, Pb^{2+}, ATP, antibiotics, amino acids, vitamins, organic dyes, peptides and proteins, additionally aptamers are not immunogenic and non-toxic, superior to antibodies [32, 33, 34, 35]. Thirty and 60 nucleotides usually comprise the length of the central region, so that the total length of the aptamer is 70 to 100 nucleotides. For selection of aptamers with higher affinity the SELEX method is used (Systematic Evolution of Ligands by Exponential Enrichment). Wherein the target molecules are incubated with a population of aptamers, which interact with the target molecule by affinity, non-interacting target molecules are removed and the oligonucleotides are amplified by PCR and characterized by sequencing, being able to maintain a stock by its introduction to bacteria using plasmids. After obtaining the individual aptamers were characterized by their interaction with the target molecule by techniques as SPR, ELISA, Western blot or slot blot [36].

3.1. Applications aptamers

The aptamers can be used in different areas of study; some of its applications are reviewed below.

Biotechnology: the aptamers can be used for protein purification [37] and also for the development of techniques such as western blot or chromatin immunoprecipitation [38], also to monitor the status of phosphorylation of proteins *in vivo* [35]. There is an aptamer with activity of inhibitor of coagulation factor IXa by the addition of antisense RNA, this is an important method to control bleeding in patients who are intolerant of heparin, the aptamer is of interest for therapeutic and diagnostic [40].

Therapy: The therapeutic targets can be divided into two classes, the intracellular targets such as transcription factors, and extracellular targets such as viruses. The aptamers can be administered intravenously or subcutaneously; there is also topical application to prevent pathogens interaction with their receptors on mucosal surfaces. The release of intracelular-aptamers to bind their targets has been made mainly by the incorporation into liposomes or by systems of viral-based expression. A technique using a liposome to release viral vector fusigenicaptamer DNA in target cells, showed sequestration of E2F (transcription factor) leading to a reduction in the growth of abnormal vascular tissue that is typically seen after angioplasty [41]. Some research groups have studied the expression of aptamers in cells. An example of this is the expression of a chimeric transcript initiating sequence, consisting of a human tRNA-Met and anti-HIV reverse transcriptase-pseudoknotaptamer under control of RNA polymerase III promoter in human 293 cells. The chimeric RNA resulted in a reduction of over 75% in viral replication, similar results were observed when carrying out the transfection in Jurkat cells [41]. The FDA (Food and Drug Administration, USA) approved the system Eyetech /Pfizer's aptamer (Macugen) for treatment of related macular degeneration. The target of Macugen is VEGF (Vascular Endothelial Growth Factor), preventing choroidal neovascularization [43, 44]. There are aptamers against amyloidogenic proteins such as peptide Aß associated with Alzheimer disease [45] and against abnormal proteins in prion diseasesand scrapie, and Creutzfeldt-Jakob disease [46, 47].

3.2. Diagnostics and biosensors

The high affinity and specificity of aptamers make them ideal as reagents for diagnosis. And also aptamers can be detected by differential staining fluorescence that results in a high sensitivity. There are an aptamers called "beacons" that have many uses ranging from detection of environmental pollutants and thus also to monitor the levels of carcinogens or drugs in the blood [48]. The development of quantum dot aptamers also could help to establish the role of aptamers as biosensors [49, 50]. The quantum dots are novel fluorophores with a different emission profile, but all they are excited in the same wavelength. In this system multiple copies of an aptamer is attached to a single quantum dot, and each aptamer base is binding to a complementary strand. The plug moves on ligand binding, leading to large increases in fluorescence emission. If different aptamers are immobilized each on a single quantum dot, multiple ligands can be detected in a single assay. The aptamers have great potential as early warning systems to detect cell surface binding to damaged or diseased cells.

3.3. Aptamers: An approach to diagnostic microbiology

It has previously been addressed different approaches to the application of aptamers. The use of aptamers in microbiology is interesting, in order to have new tools for the diagnosis of infections. Today, several research groups are involved in aptamers development aimed at the detection of microorganisms. Duan *et al.*, by means of the system evolution of ligands by exponential enrichment (SELEX) developed a DNA aptamer labeled with carboxyfluorescein (FAM) that binds specifically to *Vibrio parahaemolyticus* [51]; Zelada *et al.*, through aptamer system potentiometric biosensors based on carbon nanotubes attached to a single wall (SWCNT) were able to identify and detect *Escherichia coli* with a linear response [52]. Aptamers represent a very flexible technique for the detection of microorganisms such is the case of the determination of *E. coli* based on immunomagnetic separation and real time PCR aptamers, this technique consists of three steps, first the binding of *E. coli* to an antibody conjugated to a magnetic bead, the second RNA aptamer is captured on the surface of *E. coli* forming a sandwich and then a heat process release the aptamers and these are amplified using real time PCR. The sensitivity of this method allowed the detection of 10 *E. coli* in 1 mL of sample [53]. Aptamers have also been developed for quantum dot fluorescence assays against *Bacillus thuringiensis*, detecting up to 1000 CFU/ml [54]. Application of aptamers in the microbiological diagnosis and the advantages respect to other diagnostic techniques must be analyzed; however there is not much information about the application of aptamers in the microbiological field.

3.4. SOMAmers

SOMAmers (Slow Off-rate Modified Aptamers) are single-stranded deoxynucleotides type aptamers selected *in vitro* from large random libraries, for their ability to bind small molecules, peptides or proteins [55, 56]. SOMAmers are aptamers carrying dU residues in position 5 that are involved in interactions with target molecules [57].

SOMAmers have been created for more than 1000 protein targets of different molecular functions, including known diseases and physiological associations. The target families broadly include receptors, kinases, growth factors and hormones, and also include a diverse array of intracellular and extracellular proteins.

The core of the reagents is a SOMAmer coupled to biotin, via a photocleaveable linker allowing binding to streptavidin of the complex in the washing steps (Figure 2). A fluorophore Cy3 incorporated into the capture reagents allows quantification of protein available commercially available systems based microarray systems but not necessary for all assay formats (SomaLogic ®).

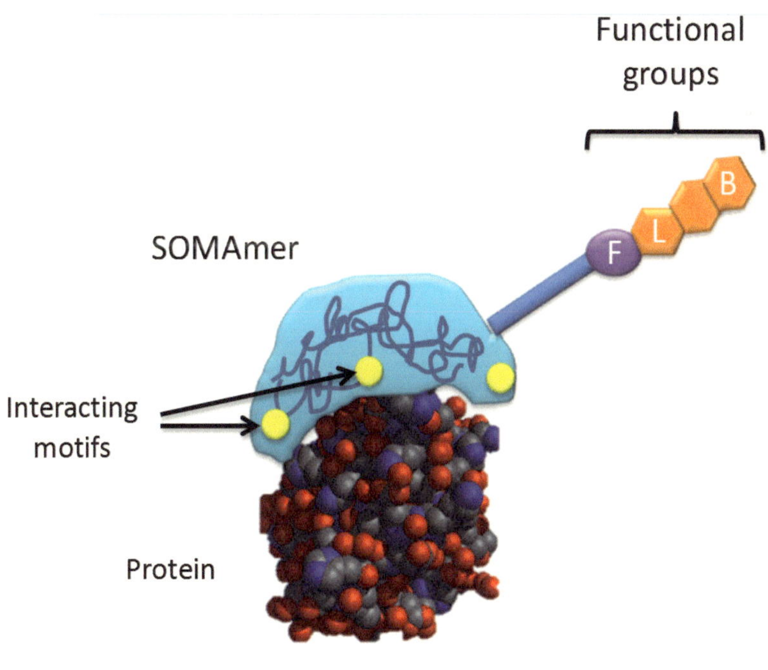

Figure 2. SOMAmer-protein complex. SOMAmer binds specifically to protein target through interacting motifs. Functional groups are: B= biotin for capture; F=Cy3 for detection and L=photocleavable linker.

3.4.1. SOMAmers applications

Comparison between proteome of healthy and diseased tissues from human using Somascan, can provide major knowledge of the biology of the disease and may lead to the discovery of new highly specific biomarkers for diagnosis, prognosis and therapeutic targets for the development of new drug treatment and it will improve personalized medicine.

Somascan premium has been used for the discovery of biomarkers for the detection of mesothelioma in the population exposed to asbestos. SOMAmers reagent showed better performance with respect to the ELISA test. Also the system is used to discover biomarkers for the detection of non-small cell lung cancer [57]. Moreover the system can be applied in tumor tissue lysate to obtain biomarkers associated with the disease as well SOMAmers same reagents can be used for histochemical evidence [58]. The SOMAmers represents an effective tool for biomarker discovery in different areas such as oncology, neurology, cardiovascular and metabolic diseases. To microbiological purposes as those related to the detection of agents in microbial infections SOMAmers represent a good alternative tool that may be applied for microbiological diagnosis in the future.

4. Mass spectrometry in microbiological diagnosis

Since its discovery, over a hundred years, mass spectrometry has been a useful tool to understanding the chemistry of proteins and biological processes involved. However, until the discovery of soft ionization techniques such as MALDI (Matrix-assisted laser desorption/ Ionization) and ESI (electrospray ionization) this methodology could be used as a routine tool in laboratories. [59].

Recently, mass spectrometry (MS) has entered to microbiology laboratories, offering a fast and reliable identification of microorganisms based on proteomic analysis.

4.1. Mass spectrometer

The mass spectrometer, in summary, is supported on the fragmentation of proteins to small peptides or other biomolecules to smaller molecules and then be ionized, these molecules are separated by the acceleration of ions in an electric field and then detected in based on their charge/mass ratio, in a gas phase state to produce a corresponding electrical signal to detect ions [60, 61].

A mass spectrometer is mainly composed of three elements in a vacuum atmosphere: an ionization source, a mass analyzer and detector.

4.1.1. Ionization source

The result of applying a source of ionization in a sample was the production of electrically charged ionized particles that gain or loss electrons in a gas phase.

There are several ionization processes that can be employed for the same purpose, to produce ionized peptides [62] among these processes are MALDI (Matrix -assisted laser desorption/Ionization) and ESI (electrospray ionization) that are most known.

4.1.2. MALDI (desorption / ionization matrix-assisted laser)

In this method, the sample is soaked in an organic matrix which is crystallized with air and is irradiated by a laser, matrix most used are the acid α-cyano-4-hydroxy-trans cinnamic acid, 2,5-dihidrobenzoic acid or sinapinic acid [59].

In MALDI, the protein or peptide of interest is coprecipitated with the organic compound which is capable of absorbing laser light of an appropriate wavelength. The laser allows to prepare the compound fragmentation and disruption of the crystalline matrix generating a cloud of particles, these particles capture electrons and therefore remain as negatively charged ions in most cases (Figure 3A) [59, 62].

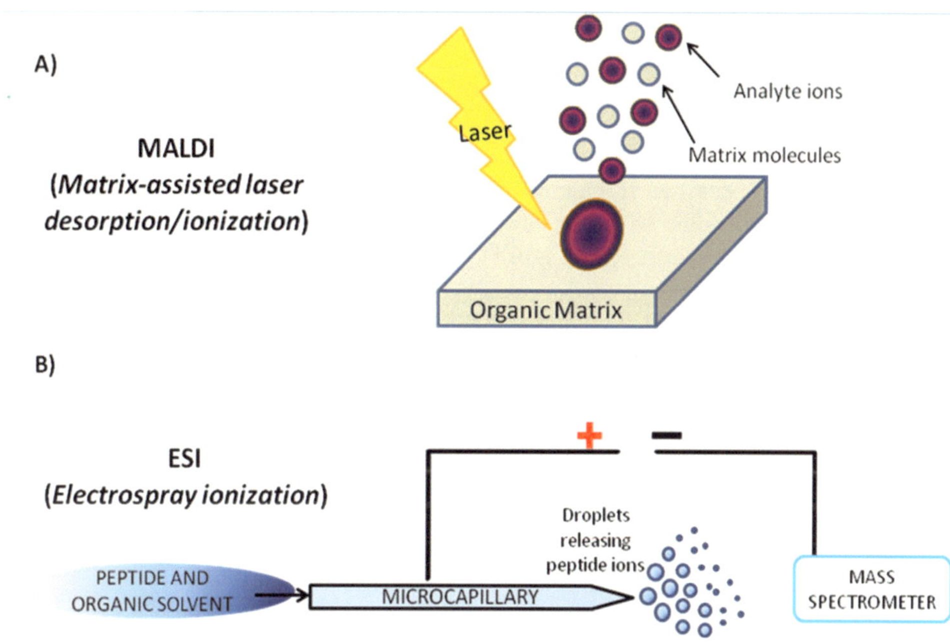

Figure 3. Schematic representation of A) MALDI (Matrix-assisted laser desorption/ionization) and B) ESI (Electrospray ionization) method. Protein samples must be ionized before they pass through mass spectrometer.

4.1.3. ESI (electrospray ionization)

In this process, the sample is dissolved in an organic solvent, this mixture passes through a fine capillary tube that is maintained in an electric field produced by an electrode near to the capillary and other on the detector, this mixture is sprayed to form high load of tiny droplets of the solvent that evaporates quickly, thus produce a series of gaseous ions that result from protonation of side chains such as Arginine and Lysine, these ions fragmented by electric field are then detected (Figure 3B) [63].

4.1.4. Mass analyzer

Is the main component of the mass spectrometer, the charged fragments (ions and radical ions), are accelerated and deflected by a strong magnetic field that affects their travel resulting in a curvilinear path. Ions and radical ions are collected, detected and quantified with high accuracy and sensitivity, depending on the mass/charge ratio (m/z). [64].

There are several analyzers; however the most common type is the TOF (Time of flight). This analyzer defines a flight zone through which the ions are accelerated by acquiring a high kinetic energy, and during this trip will be separated according to their ratio mass/ charge (m/z). Most of ions generated have a single charge (z = 1), so that the ratio m/z is equal to m. The length of time for each ion in reaching the detector is called flight of time and depends on this ratio (Figure 4) [59].

4.1.5. Ion detector

At the end of the fragmentation and separation of ions from a sample by MALDI or ESI, ions impact on the detector. The fragments after flowing through the pipe in electric field (TOF) are deflected and detected, not-charged fragments are not deflected by the field and lost in the pipe walls, but the charged fragments are recorded by the detector, and mass are calculated from the flight of time. In many cases, before the detector is the reflector, which increase the resolution of the technique (Figure 4) [65, 69].

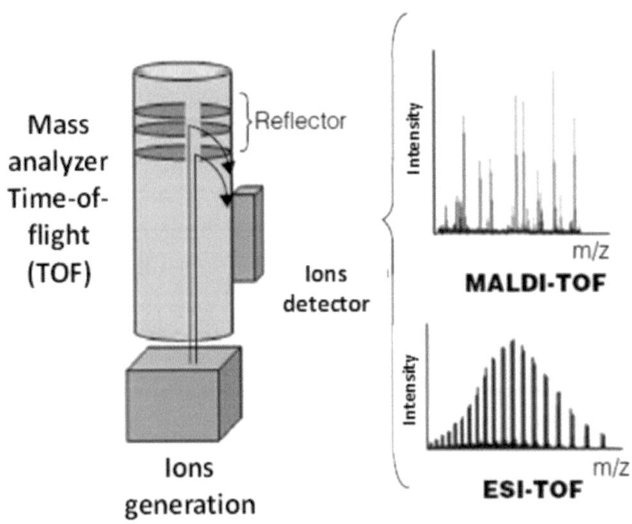

Figure 4. Scheme of Mass Spectrometer. Mass analyzer characterized and separated ions according to their mass/ charge ratio (m/z). Ions detector generate mass spectrum for every ion detected. MALDI and ESI mass spectrum obtained are shown.

The mass spectrum of a compound is typically represented as a bar graph with the masses in the X axis, and the intensity or relative abundance of the ions of the m/z reaching the detector in the Y axis. The highest peak is assigned as 100% of intensity known as the base peak, and the main peak or molecular ion is the peak corresponding to the unfragmented radical cation (Figure 4) [65].

4.2. Fingerprinter obtaining and analysis

The actual data acquisition with MALDI-TOF-MS is nowadays generally performed in an automated manner. That is, the laser focus scans the sample in a predefined pattern and accumulates a mass spectrum from a defined number of laser pulse cycles, generally several hundreds to yield a representative average mass spectrum. The raw spectrum is generally processed to yield a mass fingerprinter that contains the information about peak apex *m/z* values, thus reducing the size of individual files considerably. The essential step for species identification is the comparison of the mass fingerprinter of the sample, to be identified to a database containing reference mass fingerprints, for example MASCOT, SWISS-PROT [66].

4.3. Spectrometry in the diagnosis of microbiological specimens

The first application of this technique was the study of the chemical structures of organic compounds in the area of Structural Chemistry and also the identification of compounds in the field of organic chemistry, eventually, the use of mass spectrometry spread to biology, geology and recently the clinical and medical area.

In recent years, this technique has been applied as a routine method in the microbiology laboratory, as a useful tool for the identification of microorganisms using the bacterial colony directly and proteins extracted from the microorganism.

Once obtained mass spectrum and it is compared with a database, software assigns identification and a reliable value of such identification.

MALDI-TOF has been the most used technique in the microbiological diagnosis for bacterial identification; some databases are used for identification profiles. This technique has been useful to obtain the profile of microorganisms for diagnosis using colonies directly from the culture media [67].

One advantage of the technique results from the culture obtained from a sample or sample directly, in this connection, trials have been performed to determine the functionality of the art regarding the identification, has been performed identification of bacteria and yeast using MALDI-TOF, allows for quick low-cost diagnosis compared to conventional techniques as Vitek-II, API and biochemical tests, and it is known that these technologies are validated by comparing the technique by identifying the microorganisms from the samples at the species level and it must be matched [68].

Recently, the mass spectrometer has taken a major challenge to modernize and facilitate its use by the coupling of other techniques such as Vitek, an automated method of identifying microorganisms. In recent years several studies have been performed in routine clinical laboratory using this new technology: Vitek ® MS Biomeriuex.

This mass spectrometric technique is based on MALDI-TOF coupled to a Vitek-II and Myla, a database which receives the fingerprint of the sample from culture or sample directly and then identifies the organism. This technique has been used identifying fungi from clinical samples. Results from this study identifying 18 fungi with a quick and inexpensive strategy, since it does not require a prior extraction of proteins. These tests were perfomerd on clinical isolates from 20 patients, which were also evaluated using Vitek 2. Comparison between results from Vitek-MS and Vitek 2 correlated in 93% [69].

Ferreira *et al.*, analyzed 294 facultative anaerobic and aerobic isolates obtained from different clinical samples, using conventional microbiological methods compared to conventional microbiological methods. In the analysis they concluded that bacterial clinical isolates identification obtained by MS MALDI-TOF shows excellent correlation with identification obtained by conventional microbiological methods. Moreover, MS MALDI-TOF allows the identification of bacteria from colonies grown on agar culture plates in just a few minutes with a very simple methodology and hardly any consumable cost [70].

5. Conclusions

Ocular infections are one of the most frequent events in ophthalmology, and the treatment for these diseases must be fast, precise and effective, in order to get this goal is important to identify and characterized microorganisms involved. Clinical diagnosis of ocular infections can be confirmed by several techniques based on microbiological test of ocular samples. These techniques includes classic microbiological test, where is necessary isolate microorganisms to characterize them by biochemical analysis; molecular biology techniques, end-point PCR, real time PCR, microarrays and aptamers (e. SOMAmers) can obtain results in a short period time, as well as high sensitivity and specificity.

However, in the last years, mass spectrometry approach has dramatically changed the microbiological field. Microbiological identification by mass spectrometry has great advantages: 1) Culture and isolation of the microorganism is not necessary, so that fastidious microorganisms can be identified, 2) High sensitivity and accuracy for the microorganism identification results in a reduction of sample amount, that is common in ocular samples, and 3) Resistance markers and resistance profile can be determined at the same time of identification analysis.

In summary, the evolution of microbiological identification methods has improved treatments that impact in the prognosis of ocular infection, reducing complications and avoiding blindness cases, and as a consequence life quality of patients will be better.

Acknowledgements

This work was supported by "Fundación de Asistencia Privada Conde de Valenciana I.A.P."

http://dx.doi.org/10.5772/52468

Author details

Victor Manuel Bautista-de Lucio[1], Mariana Ortiz-Casas[1], Luis Antonio Bautista-Hernández[1], Nadia Luz López-Espinosa[1], Carolina Gaona-Juárez[1], Ángel Gustavo Salas-Lais[1,2], Dulce Aurora Frausto-del Río[1] and Herlinda Mejía-López[1]

1 Microbiology and Ocular Proteomics Department, Research Unit, Institute of Ophthalmology "Fundación de Asistencia Privada Conde de Valenciana I.A.P.", Mexico City, Mexico

2 Immunoparasitology Laboratory, Parasitology Department, Escuela Nacional de Ciencias Biológicas, Instituto Politécnico Nacional, Mexico City, Mexico

References

[1] The top 10 causes of death. 2011, World Health Organization. p. Facts sheet No. 310.

[2] Lichtinger A, Yeung SN, Kim P, *et al.* Shifting Trends in Bacterial Keratitis in Toronto: An 11-Year Review. Ophthalmology. 2012. [Epub ahead of print]PMID: 22627118.

[3] Sedó S, Iribarne Y, Fossas M, *et al.* Queratitisfúngica. Annals dÓftalmología. 2003;11(3):168-175.

[4] Robins J, Lightman S. Taylos SR. The eye in virology. Br J Hosp Med (Lond). 2011;72(12):672-676.

[5] Mackay IM. Real time PCR in the microbiology laboratory. ClinMicrobiol Infect. 2004;10(3):190-212.

[6] Valasek MA and Repa JJ. The power of real time PCR. AdvPhysiolEduc . 2005;29(3): 151-159.

[7] Espy MJ, Uhl MR, Sloan LM, *et al.* Real time PCR in clinical microbiology: applications for routine laboratory testing. ClinMicrobiol Rev. 2006;19(1):165-256.

[8] Bou G, Fernández-Olmos A, García C, *et al.* Bacterial identification methods in the microbiology laboratory. EnfermInfeccMicrobiolClin. 2011 Oct;29(8):601-608.

[9] Fleischmann RD, Adams MD, White O, *et al.* Whole-genome random sequencing and assembly of Haemophilusinfluenzae Rd. Science. 1995. 269(5223): 496-512.

[10] Torok ME and Peacock SJ. Rapid whole-genome sequencing of bacterial pathogens in the clinical microbiology laboratory--pipe dream or reality? J AntimicrobChemother. 2012. Epub ahead of print. PMID:22729921.

[11] Yeo DS, Seah SG, Chew JS. Molecular identification of coxsackievirus A24 variant, isolated from an outbreak of acute hemorrhagic conjunctivitis in Singapore in 2005. Arch Virol. 2007;152(11):2005-16.

[12] Kaleta EJ, Clark AE, Johnson DR, *et al.* Use of PCR coupled with electrospray ionization mass spectrometry for rapid identification of bacterial and yeast bloodstream pathogens from blood culture bottles. J ClinMicrobiol. 2011;49(1): 345-353.

[13] Pedreira F, Moraes H, Ecker D *et al.* ,Microbiota Evaluation of patients with Boston Type I keratoprosthesis treated with topical 0. 5% Moxifloxacin and 5% Povidone-Iodine. Cornea. 2012. Epub ahead of print. PMID: 17680326

[14] de Boer E. and Beumer, RR. Methodology for detection and typing of foodborne microorganisms. Int. J. Food Microbiol. 1999;50:119–130.

[15] Loy A, Lehner A, Lee N, *et al.* Oligonucleotide microarray for 16S rRNA gene-based detection of all recognized lineages of sulfate-reducing prokaryotes in the environment. Appl Environ Microbiol. 2002;68:5064–5081.

[16] Palmer C, Bik E, Eisen MB, *et al.* Rapid quantitative profiling of complex microbial populations. Nucleic Acids Res. 2006;34:e5.

[17] Acuna, E. 2002. math. uprm. edu/~edgar/esma683606. html

[18] He ZL, Wu LY, Li XY, *et al.* Empirical establishment of oligonucleotide probe design-criteria. Appl Environ Microbiol. 2005;71:3753–3760.

[19] Maksimov P, Zerweck J, Maksimov A, *et al.* Peptide microarray analysis of in silico-predicted epitopes for serological diagnosis of *Toxoplasma gondii* infection in humans. ClinVaccineImmunol. 2012;19(6):865-784.

[20] Guido L and Camila MA. Microarreglos: herramienta para el conocimiento de las enfermedades. REVISTA COLOMBIANA DE REUMATOLOGÍA, 2005;12(3): 263-267.

[21] Kwiatkowski P, Wierzbicki P, Kmieć A, *et al.* DNA microarray-based gene expression profiling in diagnosis, assessing prognosis and predicting response to therapy in colorectal cancer. PostepyHig Med Dosw (Online). 2012;11;66:330-338.

[22] Kim BC, Park JH and Gu MB. Development of a DNA microarray chip for the identification of sludge bacteria using an unsequenced random genomic DNA hybridization method. Environ Sci Technol. 2004;38:6767–6774.

[23] Kim BC, Park JH and Gu MB. Multiple and simultaneous detection of specific bacteria in enriched bacterial communities using a DNA microarray chip with randomly generated genomic DNA probes. Anal Chem. 2005;77:2311–2317.

[24] Cho JC and Tiedje JM. Bacterial species determination from DNA-DNA hybridization by using genome fragments and DNA microarrays. Appl Environ Microbiol. 2001;67:3677–3682.

[25] Yokoi T, Kaku Y, Suzuki H, *et al.* 'FloraArray' for screening of specific DNA probes representing the characteristics of a certain microbial community. FEMS MicrobiolLett. 2007;273:166–171.

[26] Tomohiro T, Futoshi K, Ikuro K, *et al.* Specificity of randomly generated genomic DNA fragment probes on a DNA array . FEMS MicrobiolLett. 2012;328 86–89.

[27] Chang CI, Hung PH, Wu CC, *et al.* Simultaneous Detection of Multiple Fish Pathogens Using a Naked-Eye Readable DNA Microarray. Sensors. 2012;12:2710-2728.

[28] Chiang YC, Tsen HY, Chen HY, *et Al.* Multiplex PCR and a chromogenic DNA macroarray for the detection of *Listeria monocytogens, Staphylococcus aureus, Streptococcus agalactiae, Enterobacter sakazakii, Escherichia coli* O157:H7, *Vibrio parahaemolyticus, Salmonella* spp. and *Pseudomonas fluorescens* in milk and meat samples. J Microbiol Methods. 2012;88(1):110-116.

[29] Uchida K, Yayama T, Kokubo Y, *et al.* Direct detection of pathogens in osteoarticular infections by polymerase chain reaction amplification and microarray hybridization. J Orthop Sci. 2009;14(5):471-483.

[30] Tsutomu S, Kenichi K, Akira W, *et al.* Use of DNA microarray analysis in diagnosis of bacterial and fungal endophthalmitis. Clinical Ophthalmology. 2012;6 321–326.

[31] Jayasena SD. Aptamers: An Emerging Class of Molecules That Rival Antibodies in Diagnostics. ClinChem, 1999;45(9):1628-1650.

[32] Wilson DS and Szostak JW. *In vitro* selection of functional nucleic acids. Annu. Rev. Biochem. 1999;68:611–647.

[33] Shamah SM, Healy JM and Cload ST. Complex target SELEX. AccChem Res. 2008;41:130–138.

[34] Shangguan D, Li Y, Tang Z, *et al.* Aptamers evolved from live cells as effective molecular probes for cancer study. PNAS. 2006;103:11838-11843.

[35] Stojanovic MN and Landry DW. Aptamer-Based Folding Fluorescent Sensor for Cocaine. J Am Chem Soc. 2002;124:9678.

[36] Seiwert SD, Nahreini TS, Aigner S *et al.* RNA aptamers as pathway-specific MAP kinase inhibitors. Chem Biol. 2000;7:833–843.

[37] Romig TS, Bell C. &Drolet D. W. Aptamer affinity chromatography: combinatorial chemistry applied to protein purification. J. Chromat. 1999;731:75–284

[38] Murphy MB, Fuller ST, Richardson PM *et al.* , An improved method for the in vitro evolution of aptamers and applications in protein detection and purification. Nucleic Acids Res. 2003;31: e110.

[39] Rusconi CP, Scardino E, Layzer J *et al.* Aptamers as reversible antagonists of coagulation factor IXa. Nature. 2002;419:90–94

[40] Dzau VJ, Man, MJ, Morishita R *et al.* Fusigenic viral liposome for gene therapy in cardiovascular diseases. Proc. Natl Acad. Sci. USA 1996;93:1421–11425.

[41] Chaloi, L. , Lehmann M J, Sczakiel G. *et al.* Endogenous expression of a high-affinity pseudoknot RNA aptamer suppresses replication of HIV-1. Nucleic Acid Res. 2002;30:4001–4008

[42] Ng EW, Shima DT, Calias P *et al.* ,Pegaptanib, a targeted anti-VEGF aptamer for ocular vascular disease. Nature Rev. Drug Discov. 2006;5:123–132

[43] Jellinek, D, Green, LS, Bell, C *et al.* Inhibition of receptor-binding by high-affinity RNA ligands to vascular endothelial growth-factor. Biochem. 1994;33:10450–10456

[44] Ylera, F, Lurz, R, Erdmann, VA *et al,* Selection of RNA aptamers to the Alzheimer's disease amyloid peptide. Biochem. Biophys. Res. Commun. 2002;290:1583–1588.

[45] Sayer NM, Cubin M, Rhie A *et al.* ,. Structural determinants of conformationally selective, prion-binding aptamers. J. Biol. Chem. 2004;279:13102–13109

[46] Rhie A, Kirby L, Sayer N *et al.* , Characterization of 2′-fluoro-RNA aptamers that bind preferentially to disease-associated conformations of prion protein and inhibit conversion. J. Biol. Chem. 2003;278:39697–39705

[47] Brockstedt U, Uzaroeska A, Montpetit A *et al.* , In vitro evolution of RNA aptamers recognizing carcinogenic aromatic amines. Biochem. Biophys. Res. Commun. 2003;313:1004–1008

[48] Yamamoto-Fujita R. & Kumar, P. K. R. Aptamerderived nucleic acid oligos: applications to develop nucleic acid chips to analyze proteins and small ligands. Anal. Chem. 2005;77:17:5460–5466

[49] Levy M, Cater S F & Ellington, AD. Quantum-dot aptamer beacons for the detection of proteins. Chem. Biochem. 2005;6:2163–2166

[50] Duan N, Wu S, Chen X*etal.* ,. Selection and identification of a DNA aptamer targeted to Vibrio parahemolyticus. J Agric Food Chem. 2012;60(16):4034-8.

[51] Zelada-Guillén GA, Bhosale SV, Riu J*et al.* Real time potentiometric detection of bacteria in complex samples. Anal Chem. 2010;82(22):9254-60.

[52] Lee HJ, Kim BC, Kim KW, *et al.* A sensitive method to detect Escherichia coli based on immunomagnetic separation and real time PCR amplification ofaptamers. BiosensBioelectron. 2009;24(12):3550-3555.

[53] Ikanovic M, Rudzinski WE, Bruno JG *et al.* , Fluorescence assay based on aptamer-quantum dot binding to Bacillus thuringiensis spores. J Fluoresc. 2007;17(2):193-199.

[54] Tuerk C, Gold L. Systematic evolution of ligands by exponential enrichment: RNA ligands to bacteriophage T4 DNA polymerase. Science 1990;249:505.

[55] Ellington D, Szostak JW. In vitro selection of RNA molecules that bind specific ligands. Nature 1990;346:818.

[56] Vaught JD, Bock C, Carter J *et al.* Expanding the chemistry of DNA for in vitro selection. J Am ChemSoc 2010;132:4141–4151.

[57] Ostroff RB, Franklin WL, Gold L, *et al.* ,. Unlocking Biomarker Discovery: Large Scale Use of SOMAmer Proteomic Technology for Early Detection of Lung Cancer. PLoS One. 2010;5(12): e15003.

[58] Michael M, Deborah A, Derek T *et al.* , Protein Signature of Lung Cancer Tissues. Plos One. 2012;7(4):1-15.

[59] Jordana-Lluch E, MartróCatalà E, Ausina Ruiz V. La espectrometría de masas en el laboratorio de microbiología clínica. EnfermInfeccMicrobiolClin. 2012.

[60] Abonnenc M, Qiao L, LiuB*et al.* Electrochemicalaspects of electrospray and laser desorption/ionizationformassspectrometry. AnnuRev Anal Chem 2012;3:231–254.

[61] Matteini M, Moles A. Ciencia y Restauración, métodos de Investigación. Editorial Nerea, Isla de la Cartuja, 2001;141-144

[62] Berg, Jeremy M. Bioquímica 6ta edición, Barcelona España, 2008, Editorial Reverté. Pag. 93-95

[63] Voet D. 2009. Fundamentos de bioquímica: la vida a nivel molecular. Editorial MédicaPanamericana. 2da Edición. Buenos Aires. Pag 116-118

[64] Pomilio AB, Bernatené EA, Vitale AA. Espectrometría de masas en condiciones ambientales con ionización por desorción con electrospray. Acta BioquímClínLatinoam2011;45(1):47-79

[65] McMurry J. 2008. Química Orgánica. 7a Edición. CengageEditores. Pag. 408-411

[66] Walker M. Proteomics for routine identification of microorganisms. Proteomics 2011;11:3143-3153.

[67] Ferreira L, Vega CS, Sánchez-Juanes F, *et al.* Identification of *Brucella* by MALDI-TOF Mass Spectrometry. Fast and Reliable Identification from Agar Plates and Blood Cultures. PLoS One. 2010 ;5(12):e14235.

[68] Van Veen SQ, Claas ECJ, Kuijper EJ. High-Throughput Identification of Bacteria and Yeast byMatrix-Assisted Laser Desorption Ionization–Time of Flight Mass Spectrometry in Conventional Medical Microbiology Laboratories 2010;48:3.

[69] Iriart X, Lavergne RA, Fillaux J, *et al.* ,. Routine identification of medical fungi by MALDI-TOF: performance of the new VITEK® MS using a new time-effective strategy. J. Clin. Microbiol. 2012;50(6):2107-10.

[70] Ferreira L, Vega S, Sánchez-Juanes F *et al.* ,Identificación bacteria name diantees pectrometría de masas *matriz-assited laser desorption ionization time-of-fligth.* Comparación con la metodología habitual en los laboratorios de Microbiología Clínica. EnfermInfeccMicrobiolCllin. 2010;28; (8):492-497.

Chapter 2

Infective Conjunctivitis – Its Pathogenesis, Management and Complications

Adnaan Haq, Haseebullah Wardak and
Narbeh Kraskian

Additional information is available at the end of the chapter

http://dx.doi.org/10.5772/52462

1. Introduction

The aims of this chapter are to briefly discuss infective conjunctivitis, its subtypes and its treatment. Other forms of conjunctivitis will also be considered and discussed in this chapter, namely, neonatal conjunctivitis, conjunctivitis in the immunocompromised. A comprehensive assessment of the various treatments of conjunctivitis will also be discussed.

Conjunctivitis is a term broadly used to describe an inflammation of the conjunctiva. Conjunctivitis may be split into four main aspects; bacterial, viral, allergic and irritant. Infective conjunctivitis, namely bacterial and viral will be discussed in this chapter in details.

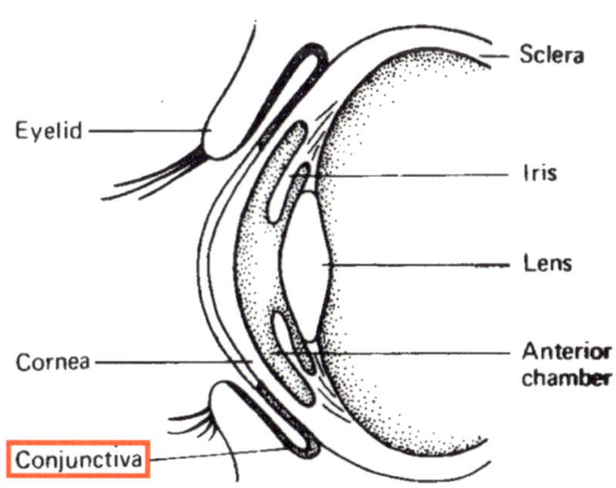

Figure 1. The conjunctiva in relation to the orbit and its structures

1.1. Anatomy of the conjunctiva

The conjunctiva is the fine mucous membrane which covers and joins the anterior surface of the eyeball to the posterior surface of eyelid. This translucent membrane lines the white part of the eye starting at the edge of the cornea (limbus) and runs behind the eye to cover the anterior part of the sclera. It then flows, loops forward, and forms the inside surface of the eyelids. At the medial canthus the conjunctiva fold thickens, which is called the semilunar fold.

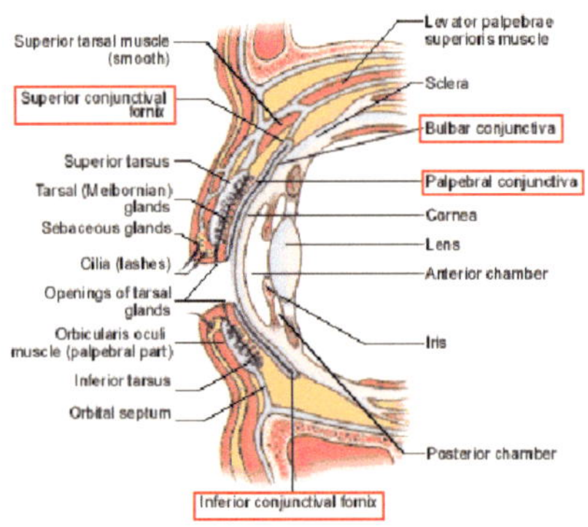

Figure 2. The different parts of the conjunctiva and its relation to other obit anatomy

The conjunctiva is subdivided into three parts depending on location: palpebral conjunctiva, bulbar conjunctiva and conjunctival fornix. Histologically the conjunctiva is divided into three layers.From superficial to deep these are epithelial, adenoid and fibrous. These conjunctival layers contain a wide range of structures that includes glands, melanocytes, langerhans cells, mast cells and lymphoid tissue.

The arterial blood supply to conjunctiva is made up of branches of ophthalmic artery, the anterior and posterior conjunctival arteries. These are branches of anterior ciliary arteries and palpebral arcades respectively. The venous drainage follows the arteries. Posterior conjunctival veins drain the veins of the lid and anterior conjunctival veins drain anterior ciliary vein to ophthalmic vein.

The lymphatic drainage of the conjunctiva depends on the region of the conjunctiva. Lymphatics in palpebral region drain into the lymphatics of eyelids. In bulbar conjunctiva, lymphatics from lateral side drain into the superficial preauricular lymph nodes & lymphatics from medial side drain to deep sub maxillary nodes.

The first division of the trigeminal provides nerve supply to the conjunctiva.

1.2. Allergic and irritant conjunctivitis

Before discussing the major contents of the chapter, it is necessary to briefly discuss allergic and irritant conjunctivitis.

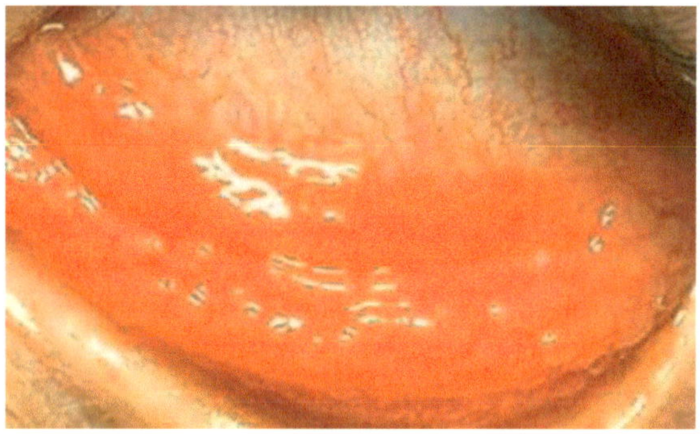

Figure 3. Allergic conjunctivitis- look for follicles and papillae which are characteristic of allergic conjunctivitis

Allergic conjunctivitis is seen in two acute disorders; seasonal allergic conjunctivitis (which is prevalent in the summer months) and perennial allergic conjunctivitis (which presents intermittently) and three chronic disorders, vernal keratoconjunctivitis, atopic keratoconjunctivitis and giant papillary conjunctivitis. Allergic conjunctivitis is considered to be a type I hypersensitivity reaction. Its treatment is largely supportive, although in severe cases, topical corticosteroids may be of some benefit 1.

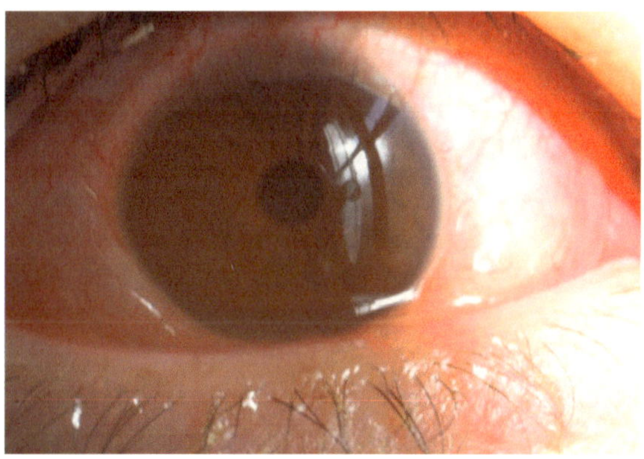

Figure 4. Irritant conjunctivitis- generalised redness around the eye and constant tearing are typical features

Irritant conjunctivitis is a form of conjunctivitis that is often bought on by an external source. The source, considered an 'irritant', directly affects the conjunctiva, causing an inflammatory response. Not all causes of irritant conjunctivitis are external however. Causes of irritant conjunctivitis are vast, though some of the more common causes are hair products (e.g. shampoos), smoke or fumes, chlorinated water used in swimming pools. A common non-external source is trapped eyelashes, which continually irritate the conjunctiva. Treatment of irritant conjunctivitis is thorough cleansing of the eye and removing the irritant.

2. Infectious conjunctivitis

Infective conjunctivitis can be caused by several bacterial and viral pathogens. Infective conjunctivitis can be further differentiated into acute infective conjunctivitis, defined as inflammation of the conjunctiva due to infection that does not last longer than 3 weeks, and chronic conjunctivitis, inflammation of the conjunctiva that lasts longer than 3 weeks.

In the developed world, acute infectious conjunctivitis is a common presentation in the primary care setting, accounting for up to 2% of consultations with the general practitioner [2]. Many general practitioners find it difficult to differentiate between bacterial and viral conjunctivitis. The uncertainty of the pathogenic cause of acute conjunctivitis has led to the routine practice of prescribing a broad spectrum antibiotic topically even though the pathogen has not been proved to be bacterial in nature. In the UK, approximately 3.4 million topical antibiotic prescriptions are issued every year, at a cost to the NHS of over £4.7 million [3].

A diagnosis of conjunctivitis is usually made on the basis of a clinical history and examination by the clinician. Other investigations of conjunctivitis, such as swabs and cultures of the conjunctiva are rarely performed as it often delays treatment and has very little prognostic benefit, as conjunctivitis is often a self limiting illness and the antibiotics currently used have a good spectrum of pathogen coverage. Swabs and cultures are mainly used in research purposes.

It is vital that a correct diagnosis is made to early to identify the cause and start treatment promptly. It is also essential to rule out more serious causes and medical emergencies that would require hospital admission. Such cases would include bacterial keratitis, acute closed angle glaucoma, corneal abrasions and others.

2.1. Bacterial conjunctivitis

Bacterial conjunctivitis is a relatively common infection and affects all people, although a higher incidence is seen in infants, school children and the elderly. Bacterial conjunctivitis has a higher prevalence in children, where a recent study by Rose et al identified 67% of 326 children as having a bacterial cause [4]. Although its incidence is continuing to decrease in developing nations, periodic rises in incidence are seen during the monsoon seasons in many countries such as Bangladesh, and thus, bacterial conjunctivitis is the most common cause of infective conjunctivitis in developing nations.

2.1.1. Types of bacterial conjunctivitis and pathogenic causes of bacterial conjunctivitis

Bacterial conjunctivitis can be broadly split into three major categories; hyperacute bacterial conjunctivitis, acute conjuncitivis and chronic conjunctivitis.

- Hyperacute bacterial conjunctivitis is commonly seen in patients affected with *N. Gonorrhoea*. The onset is often rapid with an exaggerated form of conjunctival injection, chemosis and copious purulent discharge. Prompt treatment is essential to prevent complications.

http://dx.doi.org/10.5772/52462

- Acute bacterial conjunctivitis is the most commonly seen bacterial conjunctivitis and often presents with a typical presentation, time course and prognosis. In a study done by Weiss et al, the most common pathogens in acute bacterial conjunctivitis were *Staphylococcus aureus, Haemophilus influenzae, streptococcus pneumoniae, and Moraxella catarrhalis,* whereas in an older study done by Gigilotti et al, *Chlamydia trachomatis* was also commonly found in infected patients [5, 6].
- Chronic bacterial conjunctivitis, ie, red eye with purulent discharge persisting for longer than a few weeks, is generally caused by Chlamydia trachomatis or is associated with a nidus for infection such as in dacryocystitis [7].

In certain bacterial conjunctivitis, it is essential to identify a pathogen. As mentioned, most causes of conjunctivitis are diagnosed and treated on a clinical exam basis, but in patients who are particularly susceptible such as neonates or immunodeficient patients, a microbiological diagnosis must be made to exclude harmful pathogens such as *N.gonorrheae, Listeria monocytogenes, Corynobacterium diptheriae* and certain members of the *Haemophilus* group. These pathogens contain proteolytic enzymes which may cause long term damage to the parenchyma of the conjunctiva.

2.1.2. Signs and symptoms of bacterial conjunctivitis

Although the symptoms of bacterial conjunctivitis are varied and quite vast, there are a number of key symptoms which differentiate it from other eye infections. Thick purulent discharge is seen as the major symptom that affects sufferers of bacterial conjunctivitis, compared to the watery discharge seen in viral conjunctivitis. This leads to 'glue eye' which is often the term used to describe difficulty opening the eye due to thick sticky secretions. A study done in 2004 in the Netherlands confirmed that 'early morning glue eye' was a positive predictor of bacterial conjunctivitis amongst 184 patients presenting with 'glue eye', itch or a past history of conjunctivitis [8].

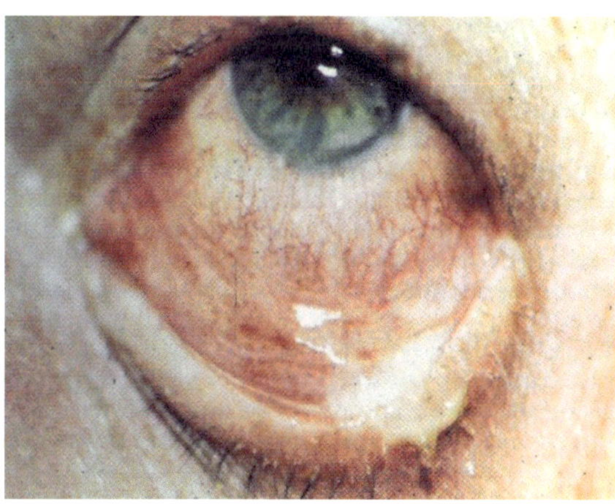

Figure 5. Mucopurulent discharge seen in bacterial conjunctivitis

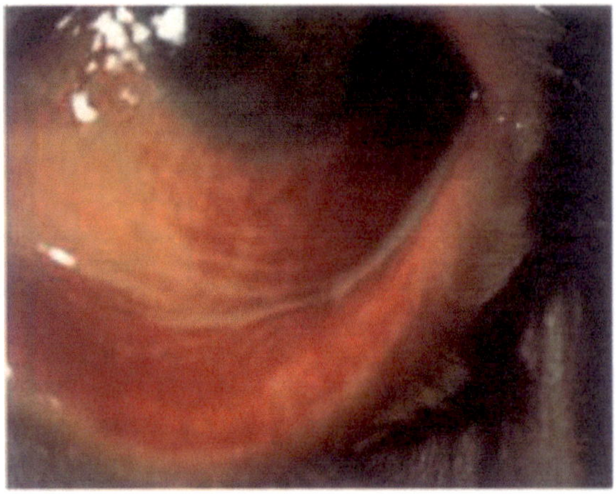

Figure 6. Injection of the conjunctiva and chemosis are two common symptoms and are demonstrated here

Other symptoms which are commonly seen in bacterial conjunctivitis is a 'foreign body' sensation, injection of the conjunctiva, chemosis (conjunctival oedema), itching, erythema of the eyelid skin and some patients also experience a slight burning or stinging sensation. In studies done by Carr et al and Wall et al almost all patients presented with injection of the conjunctiva, up to 90% of patients with bacterial conjunctivitis presented with itching and a foreign body sensation and up to 50% of patients presented with a burning or stinging sensation [9, 10]. Erythema of the eyelid was seen in 85% of patients.

2.1.3. *Complications of bacterial conjunctivitis*

Bacterial keratitis is a well known but rare complication of bacterial conjunctivitis [11]. People at particularly high risk of developing keratitis often have corneal epithelial defects or disease and patients who have particularly dry eyes are seen to be at an increased risk.

2.1.4. *Treatment of bacterial conjunctivitis*

Bacterial conjunctivitis is commonly treated empirically with broad-spectrum antibiotics. Broad-spectrum antibiotics that have good efficacy against both gram-negative and gram-positive are necessary as a diverse range of pathogens can be the cause of infections. A Cochrane systematic review found that acute bacterial conjunctivitis is often a self-limiting condition, 65% (95% confidence interval of 59% to 70%) patients treated with placebo showed significant improvement occurring by the second to fifth day of infection [12]. Patients treated with topical antibiotics were shown to have improved clinical outcome, especially when treated early (days 2 to 5) with relative risk = 1.24, 95% confidence interval = 1.05 to 1.45. Patients treated late (days 7 to 10) had reduced clinical benefit with relative risk = 1.11, 95% confidence interval = 1.02 to 1.21. Microbiological remission was also improved with treatment, early (days 2 to 5) showing relative risk = 1.77, 95% confidence interval = 1.23 to 2.54 and late (days 7 to 10) relative risk = 1.56, 95% confidence interval= 1.17 to 2.09.

An open, randomized and controlled study by Everitt et al investigated 307 adults and children with suspected infective conjunctivitis using three different treatment methods: no treatment, delayed topical treatment and immediate topical chloramphenicol treatment [13]. The varying treatments did not affect the severity of symptoms experienced within the first three days of infection. However, patients with moderate symptoms who were treated immediately with topical chloramphenicol had a reduced duration of symptoms with an average of 3.3 days whilst patients that received no treatment had 4.9 days duration.

Rietveld et al carried out a double-blind randomized and placebo controlled study in a primary care setting. The efficacy of fusidic acid gel was compared to a placebo gel in 163 adult patients presenting with a red eye and mucopurulent discharge [14]. After 7 days the treatments were evaluated with clinical cure being found in 62% of patients on fusidic acid gel and 59% of patients on placebo gel. The study found that the severity of symptoms and the duration of symptoms were not significantly different in either group. In conclusion, with the limited evidence the authors produced, they did not support the current practice of prescribing empirical antibiotics.

The majority of doctors actively treat uncomplicated acute bacterial conjunctivitis with empirical topical antibiotics at diagnosis. There are several other options available including: delaying treatment for 5 days and begin treatment if no sign of improvement and to treat patients who have clinical features associated with a bacterial cause. Studies comparing the effectiveness of different antibiotics recommended for use in suspected bacterial conjunctivitis have shown similar levels of effectiveness. Therefore, it is important to consider local bacterial resistance and cost-effectiveness of the antibiotics being prescribed [15]. All antibiotic courses should be taken for 7-10 days. Compliance with the length of time the antibioticsare prescribed for is particularly important to help prevent resistance developing.

The first line treatment in mild to moderate bacterial conjunctivitis is either Trimethoprim-Polymyxin B (Polytrim) solution, Erythromycin 0.5% ointment, or Azithromycin drops. Alternatives to these antibiotics are bacitracin ointment and sulfacetamide drops. In moderate to severe infections, or antibiotic-resistant infections and in immunocompromised patients, fluoroquinolones are recommended. These include: ofloxacin, ciprofloxacin, levofloxacin, moxifloxacin and gatifloxacin. Chlamydial conjunctivitis requires oral antibiotics alongside a topical antibiotic to treat the systemic infection alongside the ophthalmic manifestation. The oral antibiotic options include Azithromycin, doxycycline, or erythromycin. These are given in combination with Azithromycin or erythromycin drops for 2 to 3 weeks [16]. In addition, patients should be advised to take several precautions to help prevent spread of infection. Patients should wash their hands regularly and thoroughly, especially after touching any infected secretions. Furthermore, patients should avoid sharing towels, pillows, or utensils.

Studies have shown that treatment with topical antibiotics shortens the duration of disease, prevents spread of infection, reduces the rate of recurrence, and decreases the risk of complications that effect vision [17].However, there has been controversy in recent years over the use of empirical antibiotics and its role in an evidently self-limiting disease with the clinical outcome being only marginally favourable to taking no antibiotics. There has been increasing antibiotic resistance especially among the older class of antibiotics that have been used extensively such as chloramphenicol, sulphonamides, polymyxins, bacitracin, aminoglycosides and early generation fluoroquinolones. The efficacy of these drugs has reduced to a combination of resistance and narrow spectrum of activity [18, 19].The newer generation of fluoroquinolones, such as gatifloxacin and moxifloxacin, have a greater range of activity and efficacy against common pathogens of the eye [20].Specifically, they have better *in vitro* efficacy over the older generation fluoroquinolones against gram positive pathogens. However, the efficacy was not greater with *Haemophilus influenza* isolates [21]. The Ocular Tracking Resistance in the U.S. Today (TRUST) initiative annually monitors the *in vitro* susceptibility of common ocular pathogens; Staphylococcus aureus, Streptococcus pneumonia, and Haemophilus influenzae. Between 2000 and 2005 there was a 12.1% increase in the incidence of methicillin-resistant Staphylococcus aureus (MRSA). Moreover, greater than 80% of the MRSA strains were also resistant to fluoroquinolones [22, 23].

2.1.5. Prognosis of bacterial conjunctivitis

The prognosis of bacterial conjunctivitis is normally very good with the correct and prompt treatment of the infection. In many cases, spontaneous remission, without a cure, is seen. In a study done by Sheikh and Hurwitz et al, spontaneous cure occurred in 60% of patients within 1-2 weeks [24]. However, with prompt antibiotic treatment, the treatment time is significantly reduced.

2.2. Viral conjunctivitis

Viral conjunctivitis is a common infection amongst the Western population, and is often associated with other infections around the body. Due to the contiguity with the respiratory tract anatomy, viral upper respiratory tract infections are a common cause of secondary viral conjunctivitis.

Most cases of viral conjunctivitis are mild. Days 3-5 of infection are often the worst, but the infection will usually clear up in 7–14 days without treatment and without any long-term consequences. In some cases, viral conjunctivitis can take 2-3 weeks or more to clear up, especially if complications arise.

2.2.1. Pathogens causing viral conjunctivitis

Much unlike bacterial conjunctivitis, there are many pathogens associated with viral conjunctivitis, although the majority of cases of viral conjunctivitis are encompassed by a few common pathogens. The specific viruses are much dependant on the geographical area in the world. In a study done in the Far East countries of Japan, Korea and Taiwan the most common pathogens isolated from 1105 cases were *adenovirus 8* and *enterovirus 70*. Other viruses also identified were *adenoviruses 19* and *37* [25]. Similarly, the causes of viral conjunctivitis in the Western countries are mainly *adenoviruses*, though *adenovirus 13* seems to be the dominant strain in these countries.

Other rarer causes of viral conjunctivitis include *herpes simplex* virus, *herpes zoster* virus and the *measles* virus. Although less commonly seen, it is essential to identify *herpes* and *measles* viruses early to ensure prompt treatment, to prevent any long term complications associated with these viruses.

A recent study also showed outbreaks of the *avian influenza* viruses in patients, although this may possibly be linked to the recent outbreaks of the virus in humans.

2.2.2. *Signs and symptoms of viral conjunctivitis*

As with bacterial conjunctivitis, a diagnosis of viral conjunctivitis is often made by the general practitioner on the basis of a history and examination. However, due to the overlap in symptoms between viral and bacterial conjunctivitis, it is often difficult to ascertain viral from bacterial conjunctivitis.

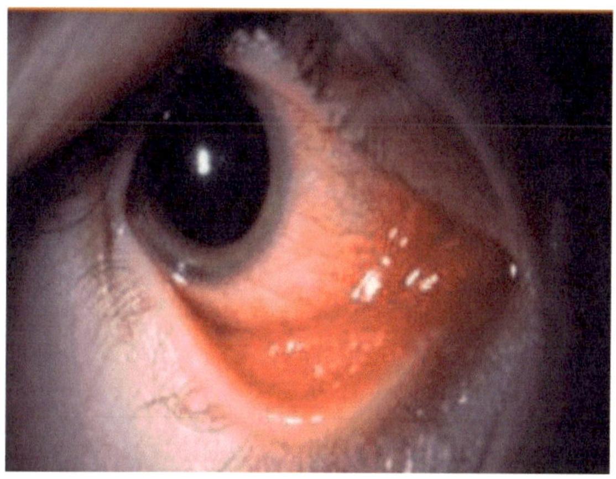

Figure 7. Classical 'pink' eye associated with conjunctival injection seen in viral conjunctivitis

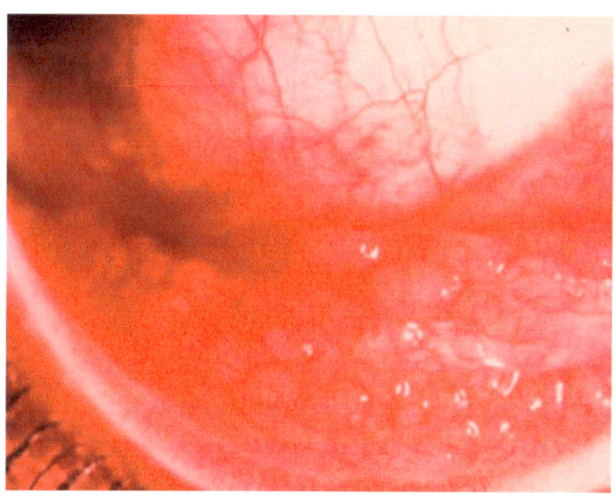

Figure 8. Classical follicles seen in the conjunctiva in a patient suffering from herpetic conjunctivitis

The key symptom of viral conjunctivitis is 'pink eye'. This shows a fine, diffuse pinkness of the conjunctiva, which is often easily mistaken for the ciliary injection of iritis. Other symptoms associated with viral conjunctivitis include discharge which is often clear and watery. This is often the most discernible difference between bacterial and viral conjunctivitis.

A history of itchy eyes is also suggestive of viral conjunctivitis, although it is a symptom also associated with irritant and allergic conjunctivitis. Rarer symptoms associated with simple *adenovirus* viral conjunctivitis include foreign body sensation, ocular discomfort, excessive tearing and sticky eyelids which are worse in the morning.

Herpes simplex conjunctivitis is usually unilateral. Symptoms include a red eye, photophobia, eye pain and mucoid discharge. There may be periorbital vesicles, and a conjunctival branching (dendritic) pattern of fluorescein staining makes the diagnosis.

Below is a table summarising the key differences between adenoviral and herpetic viral conjunctivitis.

Adenoviral	Herpetic
Watery discharge bilaterally	Usually unilateral watery discharge
Hyperaemia	Diffuse hyperaemia
Petechial hemorrhages	Vesicular eruptions on eyelid
Punctate keratitis	Follicles
Preauricular and/or submandibular lymphadenopathy	Occasional preauricularlypmphadenopathy
Serous, mucoid, or mucopurulent discharge	Serous mucoid discharge
Associated with pharyngitis	Major complication of dendritic epethilial keratitis

Table 1. A summary of the differences of adenoviral and herpetic viral conjunctivitis

Herpes zoster Ophthalmicus is shingles of the opthalmic branch of the trigeminal nerve, which innervates the cornea and the tip of the nose. It begins with unilateral neuralgia, followed by a vesicular rash in the distribution of nerve. Once spread to the eye, it may lead to an extremely painful conjunctivitis and may take several days to settle.

2.2.3. Complications of viral conjunctivitis

There are many recognised complications of viral conjunctivitis. In many cases, it may be associated with inflammation of the cornea, known as keratoconjunctivitis. There is also an increase in likelihood of a superimposed bacterial infection. Other rare complications associated with viral conjunctivitis include blepharitis, entropion and in very rare cases, scarring of the eyelid.

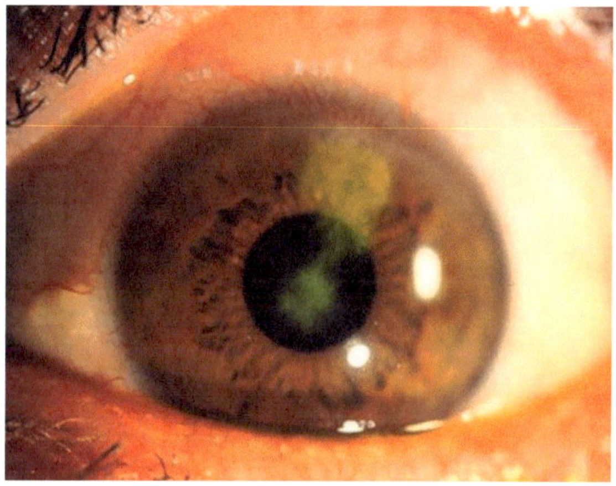

Figure 9. Herpes simplex keratitis, demonstrated here via fluorescein staining

The most serious complication of viral conjunctivitis is *herpes simplex* keratitis, a corneal ulcer, which can ultimately lead to blindness. This is an extremely rare side effect of viral conjunctivitis and requires immediate transfer to hospital and review by the ophthalmologists.

2.2.4. Treatment of viral conjunctivitis

Viral conjunctivitis is a self-limiting disease that usually resolves within two weeks of onset of symptoms and does not require treatment with antiviral medication. There is no evidence supporting the use of anti-viral medication and their efficacy has not been proven. However, as a highly contagious disease, there is a need to make infected patients aware of good hygiene practices to prevent further spread. Viral conjunctivitis is transmitted through direct contact, therefore, hands should be thoroughly washed regularly, and infected patients should not share pillows, towels and other utensils [26].The highly contagious nature of viral conjunctivitis, especially adenovirus, makes it necessary for infected patients to avoid going to work or school for 5 days to 2 weeks. Contagiousness of adenovirus conjunctivitis has been shown to be reduced in an *in vitro* study using the topical anti-viral agent povidone-iodine. Povidone-iodine at a concentration of 1:10 (0.8%) is particularly effective against free adenovirus, eradicating all of them within 10 minutes with little cytotoxicity [27]. In addition, patients with contact lenses should avoid using them until the conjunctivitis resolves and last dose of any treatment having been taken over 24 hours ago [28]. Treatment for viral conjunctivitis is supportive, involving cold compresses, ocular decongestants, and artificial tears for symptomatic relief. In patients with high susceptibility of contracting bacterial infections an antibiotic may be given to prevent a bacterial superinfection occurring.If a pseudomembrane or corneal subepithelial infiltrates develop then a topical corticosteroid may be given alongside the other non-pharmacological treatments outlined earlier. Immediate referral to an ophthalmologist should be considered in patients with a psuedomembrane or corneal subepithelial infiltrate. Immediate referral is necessary in patients with hyperacute conjunctivitis or those who have corneal involvement including ulceration and herpetic keratitis.

2.2.5. Prognosis of viral conjunctivitis

Viral conjunctivitis is extremely contagious and remains so for 14 days, which also is often how long the symptoms remain.

The prognosis is very good for viral conjunctivitis. It resolves completely within 2 weeks of the 'pink eye' onset and there are rarely any long term complications or problems associated with viral conjunctivitis [29].

3. Conjunctivitis in the immunocompromised

Conjunctivitis in the immunocompromised is something that is often overlooked by the general practioner. However, it is essential to properly investigate conjunctivitis in immunodeficient patients as they are more likely to suffer from long term complications such as dendritic ulcers and corneal damage.

3.1. Epidemiology and conjunctival microvascular disease associated with HIV

Up to 75% of HIV infected patients have suffered from conjunctivitis. Most will exhibit microvascular changes of the conjunctiva, often the inferior perilimbal bulbar conjunctiva. These changes are often seen as capillary dilations, short irregular vessels and a granular appearance of blood column within the vessels.

In some cases, there have been reports of direct infiltration of the vascular endothelial cells of the conjunctiva being infiltrated by the HIV virus, which causes a deposition of immune complexes within the conjunctiva, causing conjunctivitis.

3.2. Infections causing conjunctivitis in the immunocompromised

Most conjunctivitis reports in the immunocompromised, especially HIV, have shown *staphylococci* to be the main infective agent, with *coagulase negative staphylococci* (mostly *staphylococcal epidermidis* the majority) accounting for most of the cases. The major other normal flora organism which cause infection in immunocompromised patients include *cornybacterium pseudo/diphtherticum*(found in the nasopharynx) and certain members of the *Haemophilus* group. Isolated cases of *neisseriameningitidis*and the *measles* virus have also been found in immunocompromised patients, although no study has yet shown a direct link between these two organisms and conjunctivitis in the immunocompromised.

Opportunistic infections may also cause conjunctivitis. Below are common pathogens that have been identified as opportunistic infections causing conjunctivitis:

- Microsporidial keratoconjunctivitis- Reports of microsporidial keratoconjunctivitis in AIDS patients have been noted. This infection is caused by an intracellular protozoan parasite of the phylum *Microspora*. Patients affected with Microsporidial keratoconjunctivitis experience similar symptoms as with any other bacterial infection, but the symptoms of photophobia and extreme redness are also present. There may also be bilateral conjunctival hyperaemia with diffuse coarse white infiltrates, conjunctival hypertrophy and erosions of the corneal epithelium [30].

Microsporidial keratoconjunctivitis should not be overlooked in HIV patients because it rarely responds to conventional topical antivirals or antibacterials. In some cases, antiprotozoal medication has also been reported as ineffective. A recent study found that Fumagillin (Fumidin B) is the treatment with most positive outcome in HIV patients with Microsporidial keratoconjunctivitis [31].

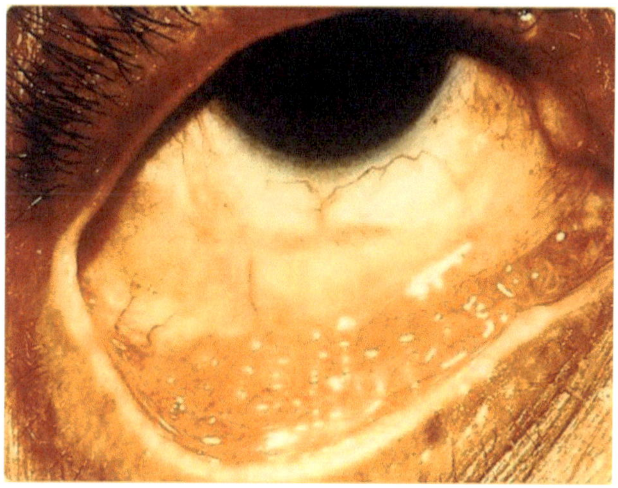

Figure 10. Conjunctivitis in a patient suffering from AIDS

- Molluscum contagiosum-Although rarely affecting the conjunctiva even in immunocompromised individuals, molluscum contagiosum has been noted to primarily affect the conjunctiva and also cause secondary conjunctival inflammation during infection. In one case report, a nodule of molluscum contagiosum was noted on the bulbar conjunctiva on a 34 year old man with AIDS [32]. However, in most cases of patients in an immunocompromised state with molluscum contagiosum, the conjunctiva is secondarily affected, causing an associated follicular conjunctivitis [33].

Treatment of primarily conjuctival infection of molluscum contagiosum is via cryotherapy and/or surgery, although this has shown to provide only limited long term correction in HIV patients.

- Fungal infections- Fungal infections affecting the conjunctiva are rare. In immunocompromised patients, the cornea is often affected, causing a keratitis to develop. This can however, cause a secondary conjunctivitis. Studies have shown that *Cryptococcus* and *Candida albicans* are the most common pathogens affecting the cornea and conjunctiva in immunocompromised patients.

Fortunately, the treatment is very effective for fungal infections. Although hospital admission is required in patients affected with keratitis, topical amphotericin B or natamycin, subconjunctival miconazole and oral ketoconazole are proven effective antifungals.

4. Neonatal conjunctivitis

Neonatal conjunctivitis also known as ophthalmia neonatorum is inflammation of the conjunctiva occurring in the first month of life. This condition is caused by a number of different pathogens. These include bacteria, viruses and chemical agents. In recent times prophylaxis has led to decreased morbidity in the developed world. However, it is still a significant cause of ocular morbidity, blindness and even death in the developing world.

4.1. Epidemiology of neonatal conjunctivitis

The incidence of ophthalmia neonatorum is dependent on many different factors. The main risk factor for ophthalmia neonatorum of infective origin is the presence of a sexually transmitted disease in the mother. The organism usually infects the neonate through direct contact as it passes through the birth canal. Therefore, incidence is high in areas with high rates of sexually transmitted disease [34]. Prolonged rupture of membranes at the time of delivery is also thought to increase the risk of infection. It is also dependent on socioeconomic factors; incidence varies in highly developed countries with good prenatal care compared to the developing parts of the world [35]. The offending pathogens vary geographically due to the differences in the prevalence of maternal infection and the use of prophylaxis. In US and Europe the incidence has been reported 1-2% depending on the socioeconomic character of the area. However in other parts of the world the incidence is reported to be as high as 17%. In recent studies in Pakistanthe incidence has been 17% and in Kenya as high 23% [36, 37].

There has been a sharp decrease in the incidence of ophthalmia neonatorum in the past few decades in the developed countries due to many reasons. In 1800s, prophylaxis (silver nitrate) for ophthalmia neonatorum in the developed countries was used for the first time. Since then there has been gradual decrease in incidence. Better prenatal care has also led to detection and treatment of sexually transmitted diseases hence reduction in the risk of transmission to new-borns during birth.

4.2. Aetiology of neonatal conjunctivitis

Ophthalmia neonatorum can be broadly divided into two types, septic and aseptic. The aseptic type (chemical conjunctivitis) is generally secondary to the instillation of silver nitrate drops for ocular prophylaxis. Septic neonatal conjunctivitis is mainly caused by bacterial and viral infections. Causes include [38]:

From maternal genital tract:

- Bacterial
  - *Neisseria gonorrhoeae*
  - *Chlamydia trachomatis*
  - *Group B beta-haemolytic streptococci*
- Viral
  - *Herpes Simplex Virus (HSV)*

From cross infection:

- *Staphylococcus aureus*
- *Coliforms*
- *Pseudomonas aeruginosa*

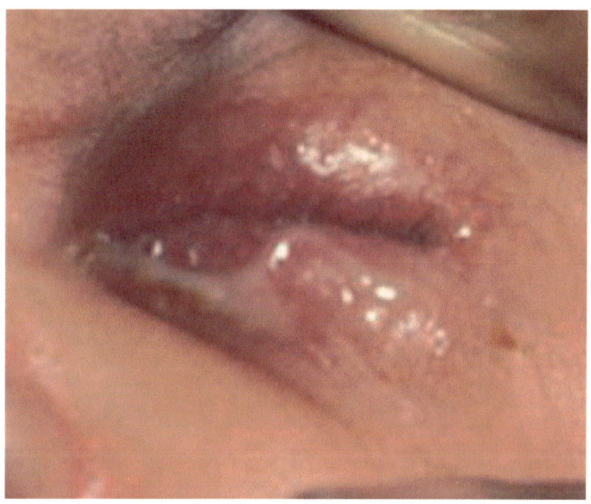

Figure 11. A neonate suffering from gonococcal conjunctivitis

Neisseria gonorrhoeae - Congenital gonorrhoea infection is acquired intrapartum and it leads to ophthalmia neonatorum. *Gonococcal* ophthalmia neonatorum presents with a severe conjunctivitis and keratitis usually in the first 48 hours of life but it can be delayed up to 3 weeks. It is frequently bilateral. If untreated, it can lead to blindness. Systemic infection can cause meningitis, arthritis and sepsis.

Chlamydia trachomatis - Also known as trachoma-inclusion conjunctivitis or TRIC.This is usually a benign, self-limiting, suppurative conjunctivitis due to *Chlamydia trachomatis* - serotypes D-K. Onset occurs around 1 week of age. Onset maybe earlier with premature rupture of membranes. It is characterised by mild swelling, hyperaemia and minimal to moderate discharge.

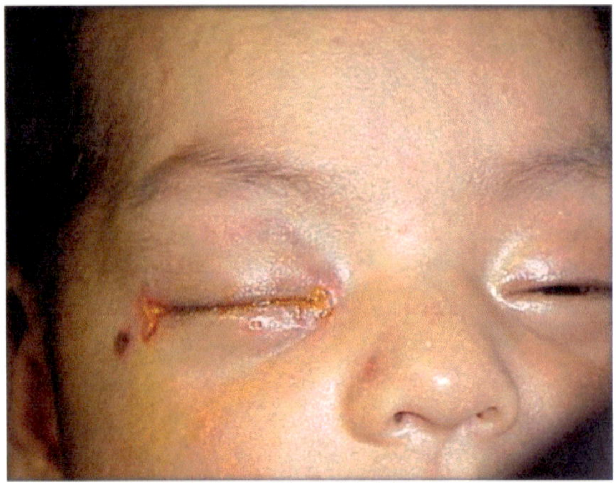

Figure 12. Typical presentation of a neonate suffering from herpetic conjunctivitis

Other bacteria -These bacteria make up 30-50% of all cases of neonatal conjunctivitis. The most commonly identified gram-positive organisms include *Staphylococcus aureus, Streptococcus pneumoniae, Streptococcus viridans,* and *Staphylococcus epidermidis.* Gram-negative organisms, such as *Escherichia coli, Klebsiella pneumoniae, Serratia marcescens,* and *Proteus, Enterobacter,* and *Pseudomonas species,* also have been implicated.

Herpes Simplex- Herpes simplex virus (HSV) can cause neonatal keratoconjunctivitis. This is a rarer form of ophthalmia neonatorum presenting in the second week of life and can be associated with a generalized herpes simplex infection.

Chemical Conjunctivitis- Classically, the most common cause of neonatal conjunctivitis is due to use of post-delivery use of ophthalmic silver nitrate used in the prophylaxis of ocular *Gonococcal* infections. There is a mild irritation, tearing and redness in a baby who has been administered prophylactic silver nitrate (used for the prevention of gonorrhoeal infection) within the preceding 24-48 hours. The incidence of chemical conjunctivitis in the United States has significantly decreased since replacement of silver nitrate with erythromycin ointment.

4.3. Presentation of neonatal conjunctivitis

Babies present with unilateral or bilateral purulent, mucopurulent or mucoid discharge from the eyes within the first month of life. Injected conjunctiva and lid swelling may also be present. There may be associated systemic infection.

- Bacterial conjunctivitis - often have a longer incubation period than for the other infective causes. Presenting with a sub-acute onset between the 4th and 28th day of life. Depending on the pathogen, there may be a mixed picture of a red eye with lid swelling and a varying amount of purulent discharge. Specific types of bacterial infection:

- *Chlamydial* infection - 5 to 14 days after birth (some report up to 28 days after birth): unilateral/bilateral watery discharge which becomes copious and purulent later on. There may be associated preseptal cellulitis and, less commonly, rhinitis, otitis and pneumonitis.
- *Gonorrhoeal* infection - typically 1-5 days after birth but may occur later: hyper-acute conjunctival injection and chemosis, lid oedema and severe purulent discharge. There may be associated corneal ulceration and perforation.
- Viral conjunctivitis
- The onset is acute usually 1-14 days after birth: unilateral/bilateral serosanguinous discharge ± vesicular skin lesions. Uncommonly it can also lead to systemic infection.

4.4. Differential diagnosis of neonatal conjunctivitis

Every other potential cause of red eye needs to be excluded. The differentials include [39]:

- Dacryocystitis
- Congenital glaucoma
- Nasolacrimal duct obstruction
- Preseptal/Orbital cellulitis
- Congenital glaucoma
- Infectious keratitis

4.5. Investigations

A definitive diagnosis of the cause of ophthalmia neonatorum is dependent on laboratory identification of the offending organism. The speed of progression of some of the causative agents makes it imperative to do a test which can identify the cause as soon as possible. Some of the laboratory tests that can be performed are as follows [40]:

- Culture on chocolate agar for *N gonorrhoeae.* Due to the rapid progression of *N gonorrhoea* conjunctivitis, it makes it imperative to perform smears, as it may be possible to identify gram-negative diplococci and initiate proper treatment within hours.
- Conjunctival scraping with Gram stain and Giemsa stain for *chlamydia.* Conjunctival specimens for *chlamydia* testing must include conjunctival epithelial cells because *C. trachomatis* is an obligate intracellular organism and exudates are not adequate for testing. Other non-culture methods such as direct fluorescent antibody testing, enzyme immunoassays and nucleic acid testing (NAT) may allow early detection of *Chlamydia* within hours rather than several days, as required for culture methods.
- Culture on blood agar for other strains of bacteria. For other viral aetiology direct cultures of the HSV vesicles can be performed. Alternatively direct antibody testing or PCR can be done. If symptoms worsen or symptoms recur after treatment cultures may have to be repeated.

4.6. Management of neonatal conjunctivitis

Prophylaxis- In 1881 for the first time silver nitrate was used as prophylactic treatment to reduce the incidence of ophthalmia neonatorum. Silver nitrate is specifically more effective against gonorrhoeal conjunctivitis. It inactivates gonococci by agglutination. It is not effective against Chlamydial conjunctivitis. However silver nitrate use also led to mild conjunctival inflammation, tearing and redness which typically resolved within 48 hours. Chemical conjunctivitis is a self-limiting condition, therefore no treatment is required. However preservative artificial tears have been used in some cases.

In recent times povidone-iodine drops are used as prophylaxis instead of silver nitrate [41]. These are shown to be more effective against *gonococcal* and *chlamydial* conjunctivitis and also less toxic. In US, erythromycin is being used as alternative to silver nitrate and povidone-iodine [42]. This is also well tolerated and effective against TRIC and gonococci agents.

Treatment -Treatment of neonatal conjunctivitis should initially be based on the history, clinical presentation and results of smears. This can later be adjusted when laboratory results become available then specific therapy can be instituted.

The risk of transmission of chlamydial, gonococcal, herpetic, and streptococcal pathogens to the foetus during the birth process should be considered. If necessary, cervical cultures should be performed and managed appropriately. To confirm the presence of a sexually transmitted disease in the neonate, examine and treat the mother and her sexual partner. If necessary, therapy can be modified when the results of culture and sensitivity are known.

Bacterial conjunctivitis- Chlamydial conjunctivitis is treated with fourteen day course of twice daily oral erythromycin(50 mg/kg/d divided qid) [43, 44]. Systemic therapy is important in Chlamydia conjunctivitis, due to the high incidence of extra-ocular infection in neonates. It has shown to eliminate Chlamydial infection in 80-100% of patients. Topical erythromycin can be used as adjunct with the oral therapy. If there is failure to respond to this course the fourteen day course can be repeated before seeking alternative antibiotics [45].

Gonococcal conjunctivitis may be treated with intramascular or intravenous ceftriaxone 50 mg/kg/day or as a single dose treatment of 125mg [46]. Alternatively, cefotaxime 100mg can be given intramuscularly or 25 mg/kg given either intramuscularly or intravenously every 12 hours for 7 days [47].

Neonates with conjunctivitis caused by herpetic simplex virus should be treated with systemic acyclovir to reduce the chance of a systemic infection [48]. An effective dose is 60 mg/kg/day IV divided.The recommended minimal duration is 14 days, but a course as long as 21 days may be required.Infants with neonatal HSV keratitis should receive a topical ophthalmic drug, most commonly 1% trifluridine drops or 3% vidarabine ointment.

4.7. Complications of neonatal conjunctivitis

Complications of neonatal conjunctivitis vary. There are two main types of complications, ocular and systemic complications. These can be prevented with prompt diagnosis and treatment. Ocular complications include pseudomembrane formation, peripheral pannus formation, thickened palpebral conjunctiva, cornealoedema, corneal opacification, corneal perforation, staphyloma, endophthalmitis, loss of eye, and blindness [49].

Systemic complications of chlamydia conjunctivitis include pneumonitis, otitis, and pharyngeal and rectal colonization. Pneumonia has been reported in 10-20% of infants with chlamydial conjunctivitis. Complications of gonococcal conjunctivitis and subsequent systemic involvement include arthritis, meningitis, anorectal infection, septicaemia, and death.

Ophthalmia neonatorum is a preventable cause of childhood blindness and with prompt diagnosis, treatment and efforts on all levels, this can be eradicated.

5. Prevention of conjunctivitis

Infective conjunctivitis is a condition which affects people of all ages. Its spread is something that can be effectively controlled via good personal hygiene and adequate education. Once an individual is affected, rapid measures must be taken to ensure that the spread is limited.

Good personal hygiene is primarily achieved via effective hand washing and eye care. Where an outbreak of the highly contagious viral conjunctivitis has occurred, stringent measures to control the spread must be undertaken immediately. Simple measures such as removal of possible contaminated materials (hand cloth, towels and face cloths) are very effective in reducing spread.

For specialist cases of conjunctivitis, i.e. neonatal conjunctivitis and conjunctivitis in the immunocompromised, immediate action must be undertaken to ensure no long term complications and quick recovery. Should there be any delay in treatment, the potential for long term damage, and even blindness, is very high. Prevention of such conditions can be attained by immediate and frequent treatment via hospital admissions, prophylactic medication and good eye hygiene.

6. Conclusion

Conjunctivitis can be a very irritating and frustrating condition to suffer from. Not only does it have profound social implications, it can also affect education and finances if social exclusion is required. General practitioners must remain vigilant when diagnosing viral from bacterial conjunctivitis and try to ensure that patient education of the condition is at an optimum level to prevent spread. Special care must also be taken into consideration in neonatal conjunctivitis and conjunctivitis in the immunocompromised.

Although conjunctivitis is mostly a mild condition, GPs must also be aware of other more serious conditions and be able to differentiate mild conditions from more serious underlying and emergency conditions. This is only achieved via being able to create a list of differentials from a thorough patient history, examination and referral to an ophthalmologist if required.

Author details

Adnaan Haq, Haseebullah Wardak and Narbeh Kraskian

St. George's University of London, UK

References

[1] Santa JO, Mark BA. Allergic conjunctivitis: Update on pathophysiology and prospects for future treatment. The Journal of Allergy and Clinical Immunology. 2004; 115: 118-122.

[2] Sheikh A, Hurwitz B. Topical antibiotics for acute bacterial conjunctivitis: a systematic review. Br J Gen Pract. 2001; 51:473–7.

[3] Department of Health, Prescription cost analysis data. Leeds: Department of Health, 1998.

[4] Rose PW, Harnden A, Brueggemann AB, Perera R, Sheikh A, Crook D, Mant D. Chloramphenicol treatment for acute infective conjunctivitis in children in primary care: a randomised double-blind placebo-controlled study. Lancet. 2005; 366: 37–43.

[5] Weiss A, Brinser JH, Nazar-Stewart V. Acute conjunctivitis in childhood. J Pediatr. 1993; 122: 10–14.

[6] Gigliotti F, Williams WT, Hayden FG, Hendley JO. Etiology of acute conjunctivitis in children. J Pediatr. 1981; 98: 531–536.

[7] Tarabishy BA, Jeng HB. Bacterial conjuntivitis: A review for internists. Cleveland Clinic Journal of Medicine. 2008; 75: 508-512.

[8] Genees en hulpmiddelen Informatie Project. Annual report prescription data. Collegevoorzorg verzekeringen, Amstelveen, 2001.

[9] Carr WD. Comparison of Fucithalmic® (fusidic acid viscous eye drops 1%) and Chloromycetin Redidrops® (chloramphenicol eye drops 0. 5%) in the treatment of acute bacterial conjunctivitis. J Clin Res. 1998; 1: 403–411.

[10] Wall AR, Sinclair N, Adenis JP. Comparison of Fucithalmic® (fusidic acid viscous eye drops 1%) and Noroxin (norfloxacin ophthalmic solution 0. 3%) in the treatment of acute bacterial conjunctivitis. J Drug Assess. 1998; 1: 549–558.

[11] Schiebel N: Use of antibiotics in patients with acute bacterial conjunctivitis. Ann Emerg Med. 2003; 41: 407–409.

[12] Sheikh A, Hurwitz B. Topical antibiotics for acute bacterial conjunctivitis: Cochrane systematic review and meta-analysis update. British Journal of General Practice. 2005; 55: 962-964.

[13] Everitt HA, Little PS, Smith PW. A randomised controlled trial of management strategies for acute infective conjunctivitis in general practice. BMJ. 2006; 333: 321.

[14] Rietveld RP, Bindels PJE, Sloos JH, van Weert HCPM. The treatment of acute infectious conjunctivitis with fusidic acid: a randomised controlled trial. Br J Gen Pract. 2005; 55: 924–930.

[15] Cronau H, Kankanala RR, Mauger T. Diagnosis and management of red eye in primary care. Am Fam Physician. 2010; 81: 137-44.

[16] Anon. Acute Conjunctivitis. Best Medical Practice, BMJ [serial online]. Available from:http://bestpractice. bmj. com/best-practice/monograph/68/treatment/details. html

[17] Sheikh A, Hurwitz B. Topical antibiotics for acute bacterial conjunctivitis: Cochrane systematic review and meta-analysis update. British Journal of General Practice. 2005; 55: 962-964

[18] Fraunfelder FW. Corneal toxicity from topical ocular and systemic medications. Cornea. 2006; 25: 1133-8

[19] Schlech BA, Blondeau J. Future of ophthalmic anti-infective therapy and the role of moxifloxacin ophthalmic solution 0. 5% (VIGAMOX) . SurvOphthalmol. 2005; 50: 64-7.

[20] Kowalski RP, Dhaliwal DK, Karenchak LM, Romanowski EG, Mah FS, Ritterband DC, Gordon YJ. Gatifloxacin and moxifloxacin: an in vitro susceptibility comparison to levofloxacin, ciprofloxacin, and ofloxacin using bacterial keratitis isolates. Am J Ophthalmol. 2003; 136: 500-5.

[21] Kowalski RP, Yates KA, Romanowski EG, Karenchak LM, Mah FS, Gordon YJ. An ophthalmologist's guide to understanding antibiotic susceptibility and minimum inhibitory concentration data. Ophthalmology. 2005; 112: 1987.

[22] Asbell PA, Colby KA, Deng S, McDonnell P, Meisler DM, Raizman MB, Sheppard JD Jr, Sahm DF. Ocular TRUST: nationwide antimicrobial susceptibility patterns in ocular isolates. Am J Ophthalmol. 2008; 145: 951-958.

[23] Asbell PA, Sahm DF, Shaw M, Draghi DC, Brown NP. Increasing prevalence of methicillin resistance in serious ocular infections caused by Staphylococcus aureus in the United States: 2000 to 2005. J Cataract Refract Surg. 2008; 34: 814-8

[24] Sheikh A & Hurwitz B: Topical antibiotics for acute bacterial conjunctivitis: a systematic review. Br J General Prac. 2001; 51: 473–477.

[25] Ishii K, Nakazono N, FujinagaK, Fujji S, Kato M, Ohtusaka H, Aoki K, Chen CW, Lin CC, Sheu MM, Lin KH, Oum BS, Lee SH, Chun CH, Yoshii T, Yamazaki S. Comparative Studies on Aetiology and Epidemiology of Viral Conjunctivitis in Three Countries of East Asia—Japan, Taiwan and South Korea. International Journal of Epidemiology. 1986; 16: 98-103.

[26] Donahue, S. P. , Khoury, J. M. , Kowalski, R. P. (1996) Common ocular infections: a prescriber's guide. Drugs. 52 (4) , pp. 528-529.

[27] Monnerat, N. , Bossart, W. , Thiel, M. A. (2006) Povidone-iodine for treatment of adenoviral conjunctivitis: an in vitro study. Klinische Monatsblätterfür Augenheilkunde. 223 (5) , pp. 349-52.

[28] Cronau, H. , Kankanala, R. R. , Mauger, T. (2010) Diagnosis and management of red eye in primary care. American Academy of Family Physicians. 81(2) , pp. 137-44.

[29] Schueler, S. J. , Beckett, J. H. , Gettings, D. S. (2008) Viral Conjunctivitis: Outlook. Available: http://www. freemd. com/viral-conjunctivitis/outlook. htm. Last accessed 8th August 2012.

[30] Chronister, C. L. (1996) Review of External Ocular Disease Associated with AIDS and HIV infection. American Academy of Optometry. 73 (4) , pp. 225-230.

[31] Diesenhouse, M. C. , Wilson, L. A. , Corrent, G. F. , Visvesvara, G. C. (1993) Treatment of Microsporidial keratoconjunctivitis with topical fumagillin. American Journal of Ophthalmology. 115 (1) , pp. 293-298.

[32] Charles, N. C. , Freidberg, D. N. (1992) Molluscum Contagiosum in AIDS. Ophthalmology (Rochester) . 99 (7) , pp. 1123-1126.

[33] Kohn, S. R. (1987) MolluscumContagiosum in patients with AIDS. American Medical Association: Archives of Ophthalmology. 105 (4) , p. 458.

[34] Schryver, A. D. , Meheus, A. (1990) Epidemiology of sexually transmitted diseases: the global picture. Bulletin of the World Health Organization. 68(5) , pp. 639–654.

[35] Verma, M. , Chaatwal, J. , Varughese, P. (1994) Neonatal Conjunctivitis: A Profile. Indian Paediatrics. 31(11) , pp. 1357-61.

[36] Jamal, L. , Khan, M. (2010) Ophthalmianeonatorum. Journal of College Physicians and Surgeons Pakistan. 20(9) , pp. 595-8.

[37] Laga, M. , Plummer, F. A. , Nzanze, H. , Namaara, W. , Brunham, R. C. , Ndinya-Achola, J. O. , Maitha, G. , Ronald, A. R. , D'Costa, L. J. , Bhullar, V. B. , Fransen, L. , Piot, P. , (1986) Epidemiology of Opthalmia Neonatorum in Kenya. The Lancet. 328(8516) , pp. 1145-1149.

[38] Enzenauer R. W. , (2011) Neonatal Conjunctivitis. Available at: http://emedicine. medscape. com/article/1192190-overview(Accessed: 5th August 2012) .

[39] Scott, O. , (2011) OphtalmiaNeonatorum Available at: http://www. patient. co. uk/doctor/Ophthalmia-Neonatorum. htm(Accessed 5th August 2012) .

[40] Gregory, S. , Cantor, L. , Louis, B. , Weiss, J. S. , (2011) Paediatric Opthalmology and Strabismus. In The American Academy of Ophthalmology, ed, Basic and clinical science course. 1st edn. Singapore: American Academy of Ophthalmology, pp. 186-188.

[41] Sherwin, J. , Isenberg, A. P. T. , Leonard, A. P. T. , Wood, M. , (1995) A Controlled Trial of Povidone–Iodine as Prophylaxis against OphthalmiaNeonatorum. The New England Journal of Medicine. 332 (9) , pp. 562-566.

[42] Darling, E. , McDonald, H. , (2010) A meta-analysis of the efficacy of ocular prophylactic agents used for the prevention of gonococcal and chlamydial ophthalmianeonatorum. Journal of Midwifery and Women's Health. 55(4) , pp. 319-27.

[43] Heggie, A. D. , Jaffe, A. C. , Stuart, L. A. , Thombre, P. S. , Sorensen, R. U. (1985) Topical Sulfacetamidevs Oral Erythromycin for Neonatal Chlamydial Conjunctivitis. American Journal of diseases of children. 139(6) , pp. 564-566.

[44] Zar H. J. , (2005) Neonatal Chlamydial Infections: Prevention and Treatment. Pediatric Drugs. 7(2) , pp. 103-110.

[45] Stenberg, K. , Mardhip, A. , (1991) Treatment of chlamydial conjunctivitis in newborns and adults with erythromycin and roxithromycin. Journal of Antimicrobial Chemotherapy. 28(2) , pp. 301-307.

[46] Laga, M. , Naamara, W. , Brunham, R. C. , D'Costa, L. , Nsanze, H. , Piot, P. , Kunimoto, D. , Ndinya-Achola, J. , Slaney, L. , Ronald, A. R. , Plummer, F. A. (1986) Single-Dose Therapy of Gonococcal Ophthalmia Neonatorum with Ceftriaxone. The New England Journal of Medicine. 315(22) , pp. 1382-1385.

[47] Pierce, J. M. , Ward, M. E. , Seal, D. V. (1982) Ophthalmianeonatorum in the 1980s: incidence, aetiology and treatment. British Journal of Ophthalmology. 66 (11) , pp. 728-731.

[48] Whitley, R. , (2004) Neonatal herpes simplex virus infection. Current Opinion in Infectious Diseases. 17(3) , pp. 243-246.

[49] Gogate, P. , Gilbert, C. , Zin, A. (2011) Severe Visual Impairment and Blindness in Infants: Causes and Opportunities for Control. Middle East African Journal of Ophthalmology. 18(2) , pp. 109-114.

Chapter 3

Treatments in Infectious and Allergic Conjunctivitis: Is Immunomodulation the Future?

Concepcion Santacruz, Sonia Mayra Perez-Tapia, Angel Nava-Castañeda, Sergio Estrada-Parra and Maria C. Jimenez-Martinez

Additional information is available at the end of the chapter

http://dx.doi.org/10.5772/52263

1. Introduction

The ocular surface is a functional unit mainly formed by the conjunctival and corneal epithelium (structural component), and tear film (soluble component). Microorganisms and environmental allergens can interact with the tear film, reach the structural component and generate an immune response against them. Understanding the cellular and soluble mediators that are involved in these inflammatory responses not only helps in understanding the mechanisms of current treatments, but also is needed to identification and development of new therapeutics targets. The aim of this review was to investigate the novel and developing therapies, with special emphasis in immunomodulatory drugs/ molecules that could have some clinical indication in the treatment of infectious and allergic conjunctivitis in few years.

2. Novel therapies in infectious keratoconjunctivitis

2.1. Interferons (IFN) and adenoviral conjunctivitis

Interferons were first described as the major effector cytokines of the host immune response against viral infections. IFN are well recognized by their potent antiviral properties, however IFN production is also induced in response to bacterial ligands of innate immune receptors and/or bacterial infections, indicating a broader physiological role for these cytokines in host defence and homeostasis than was originally described.

Three main types of cytokines compose the IFN family: type I, type II and type III IFN. Type I IFN family is composed of 16 members, namely 12 IFNα subtypes, IFNβ, IFNε, IFNκ and IFNω. By contrast, the type II IFN family includes only one cytokine: IFNγ, which also exhibits antiviral activities. The third type of IFN is the IFNλ family, which includes IFNλ1 (also known as IL-29), IFNλ2 (also known as IL-28A) and IFNλ3 (also known as IL-28B). On the basis of protein sequence and structure, type III IFN are markedly different from type I and type II IFN and are more similar to members of the interleukin-10 (IL-10) family; however, they provoke antiviral responses and induce the activation of IFN-stimulated genes. [1]

Epidemic keratoconjunctivitis (EKC) is a severe ocular infection, caused by highly contagious adenoviruses Ad8, Ad19, and Ad37. Adenoviral infection of the eye induces keratitis and conjunctivitis, accompanied by pain, lacrimation, red and swollen eye, as well as decreased vision that may last for months or even years. No specific antiviral drugs are currently available for the treatment of EKC or any other infection caused by adenoviruses. Interestingly, it has been suggested that five strains of different serotypes of adenovirus, types 3 (AdV3; species B), 4 (species E), 8, 19a and 37 (species D) involved in acute keratoconjunctivitis are highly inhibited by IFN-b and IFN-g in the A549 cell line, [2] However, IFN therapy in adenoviral keratoconjunctivitis has not been evaluated in clinical trials yet.

2.2. Glycan interactions and EKC

The initial event leading to EKC is binding of the viruses to glycans that contain sialic acid moieties on epithelial cells in the cornea or conjunctiva through trimeric fiber structures extending from the viral particles. The receptor-binding domain is located at the C terminus of each fiber and contains three separate pockets that each can accommodate one sialic acid residue. Ad37 was recently shown to bind to cell-surface glycoproteins carrying a glycan structure named GD1a due to similitude to GD1a ganglioside. The GD1a glycan is a branched hexasaccharide with a terminal sialic acid residue on each of its two arms. Structural studies showed that the two sialic acid moieties dock into two of three sialic acid binding sites in the trimeric knob of the Ad37 fiber protein. Most likely, multiple fiber proteins simultaneously engage several host-cell epitopes containing terminal sialic acids; internalization and subsequent infection follow. In this context, the molecules named ME0322, ME0323, and ME0324 were synthetized as a tri- and tetravalent sialic acid compounds, and interestingly all of theses molecules inhibited the attachment of Ad37 virions to HCE cells in a dose-dependent manner and were at least two orders of magnitude more effective than sialic acid, suggesting a promissory inhibitor of Ad37 infection on corneal cells, composed by a multivalent sialic acid conjugate. If these compounds could be useful as a topical treatment is not known and needs further investigation. [3]

2.3. Vaccines and Herpetic Stromal Keratitis (HSK)

The disease course in herpetic stromal keratitis (HSK) begins with a primary infection by herpes simplex virus (HSV) followed by a period during which the virus enters latency in sensory and autonomic ganglia, after that a reactivation from the trigeminal ganglia following primary infection induce virus transportation to the ocular mucosa via antero-grade movement from the ganglia, ultimately causing herpetic keratitis, conjunctivitis and other ocular sequelae [4]

Many studies have shown that clinical disease is the result of a recruitment of inflammatory cells, mainly polymorphonuclear cells (PMN), macrophages, and T cells to the corneas of patients with HSK. [5] Due to HSK could lead to a potentially blinding disease; several therapeutical strategies are in development to control ocular damage at initial steps of inflammatory process, i.e. vaccination with different HSV epitopes.

Since the early nineties many attempts have been made to develop a vaccine that would be effective in preventing HSK. Most of these vaccines were useful to prevent primary HSK when given prior to HSV infection however failed to prevent recurrent HSK lesions. [6, 7, 8] Recently, a novel construct with a DNA vaccine expressing herpes simplex virus type 1gD and IL-21, appears to be effective in protect from primary lesions, and also ameliorates herpes keratitis severity and time course after corneal infection with HSV-1 in the animal model [9] Nevertheles, future studies are needed in humans HSK to study efficacy of this vaccine.

2.4. Lipids mediators and HSK

Resolvins are lipid mediators that are derived from the v-3 polyunsaturated fatty acids eicosapentaenoic acid and do- cosahexaenoic acid [10] The name of these lipid mediators is related to their main function, control of inflammation. Resolvins are involved in prevention of diapedesis, regulation of dendritic cell costimulatory factors, [11], increased macrophage phagocytosis of apoptotic neutrophils, inhibition of host tissue inflammatory responses, with the release of chemokines and cytokines, [12] promotion of tissue repair, and prevention of host tissue cell death during stress. [13] Interestingly, topical therapy with resolvins in corneas infected with HSV showed a diminished lesion severity and corneal neovascularization when compared with non-treated eyes. Therapy with resolvins, induced a decreased influx of effector CD4+ T cells and neutrophils to corneal tissue; a diminished production of proinflammatory cytokines and molecules involved in ocular neovascularization were also observed during this treatment in the animal model, suggesting resolvins as promissory molecules in the treatment of HSK.

2.5. Dialyzable Leuckocyte Extracts (DLE) and HSK

DLE were described by Lawrence in 1955, who proved that the extract obtained from a dialyzed of viable leukocytes from a health donor presenting a positive percutaneous tuberculin test was able to transfer to a healthy receptor the ability to respond to this test [14] DLE are constituted by a group of numerous molecules all of them with a molecular weight between 1-12 KDa. DLE have been widely used as adjuvant for treating patients with infectious diseases, and deficient cell-mediated immune response. [15]

The most consistent effects of DLE on the immune system are expression of delayed-type hypersensitivity (DTH) and production of cytokines. [16] Despite DLE have been extensively studied in worldwide, in our country, only Transferon® has been approved for human use by the federal regulatory authorities of health (COFEPRIS), this clarification is relevant, since the following immunological activities correspond exclusively to preclinical and clinical research related to Transferon®. Immunomodulation by Transferon® has been demonstrated by restoration of iNOS expression in a mouse model of tuberculosis, provoking inhibition of bacterial proliferation and significant increase of DTH [17] Transferon® also induces mRNA expression and IFN-γ secretion in peripheral blood mononuclear cells (PBMC) in animals with experimental glioma when compared with non-treated animals. [18] Due to Transferon® induces a Th1 response a clinical study comparing acyclovir treatment and Transferon® during human herpes virus infection was conducted; in that study patients treated with Transferon® had low incidence of clinical complications, better pain control, and also IFN-g was significant increased in serum when compared with patients treated only with acyclovir. [19] Then, our group conducted a second clinical trial to evaluate immunological data and clinical outcome of patients with HSK treated with acyclovir or acyclovir and Transferon® as adjuvant therapy in patients with herpetic keratitis. Interestingly, patients treated with acyclovir and Transferon® showed higher frequency of circulating CD4+IFN-g+ T cells and lower frequency of circulating CD4+IL4+ T cells after treatment; [20], when clinical outcome was evaluated, patients who received acyclovir and Transferon® as adjuvant showed a significant better clinical outcome than patients treated only with Acyclovir after three months of treatment. (Figure 1)

Despite conclusion of this study was that Transferon® could be used as therapeutical tool as adjuvant treatment in herpetic keratitis, additional clinical studies with more number of patients are needed to confirm these results.

2.6. Amniotic membrane as immunomodulator in infectious keratitis

Amniotic membrane (AM) is the inner layer of the fetal membranes that is in contact with the fetus. An avascular stroma and single epithelial cells constitute the amniotic membrane [21] It has been documented in various clinical trials that transplantation of amniotic membrane is therapeutically useful in different superficial ocular pathologies [22, 23, 24, 25] Its beneficial effects for transplantation are due to the following characteristics: amniotic membrane promotes epithelialization, [26] inhibits angiogenesis [27] and has been used as a carrier for ex-vivo expansion of corneal epithelial [28] and endothelial cells [29] Recently, we demonstrated that AM is able to induce apoptosis, inhibit cell proliferation of human PBMC, and abolish the synthesis and the secretion of pro-inflammatory cytokines even when they are LPS stimulated in vitro. [30] Similarly to us, Bauer *et. al.* demonstrated that amniotic membrane transplantation (AMT) in a mouse model of necrotizing HSK, induced an increased rate of local macrophages apoptosis, with decrement in proinflammatory cytokines IL-6, IL-10, IL-12, TNF-α. Nevertheless, in this animal model, the authors suggest that corneas treated with AMT induced peroxisome proliferator-activated receptor-γ (PPAR- γ) which is associated to phenotypical change in macrophages, turning them from classically activated into alternatively activated macrophages or macrophage cell death, through lipid metabolism and PPAR-γ pathway. [31] In the other hand, animal models of *Staphylococcus aureus* keratitis treated with AMT, have suggested that AM improved the healing process,

http://dx.doi.org/10.5772/52263

resulting in decreased corneal haze and less neovascularization.[32] however the exact molecular mechanism remains unknown and needs investigation. Due to a lack in this molecular aspects clinical use of AM is limited and only in certain cases immunomodulation function of AM could be exploited, i.e. keratitis with secondary ocular surface damage. (Figure 2)

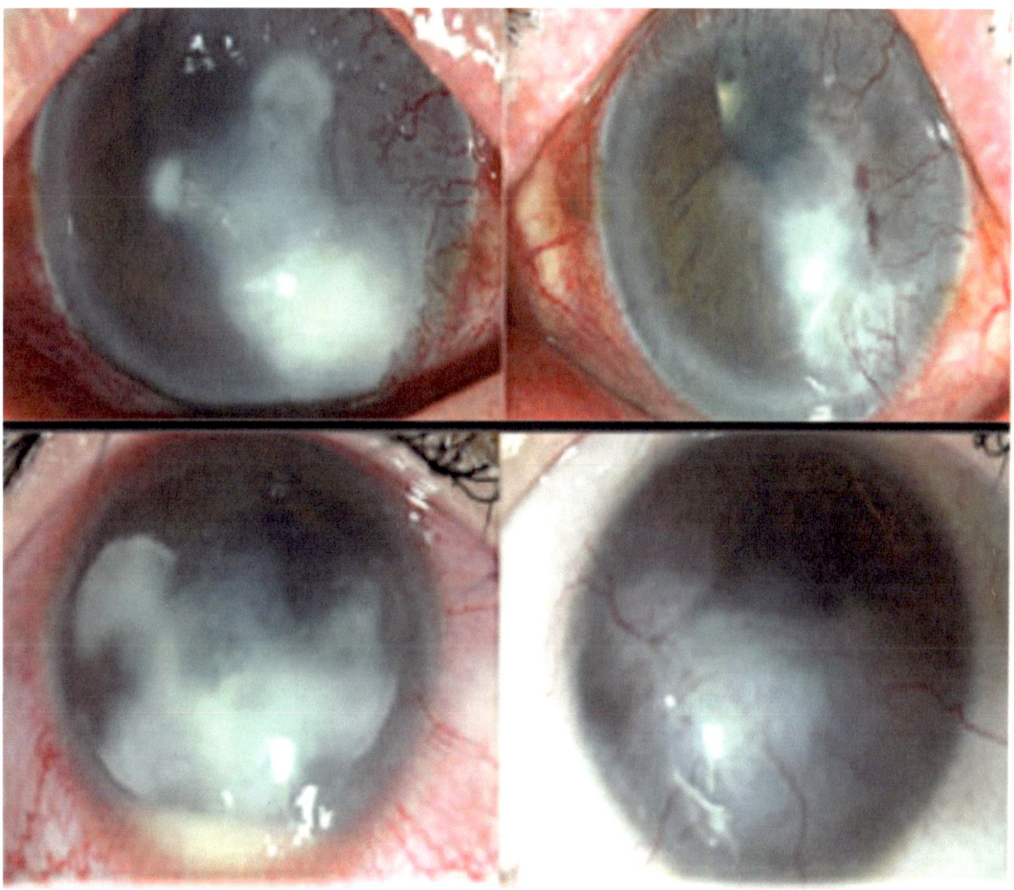

Figure 1. Representative clinical photographs of patients with herpetic keratitis treated with Acyclovir or treated with acyclovir and Transferon®. Upper left, Before treatment; Upper right, Same patient, at 3 months of treatment with acyclovir; Low left, Before treatment; Low right, Same patient, at 3 months of treatment with acyclovir and Transferon®

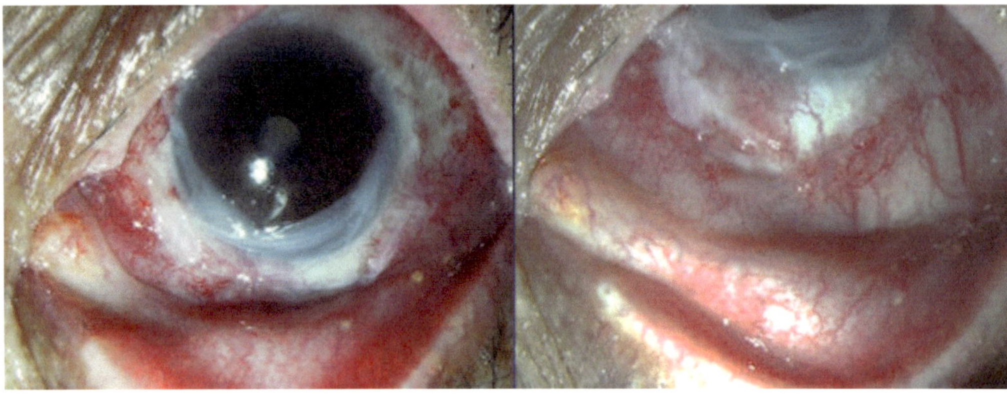

Figure 2. Clinical photographs of AMT in 67 year old female patient with a history of peripheral infectious keratitis secondary to trichiasis. Left, AMT covering the lower peripheral corneal defect. Amniotic membrane was folded several times over the cornea to increase their anti-inflammatory properties. Right, Same patient, 15 days after AMT, clinical photograph showing apparent control of hyperaemia and inflammation

2.7. MIF-CD74 blockade in *Pseudomona aeurginosa* keratitis

Macrophage migration inhibitory factor (MIF) is an integral component of inflammatory responses. MIF induces and sustains expression of several pro-inflammatory cytokines.[33] trough interaction with a receptor complex composed by CD74/CD44 [34] CD74 was first described as class II invariant chain, while CD44 is an adhesion molecule that binds hyaluronic acid and other matrix metalloproteinases. Interaction of MIF with CD74/CD44 results in activation of Mitogen-Activated Protein Kinase (MAPK), production of PGE214 and further induction of inflammatory mediators [35]

Corneal infections by *Pseudomonas aeruginosa* are more difficult to treat and result in worse visual outcome than other bacterial corneal ulcers. Unfortunately the existing therapies fail to control the inflammation secondary to P. aeruginosa keratitis and novel interventions are needed to alleviate tissue damage resulting from local inflammation, recently two studies suggest that blockade of MIF-CD74 ligation ameliorate the disease-associated pathology by decreased proinflammatory mediators and reduced bacterial presence in the cornea [36, 37]

3. Novel therapies in allergic conjunctivitis

Treatment of allergic conjunctivitis can be a challenge by the diverse immunological mechanisms of damage involved in ocular allergic diseases, reviewed in [38]. To date, a wide range of antiallergic drops treatments are available and can be confusing due to lack of improvement at the ocular surface in terms of avoiding anatomical changes in severe cases and control of symptoms in the long time period, reviewed in [39, 40, 41]

Hence our primary goal for treating allergic patients should be preferently to recognize allergy background and ocular inflammation status at the time visit to better establish the

http://dx.doi.org/10.5772/52263

type and source of antigenic stimuli. In this way, primary action such as avoidance and clearance of antigen with lubrication is recommended preferently in acute but also in the late stage of the chronic forms when dry eye could be implicated. Secondary treatment algorithm includes topical antiallergic agents, which are used towards the reaction characterized by mast cell activation, release of preformed and newly formed mediators such as histamine, prostaglandins, leukotrienes, production of chemokines and expression of adhesion molecules. The aim of treatment in seasonal allergic conjunctivitis and perennial allergic conjunctivitis is directed to symptom relief and control, whereas the objective in the chronic forms of vernal keratoconjunctivitis and atopic keratoconjuctivitis will be also to prevent visual complications or try to identify in early stages possible implication of cornea injury. Therefore the efficacy of therapeutic agents varies from patient to patient in terms of grade of severity at the ocular surface, reviewed in [38] and actual local and systemic status activity of the immune system making the choice of treatment depending on multiple variables, each case must be individualized. In general ocular allergic diseases involve mast cell degranulation that will initiate through inflammatory mediators activation of enzymatic cascades, giving rise to pro-inflammatory mediators and in consequence antihistamines, mast cell stabilizers, non-steroidal anti-inflammatory agents, corticosteroids are agents of common use for acute and chronic conjunctivitis.

Nonetheless this wide range of drugs, management of allergic conjunctivits is still a challenge and immune modulation could be the missing link in the therapeutical approach of ocular allergic diseases.

3.1. Calcineurin inhibitors and atopic keratoconjunctivitis

Calcineurin inhibitors are capable of inducing local immunosuppression more than immunomodulation. Topical [42] and systemic cyclosporine a (CsA) [43] have been suggested in the treatment of severe atopic keratoconjunctivitis. Cyclosporine is effective in controlling ocular allergic inflammation by blocking Th2 lymphocyte proliferation and IL-2 production. It also reduces eosinophils production via inhibition of IL-5 production. Use of CsA appears to be safe and the clinical goal for its use is to eliminate the need/dependence of steroids and favourably alter the long-term prognosis of patients with AKC.

Others calcineurins inhibitors that appears to be well tolerated by patients with severe atopic blepharoconjunctivitis [44] and severe atopic keratoconjunctivitis [45] and acceptable clinical outcome are tacrolimus and pimecrolimus, both of them were used first in atopic dermatitis treatment [46]. To date the real impact of anti-allergic treatment with calcineurin inhibitors is unknown.

3.2. Mapracorat and eosinophils in ocular allergy

Mapracorat is a novel selective glucocorticoid receptor agonist that maintains a beneficial anti-inflammatory activity but seems to be less effective in transactivation, resulting in a lower potential for side effect; it has been proposed for the topical treatment of inflammatory skin disorders. In vitro, Mapracorat inhibited eosinophil migration and IL-8 release from eosinophils or the release of IL-6, IL-8, CCL5/RANTES, and TNF-α from a human mast cell line with equal potency as dexamethasone, whereas it was clearly less potent than this glucocorticoid in inducing annexin I and CXCR4 expression on the human eosinophil surface; in other hand, animal model of allergic conjunctivitis showed that mapracorat was similar to dexamethasone eye drops in analogous reduction in clinical symptoms of allergic conjunctivitis and conjunctival eosinophil accumulation. [47] The authors suggest this novel glucocorticoid receptor agonist as a candidate to be used in clinical trials of ocular allergy.

3.3. Omalizumab and allergic diseases

Omalizumab is a biological engineered molecule, targeting the Cε3 domain of the IgE molecule. It binds with free IgE and prevents free IgE from attaching to high-affinity IgE receptor (FcεRI) on effector cells such as mast cells, basophils and also on dendritic cells. An IgE-anti-IgE complex is formed, and as a result, free IgE is decreased. [48] Omalizumab has been well studied and used in treatment of asthma [49, 50, 51] and other allergic diseases such as uriticaria and and stational rhinitis [52] Like other immunomodulators mentioned above, clinical trials with allergic conjunctivitis patients are needed to asses the real impact in ocular allergic diseases.

4. Ocular complications with topical or systemic treatments

Allergic reactions to medication could generate ocular manifestations ranging from mild to severe and it would not be considered infrequent. Demonstration of allergy to topical medications could not be easily evaluated by allergen test, but give some information. Direct provocation in conjunctiva with suspicious drug has been reported, [53] the authors of this review do not recommend this method as a diagnostic protocol, however this test could be used as a research tool to investigate immune responses during allergy to topical medication. To evaluate ocular allergy to drug medications, epicutaneous allergen test and immediate-reading intradermal tests are carried out to diagnose immediate hypersensitivity reactions, while atopy patch tests are usually performed to evaluate delayed reactions, reviewed in [38, 54] with this diagnostic methodology, Wijnmaalen et al reported that the most frequent medication-associated allergies were directed against tobramycin, neomycin sulphate and thimerosal. [55]

Mild to severe ocular reactions to drug-medications are also associated with systemic medications (Figure 3) and in some extreme cases could be life threatening or lead to blinding disease such Stevens Johnson syndrome. If Systemic reactions to medications are mediated by IgE hypersensitivity, it could be easy evaluated by flow cytometry with the Basophil Activation Test. (Figure 4)

Principle of this test is simple, basophils are activated in vitro by suspicious medication, if basophils are sensitized to the drug, basophils became active and up regulate on its surface a molecule named CD63. [56] CD63 is an intracellular lysosomal protein whose surface expression is up regulated also on activated platelets, degranulated neutrophils, monocytes,

http://dx.doi.org/10.5772/52263

macrophages, and endothelium. To be sure that CD63 expressing cells are basophils, analysed cells are also labelled against CD123 and HLA-DR. CD123 is the IL-3Rα, the granulocytic line, including basophils, express constitutively this cluster of differentiation; [57] while HLA-DR is expressed on B lymphocytes, monocytes, macrophages, activated T lymphocytes, activated natural killer (NK) lymphocytes, but is absent in Basophils. Altogether means that by flow cytometry basophils would be CD123+HLA-DR- and only if they were activated by IgE-allergen or drug-medication basophils would be CD63+ [58] (Figure 4).

A

B

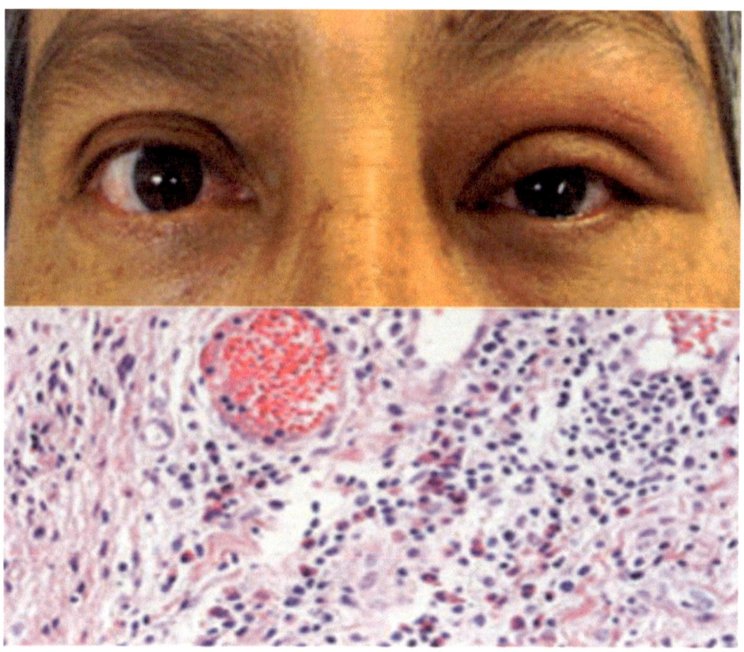

Figure 3. Clinical photograph of a patient with ocular reaction against systemic steroids. Excisional biopsy revealed an extensive eosinophilic infiltrate remaining angiocentric eosinophilic fibrosis. Demonstration of drug allergy was performed by flow cytometry.

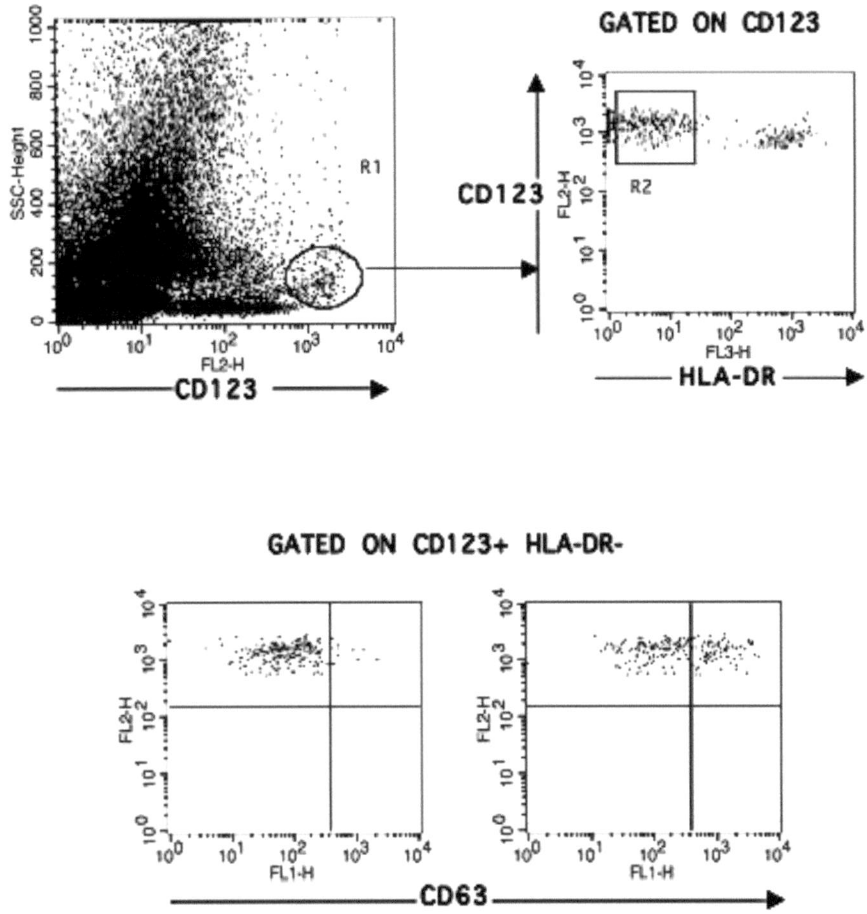

Figure 4. Representative cytometer data of Basophil activation test. Analysis gates are shown at upper dot plots. Upper left, a gate was drawn on CD123 positive cells according to SSC characteristics; these cells correspond mainly to basophils. Upper right, A second gate is performed on HLA-DR negative cells; Dot plots of gated CD123+HLA-DR- cells (basophils) are displayed. Low left, negative test; Low right, Positive test, markedly up regulated expression of CD63 is observed.

5. Conclusions

As the prevalence of allergic disease increases around the world, resistance to antibiotics/antivirals/or antimicotic drugs grows, and virulence of microorganisms improves its capacity of infection, it is clear that more effective therapies and disease-modifying agents are needed. Only treatment evolution will be obtained understanding immune pathophysiological mechanism underlying infectious and allergic diseases. The authors of this review are convinced that immunomodulation is part of our future as health professionals and are working today to make it posible as soon as posible.

Acknowledgments

C Santacruz and SM Perez-Tapia should be considerer as a first authors indistinctly. This work was supported in part by "Fundación Conde de Valenciana" and Transfer Factor Project.

Author details

Concepcion Santacruz[1], Sonia Mayra Perez-Tapia[2], Angel Nava-Castañeda[1], Sergio Estrada-Parra[2] and Maria C. Jimenez-Martinez[3*]

1 Research Unit, Institute of Ophthalmology "Conde de Valenciana", Mexico City, Mexico

2 National School of Biological Sciences, IPN, Mexico City, Mexico

3 Faculty of Medicine, UNAM and Research Unit, Institute of Ophthalmology "Conde de Valenciana", Mexico City, Mexico

References

[1] González-Navajas JM, Lee J, David M, Raz E. Immunomodulatory functions of type I interferons. Nat Rev Immunol. 2012 Jan 6;12(2):125-35. doi: 10.1038/nri3133.

[2] Uchio E, Inoue H, Fuchigami A, Kadonosono K. Anti-adenoviral effect of interferon-β and interferon-γ in serotypes that cause acute keratoconjunctivitis. Clin Experiment Ophthalmol 2011 May-Jun;39(4):358-63. doi: 10.1111/j.1442-9071.2010.02457.x. Epub 2011 Jan 14.

[3] Sara Spjut, Weixing Qian, Johannes Bauer, Rickard Storm, Lars Frängsmyr, Thilo Stehle, Niklas Arnberg, and Mikael Elofsson A Potent Trivalent Sialic Acid Inhibitor of Adenovirus Type 37 Infection of Human Corneal Cells. Angew Chem Int Ed Engl. 2011 July 11; 50(29): 6519–6521.

[4] Labetoulle M, Kucera P, Ugolini G, et al. Neuronal propagation of HSV1 from the oral mucosa to the eye. Invest. Ophthalmol. Vis. Sci 2000;41(9):2600–2606.

[5] Divito SJ, Hendricks RL. Activated inflammatory infiltrate in HSV-1-infected corneas without herpes stromal keratitis. Investigative Ophthalmology and Visual Science. 2008;49(4):1488–1495

[6] Inoue Y, Ohashi Y, Shimomura Y, et al. Herpes simplex virus glycoprotein D. Protective immunity against murine herpetic keratitis. Investigative Ophthalmology and Visual Science. 1990;31(3):411–418

[7] Heiligenhaus, Wells PA, Foster CS. Immunisation against HSV-1 keratitis with a synthetic gD peptide. Eye. 1995;9(1):89–95.

[8] Walker J, Leib DA. Protection from primary infection and establishment of latency by vaccination with a herpes simplex virus type 1 recombinant deficient in the virion host shutoff (vhs) function. Vaccine. 1998;16(1):1–5.

[9] Hu K, He X, Yu F, Yuan X, Hu W, Liu C, Zhao F, Dou J. Immunization with DNA vaccine expressing herpes simplex virus type 1 gD and IL-21 protects against mouse herpes keratitis. Immunol Invest. 2011;40(3):265-78. Epub 2011 Jan 4.

[10] Serhan, C. N., N. Chiang, and T. E. Van Dyke. 2008. Resolving inflammation: dual anti-inflammatory and pro-resolution lipid mediators. Nat. Rev. Immunol. 8: 349–361.

[11] Vassiliou, E. K., O. M. Kesler, J. H. Tadros, and D. Ganea. 2008. Bone marrow- derived dendritic cells generated in the presence of resolvin E1 induce apoptosis of activated CD4+ T cells. J. Immunol. 181: 4534–4544

[12] Bannenberg, G., and C. N. Serhan. 2010. Specialized pro-resolving lipid mediators in the inflammatory response: an update. Biochim. Biophys. Acta 1801: 1260–1273.

[13] Zhang, F., H. Yang, Z. Pan, Z. Wang, J. M. Wolosin, P. Gjorstrup, and P. S. Reinach. 2010. Dependence of resolvin-induced increases in corneal epithelial cell migration on EGF receptor transactivation. Invest. Ophthalmol. Vis. Sci. 51: 5601–5609.

[14] Lawrence, HS. (1955). The transfer in humans of delayed skin sensitivity to streptococcal M substance and to tuberculin with disrupted leucocytes. J Clin Invest. pp. 219- 230.

[15] Wilson, GB., Fudenberg, HH. & Keller, RH. (1984). Guidelines for immunotherapy of antigen-specific defects with transfer factor. J Clin Lab Immunol. pp. 51-58. Berrón-Pérez, R., Chávez-Sánchez, R., Estrada-García, I., Espinosa-Padilla, S., Cortez-Gómez, R. et al. (2007). Indications, usage, and dosage of the transfer factor. Rev Alerg Mex. pp. 134-139.

[16] Kirkpatrick, CH. (1993) Structural nature and functions of transfer factors. Ann N Y Acad Sci. pp. 362-368.

[17] Fabre, RA., Pérez, TM., Aguilar, LD., Rangel, MJ., Estrada-Garcìa, I., et al.(2004) Transfer factors as immunotherapy and supplement of chemotherapy in experimental pulmonary tuberculosis. Clin Exp Immunol. pp. 215-23.

[18] Pineda B, Estrada-Parra S, Pedraza-Medina B, Rodriguez-Ropon A, Pérez R, Arrieta O. Interstitial transfer factor as adjuvant immunotherapy for experimental glioma. J Exp Clin Cancer Res. 2005 Dec;24(4):575-83.

[19] Estrada-Parra S, Nagaya A, Serrano E, Rodriguez O, Santamaria V, Ondarza R, Chavez R, Correa B, Monges A, Cabezas R, Calva C, Estrada-Garcia I. Comparative study of transfer factor and acyclovir in the treatment of herpes zoster. Int J Immunopharmacol. 1998 Oct;20(10):521-35.

[20] Luna-Baca GA, Linares M, Santacruz-Valdes C, Aguilar-Velazquez G, Chavez R, Perez-Tapia M, Estrada-Garcia I, Estrada-Parra S, Jimenez-Martinez MC. Immunological study of patients with herpetic stromal keratitis treated with Dialyzable Leukocyte Extracts. In 13th International Congress of Immunology – ICI. Proceedings Immunology 2007, CD: ISBN:978-88-7587-380-6, Book: ISBN:978-88-7587-379-0

[21] Ellies, P., Anderson, D., Dighiero, P., Legeais, J. M., Renard, G., Tseng, S. G. (2001). Mise au point sur la membrane amniotique humaine dans la prise en charge des pathologies de la surface oculaire. J. Fr. Opthalmol. 24(5):546–556.

[22] Burman, S., Tejwani, S., Vemuganti, G.K., Gopinathan, U., Sangwan, V.S. (2004). Ophthalmic application of preserved human amniotic membrane: A review of current indications. Cell Tissue Bank 5(3):161–175

[23] Dua, H. S., Gomes, J. A. P., King, A. J., Maharajan, V. S. (2004). The amniotic membrane in ophthalmology. Surv. Ophthalmol. 49(1):510–577.

[24] Dua, H. S., Gomes, J. A. P., King, A. J., Maharajan, V. S. (2004). The amniotic membrane in ophthalmology. Surv. Ophthalmol. 49(1):510–577.

[25] Giasson, C. J., Bouchard, C., Boisjoly, H., Germain, L. (2006). Amnios et problèmes de surface oculaire. Med. Sci. 22(6–7):639–644.

[26] Grueterich, M., Espana, E. M., Tseng, S. C. G. (2003). Ex vivo expansion of limbal epithelial stem cells: Amniotic membrane serving as a stem cell niche. Surv. Ophthalmic- mol. 48(6):631–646.

[27] Ma, D. H. K., Yao, J. Y., Yeh, L. K., et al. (2004). In vitro antiangiogenic activity in ex vivo expanded human limbocorneal epithelial cells cultivated on human amniotic membrane. Invest. Ophthalmol. Vis. Sci. 45(8):2586–2595.,

[28] Koizumi, N., Fullwood, N. J., Bairaktaris, G., Inatomi, T., Kinoshita, S., Quantock, A. J. (2000). Cultivation of corneal epithelial cells on intact and denuded human amniotic membrane. Invest. Ophthalmol. Vis. Sci. 41(9):2506–2513.

[29] Ishino, Y., Sano, Y., Nakamura, T., Connon, C. H., Rigby, H., Fullwood, N. J., Kinoshita, S. (2004). Amniotic membrane as a carrier for cultivated human corneal endothelial cell transplantation. Invest. Ophthalmol. Vis. Sci. 45(3):800–806.

[30] Garfias Y, Zaga-Clavellina V, Vadillo-Ortega F, Osorio M, Jiménez-Martinez MC. Amniotic Membrane is an immunosuppressor of peripheral blood mononuclear cells. Immunological Investigations 2011, 40(2): 1-14.

[31] Bauer D, Hennig M, Wasmuth S, Baehler H, Busch M, Steuhl KP, Thanos S, Heiligenhaus A. Amniotic membrane induces peroxisome proliferator-activated receptor-γ

positive alternatively activated macrophages. Invest Ophthalmol Vis Sci. 2012 Feb 21;53(2):799-810.

[32] Barequet IS, Habot-Wilner Z, Keller N, Smollan G, Ziv H, Belkin M, Rosner M. Effect of amniotic membrane transplantation on the healing of bacterial keratitis. Invest Ophthalmol Vis Sci. 2008 Jan;49(1):163-7.

[33] Bernhagen, J., Calandra, T., & Bucala, R. The emerging role of MIF in septic shock and infection. Biotherapy 8, 123–127 (1994).

[34] Leng, L. et al. MIF signal transduction initiated by binding to CD74. The Journal of experimental medicine 197, 1467–1476 (2003).

[35] Shi, X. et al. CD44 is the signalling component of the macrophage migration inhibitory factor-CD74 receptor complex. Immunity 25, 595–606 (2006).

[36] Gadjeva M, Nagashima J, Zaidi T, Mitchell RA, Pier GB. Inhibition of macrophage migration inhibitory factor ameliorates ocular Pseudomonas aeruginosa-induced keratitis. PLoS Pathog. 2010 Mar 26;6(3):e1000826.

[37] Zaidi T, Reidy T, D'Ortona S, Fichorova R, Pier G, Gadjeva M. CD74 deficiency ameliorates Pseudomonas aeruginosa-induced ocular infection. Sci Rep. 2011;1:58.

[38] Robles-Contreras A, Santacruz C, Ayala J, Bracamontes E, Godinez V, Estrada-García I, Estrada-Parra S, Chávez R, Perez-Tapia M, Bautista-De Lucio V, Jimenez-Martínez MC. Allergic conjunctivitis: an immunological point of view. Book: Conjunctivitis: A Complex and Multifaceted Disorder. 2011, InTech. ISBN 978-953-307-750-5

[39] Bielory Leonard, Lien WK,Bigelsen S. Allergic conjunctivitis Drugs 2005:65 (2): 215-228.

[40] Manzouri B, H Flynn T, Larkin Frank, J Ono S, Wyse R. Pharmacotherapy of allergic eye disease. Expert Opin Pharmacother. (2006) 7 (9): 1191-1200

[41] Abelson MB, McLaughlin JT, Gomes PJ. Antihistamines in ocular allergy: are they all created equal? Curr Allergy Asthma Rep. 2011 Jun;11(3):205-11.

[42] Tzu JH, Utine CA, Stern ME, Akpek EK. Topical calcineurin inhibitors in the treatment of steroid-dependent atopic keratoconjunctivitis Cornea. 2012 Jun;31(6):649-54.

[43] Cornish KS, Gregory ME, Ramaesh K. Systemic cyclosporin A in severe atopic keratoconjunctivitis. Eur J Ophthalmol. 2010 Sep-Oct;20(5):844-51.

[44] Virtanen HM, Reitamo S, Kari M, Kari O. Effect of 0.03% tacrolimus ointment on conjunctival cytology in patients with severe atopic blepharoconjunctivitis: a retrospective study. Acta Ophtalmol Scand. 2006;84(5):693–695

[45] García DP, Alperte JI, Cristóbal JA, Mateo Orobia AJ, Muro EM, Valyi Z, Del Rio BJ, Arnao MR. Topical tacrolimus ointment for treatment of intractable atopic keratoconjunctivitis: a case report and review of the literature. Cornea. 2011 Apr;30(4):462-5.

[46] Reynolds NJ, Al-Daraji WI. Calcineurin inhibitors and sirolimus: mechanism of action and applications in dermatology. Clin Exp Dermatol. 2002;27(7):555–561 Reitamo S. Tacrolimus: a new topical immunomodulatory therapy for atopic dermatitis. J Allergy Clin Immunol. 2001;107(3):445–448.

[47] Baiula M, Spartà A, Bedini A, Carbonari G, Bucolo C, Ward KW, Zhang JZ, Govoni P, Spampinato S. Eosinophil as a cellular target of the ocular anti-allergic action of mapracorat, a novel selective glucocorticoid receptor agonist. Mol Vis. 2011;17:3208-23. Epub 2011 Dec 14.

[48] Vichyanond P. Omalizumab in allergic diseases, a recent review. Asian Pac J Allergy Immunol. 2011 Sep;29(3):209-19.

[49] Fahy JV, Fleming HE, Wong HH, Liu JT, Su JQ, Reimann J, et al. The effect of an anti-IgE monoclonal antibody on the early- and late-phase responses to allergen inhalation in asthmatic subjects. Am J Respir Crit Care Med. 1997;155:1828-34.

[50] Holgate S, Buhl R, Bousquet J, Smith N, Panahloo Z, Jimenez P. The use of omalizumab in the treatment of severe allergic asthma: A clinical experience update. Respir Med. 2009;103:1098-113.

[51] Humbert M, Beasley R, Ayres J, Slavin R, Hebert J, Bousquet J, et al. Benefits of omalizumab as add-on therapy in patients with severe persistent asthma who are inadequately controlled despite best available therapy (GINA 2002 step 4 treatment): INNOVATE. Allergy. 2005;60:309-16.

[52] Casale TB, Busse WW, Kline JN, Ballas ZK, Moss MH, Townley RG, et al. Omalizumab pretreatment decreases acute reactions after rush immunotherapy for ragweed-induced seasonal allergic rhinitis. J Allergy Clin Immunol. 2006;117:134-40.

[53] Petersen PE, Evans RB, Johnstone MA, Henderson WR Jr. Evaluation of ocular hypersensitivity to dipivalyl epinephrine by component eye-drop testing. J Allergy Clin Immunol. 1990 May;85(5):954-8

[54] Ventura MT, Viola M, Gaeta F, Di Leo E, Buquicchio R, Romano A. Hypersensitivity reactions to ophthalmic products. Curr Pharm Des. 2006;12(26):3401-10.

[55] Wijnmaalen AL, van Zuuren EJ, de Keizer RJ, Jager MJ. Ophthalmic Res. 2009;41(4): 225-9. Epub 2009 May 15. Cutaneous allergy testing in patients suspected of an allergic reaction to eye medication.

[56] Stain C, Stockinger H, Scharf M, et al. Human blood basophils display a unique phenotype including activation linked membrane structures. Blood. 1987;70:1872-1879

[57] Smith WB, Guida L, Sun Q, et al. Neutrophils activated by granulocyte-macrophage colony-stimulating factor express receptors for Interleukin-3 which mediate class II expression. Blood. 1995;86:3938-3944.

[58] Sainte-Laudy J, Vallon C, Guerin JC. Diagnosis of latex allergy: comparison of histamine release and flow cytometric
analysis of basophil activation. Inflamm Res. 1996;45:S35-S36.

Chapter 4

Laboratory in the Diagnosis of Bacterial and Fungal Keratitis

Virginia Vanzzini Zago and
Ana Lilia Perez-Balbuena

Additional information is available at the end of the chapter

http://dx.doi.org/10.5772/52383

1. Introduction

Bacterial and fungal corneal infections are characterized by the presence of a replicating microorganism as the cause of inflammation, and loss of corneal epithelial cells and ulcers, as the last expression of inflammatory phenomenon [1]. Clinically, it is difficult to establish a diagnosis of bacterial keratitis specifically the causal agent. For this reason, the use of laboratory techniques is extremely important to establish a diagnosis. Clinical data created a suspected diagnosis, but results from the laboratory, particularly crops, studies represent the fundamental basis for a definitive diagnosis. Microbiological culture is the only way to determine the sensitivity to antibiotics and guide therapy to achieve optimal management of these conditions [2].

The active replication agents of the infectious ulcers can be viruses, bacteria, fungus *Acanthamoeba* or *Microsporidium*. An early detection of causative of microorganism helps to a better and specific medical treatment in order to reach a better prognosis, visual acuity and even preservation of the ocular integrity.

2. Natural history of a corneal infection

Colonization: Colonization is the first step after the arrival of pathogenic bacteria to corneal surface. The ability of bacteria or fungi for its adhesion to corneal epithelial cells defines its pathogenesis. After the adhesion phase, fungus or bacteria start an active replication supported by nutritional and temperature conditions of the tissue, reaching a bunch of living microorganism over the corneal epithelial cells.

Invasion: By means of proteases, lipopolysaccharides, streptolisines, dermonecrotic staphylolisines, the microorganism can breakdown the epithelium layer cells and originate a corneal epithelial ulcer or crossing Bauman layer, in some cases reaching corneal stroma. This tissue invasion can be observed in the slit lamp and itis described as desepithelization due to the loss of surface epithelial cells.

Multiplication: In the surface of epithelial layers, or because a traumatism some microorganism reach corneal stroma, finding good conditions in nutrients and temperature for an active multiplication and liberation of harmful substances that initiate the inflammatory phenomenon.

Inflammatory response: As a response of the invasion of pathogenic microorganism, the corneal tissue elaborates some potent mediators substances for inflammatory and immune response named cytokines, synthesized mainly by lymphocyte cells, chemo tactic,and tumor necrotic factors (TNF). The first sign of inflammatory response is edema by accumulation of interstitial water between epithelial cells itself and keratocytes.

Migration of leukocytes. By diapedesis phenomenon, the migrating leukocytes arrive to inflicted corneal tissue, from new vessels formed on clear cornea or from limbus, after this fibrin and collagen IV accumulation into deep corneal stroma form an evident infiltrate. The role of polymorphonuclear leukocytesis part of innate immune defense, mainly is based on his ability of ingest bacteria and digest it, by the oxygen dependent killing pathway or by potent oxidants like hydrogen-peroxide, hydroxyl radicals, chloramines and hipoclorous acid. In fungal keratitis, extensive migration of polymorphonuclear neutrophils (PN), around fungal hyphae in order to destroy it, plasma cell and in some cases eosinophils are observed. The dead of inflammatory cells (PN) contribute to the destruction of surrounding corneal tissue because the release of lysosomal enzymes and oxygen metabolites.

Anterior chamber inflammatory reaction: The arrival of leucocytes and fibrin to anterior chamber is called flare and the accumulation of inflammatory cells (PN)is visualized like hypopyon, this phenomenon can be accompanied by inflammation of the endothelial tissue with fibrin small spots named retrokeratic deposit.

Scar: The last step of an infectious keratitis is the accumulation of fibrin in the site of corneal wound or where invasive infectious process has begun, and form a permanent scar that, depending on its size and localization, can permanently low the visual acuity. [3]

3. Corneal predisposing factors in corneal infections

a. **Local corneal and systemic factor.** The risk factors that predispose to corneal infection involve a breakdown of normal defense mechanism like in diabetes, Sjögren or any kind of systemic immunosuppressant that helps the invasion of pathogenic microorganism.

b. **Corneal trauma.** It is one of the most frequent predisposing factors for bacterial and fungal keratitis. Ocular surface disorders like, dysfunctional tear film and dry eye syn-

http://dx.doi.org/10.5772/52383

drome, epithelial abrasion with mineral or organic foreign body, trauma due to surgeries, long lasting use of contaminated contact lens and toxic agent are considered as local risk factor for both corneal infections, and with the presence of one or more of these events, even local conjunctiva microbioma as coagulase negative *Staphylococcus* are capable of causing corneal inflammatory response.

c. **Erosions and dry eye.** Preexisting ocular disorders located in the eye lids as *Staphylococcus aureus* blepharitis or apposition of eyelashes can cause erosions in corneal epithelium. Corneal exposures for old scars in the palpebral border may affect the perfect ocular occlusion and may be the cause of corneal epithelial desiccation and micro-erosions. Tear film dysfunction and dry eye syndrome after the 5th decade of life are the main cause of epithelial irregularities in corneal surface in males and females.

d. **Corneal wounds and scars.** The corneal surgeries like penetrating or lamellar keratoplasty, kerato-refractive (Laser In Situ Keratomileusis, Photo Refractive Keratoplasty or any other surgery), corneal sutures or limbus wounds may open the corneal tissue to microbial entry of bacteria or fungus to epithelium or stroma, the subsequent microbial proliferation and tissue inflammation leads to the infectious keratitis.

4. Bacterial pathogenesis

a. **Adherence:** Bacterial adherence occurs when the pathogenic or non pathogenic bacteria adheres over the corneal wounded or normal epithelial cells, using their bacterial adhesin for attachment and beginning the colonization on the glicocalix; one glycoprotein located over the epithelial corneal cells. After this step the bacterial multiplication and subsequent invasion can cause an inflammatory response and severe ulceration as is observed in corneal keratitis caused mainly by pathogenic species of *Listeria monocytogenes, Streptococcus pneumoniae* and *Neisseria gonhorroae.*

b. **Evasion of corneal defense.** Some indigenous bacteria of the conjunctiva, like coagulasa negative *Staphylococcus, Corynebacterium,* and *Propionibacterium* lives in conjunctiva attached by means of adhesines evading the antibodies and multiple defense substances solute in ocular tears film and ocular blinking because the conjunctiva is his own habitat [4].

c. **Toxins and proteases.** Bacterial exotoxin and endotoxin can cause severe inflammation like the endotoxin in *Pseudomonas aeruginosa, Serratiamarcescens, Enterobacter cloacae* and exotoxin staphylolisin of *Staphylococcus aureus.*

d. *Pseudomonas aeruginosa* produce an exotoxin A, capable of causing inhibition in protein synthesis in mammalian cells by the same mechanism as diphtheria toxin. It also produces two extracellular proteases (elastase and alkaline protease) that have tissue-damaging activity capable of degrading complement and coagulation factors [5]. Experimentally in corneas of mice and rabbits, it was described a novel *Pseudomonas* protease IV (exoprotein) that contribute to corneal surface and stroma virulence [6].

e. **Multiplication capability.***Streptoccoccus penumoniae* shows an accelerated multiplication rate and leukocytes chemotactic factors synthesis that may originate a huge inflammatory cell accumulation in anterior chamber. *Enterobacteriaceae* like *Serratia, Enterobacter, Escherichia* etc. have a multiplication rate of two hours for each generation cell, and its growth is exponential. Depending on the adaptability and the capability of the invading microorganism, like quick reproduction and production of toxic substances as results of his own metabolism, both factors known as virulence, the keratitis caused by the bacterium mentioned above rapidly progress to corneal edema,epithelial ulcer, and dense infiltrate. [7]

f. **Bacterial corneal invasion.** The bacterial invasion to corneal epithelium or corneal stroma is the first step to a severe inflammatory process, with the attraction of inflammatory substances and the initiation of edema and disruption of cellular union on the corneal epithelial cells. Yi [8] demonstrated that Gram negative bacteria lipopolysaccharide attaches on Occludin ZO-1 and ZO-2 disrupting the tight cellular junction in rat corneal epithelium and human cultured cells.

5. Fungal pathogenesis

a. **Fungal adhesive mannoproteins.** The mannoproteins regulate the attachment of yeast and filamentous fungi to corneal epithelial cells. The cell wall of Candida albicans is composed mainly by the polysaccharides mannan, glycan and chitin, in this yeast the ligands proteins for the attachment cell are mannoproteins too. The presence of large quantities of mannoprotein reveals its pathogenic capability.

The outer fibrilar layer in filamentous fungi and yeast is composed by mannoprotein described as an external coat, which regulates the attachment; this coat is sloughed off during the invasive phase in a corneal infection.

In *Aspergillus fumigatus* keratitis have been demonstrated toll-like2 and 4 (TLR2, TLR4) cell receptors as participants in inflammatory response as key of innate immune system that triggers host defensive responses inducing interleukins IL-1β and IL-6. [9]

b. **Fungal corneal penetration.** Fungal corneal infections always begin in the surface where traumatic events happen, then the fungal cells grow in the surface because the fungi are mainly aerobic microorganism; however, pathogenic Candida can reach deep corneal stroma in his hyphae cell form. In some cases, contaminated trauma involve deep cornea, the fungal cells reach the corneal surface after, in both cases the arrival of polymorphonuclear leukocytes and fibrin make a dense infiltrate after the third week of the inflicted cornea.

c. **Fungal toxins.** The investigations about the harmful action of fungal toxins or micotoxines in corneal infections are beginning nowadays. In keratitis due to *Aspergillus flavus* have been demonstrated aflatoxin B1 in 80% of strains isolated from human corneal infection, and only in 40 % of *Aspergillus flavus* strains isolated from the environment. [10]

6. Corneal innate defense

a. **Epithelial integrity.** The intact cornea epithelium cells act as an effective barrier that avoids the entrance of bacteria and fungi. Trauma and hypoxia caused by contact lenses or dry eye may cause corneal epithelial cells loss opening the sites for a bacterial or fungal infection.

b. **Limbo stem cells.** The constant renovation of corneal cells, moving across the epithelium surface to the corneal center, is a renewal system of cells on the outer layer making new and strong unions between them; this renewal mechanism is also important for the wound reconstruction.

c. **Phagocyte phenomenon.** It is a non specific, innate immune system form for clear bacteria, and it is very important in acute bacterial infections (Figure 1) diminishing bacterial multiplication by digesting it by several ways as mentioned before.

d. **Tear layer.** This important aqueous-lipidic layer is a rich water soluble components barrier, it have immunoprotein mainly secretory IgA, immunoglobulin G, complement, lisozime and ferritin that affect bacterial cell wall.

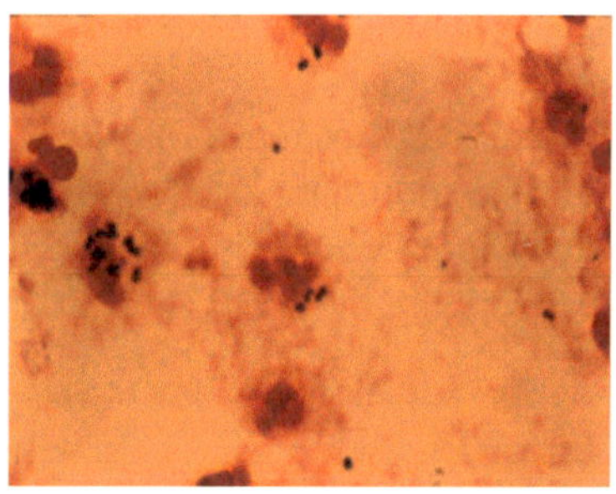

Figure 1. *Streptococcus pneumoniae* fagocitized in the protoplasm of Polymorphonuclear leucocyte in Gram stained smear of corneal ulcer. 1000 X magnification.

7. Problem statement

Viral keratitis is more often diagnosed in any ages in developed countries. Bacterial keratitis related to contact lens use and subsequent to a conjunctivitis are more frequent than fungal corneal ulceration often caused by trauma contaminated with organic soil in patients with agricultural or related activities, in developing and undeveloped countries.

All this corneal infections are important cause of visual loss in children or in males and females in productive ages; for these reasons, itis very important an early clinical and microbiological diagnoses and specific medical or surgical treatment in order to reach a better visual prognosis for those affected patients.

8. Application area

The area of application of this descriptive study, is in the diagnosis of corneal infections, and specifically related to the support of the laboratory in the diagnosis of bacterial and fungal keratitis.

9. Laboratory methods: The support of the diagnosis in bacterial and fungal keratitis

In all inflammatory corneal infection it is recommended in the first consultation, for diagnostic purposes, to take a small sample of corneal secretion of the surrounding or central zone of the ulcer, taking care of avoiding being so invasive. In imminent perforation risk keratitis, the best site is in the edges of the ulcer, and it is the best to take the sample with cotton swab, alginate [11] or Kimura spatula for seeding the sample in the cultures mediums.

Before taking the corneal sample, 2 drops of topical anesthetic (tetracaine 5 mgs/ml) are applied before obtaining smears from the corneal ulcer with heat sterilized and cold Kimura spatula, or with the sterile cotton or alginate swab as mentioned before, in order to be seeded in Petri dishes with culture medium in C streaks, in a wide variety of medium; blood agar (5% sheep blood in brain heart agar base), chocolate agar (1% enrichment supplemented) incubated in 4-5% CO_2 ambient at 37º centigrade for bacterial growth. For fungus cultures, Biggy agar slant for *Candida;*Sabouraud dextrose 2%, or Sabouraud Emmons both with 0.01% cloramphenicol and without cycloheximide inhibitor agar slant, with incubation at 27º centigrade and daily observation for a minimum of 3 weeks [12].

In the same way, three samples it have to be taken for making three smears in the center of each previously cleaned slide marked with a circle made with glass pencil for staining and microscopic observation.

Microscopic examination to search bacteria and fungi was made in each case by periodic-acid Schiff (PAS), Giemsa and Gram or in some cases by Zihel-Neelsen for acid-fast bacilli according to Prophet [13], and in few cases with calcofluor-Evans Blue(Cellfluor) and epifluorescent light microscopy. (Figure 2)

In keratitis cases diagnosed with concomitant anterior or posterior endophtalmitis, the samples of aqueous and vitreous humors, can be taken in the surgical room by an ophthalmologist and sent to the laboratory in the same syringe, in which the samples were collected. These samples will be seeded in the cultures mediums as described before and in conventional mediums for anaerobic incubation. The isolated bacteria can be identified by conventional, automated or semi automated test.

The fungal yeast isolated from corneal scrap samples may be identified by AUXACOLOR ® 2 (Biorad® France) absorption sugars kit for *Candida,* cell germination forming pseudomyicelium (Figure 3) and microcultures in corn meal agar with cover glass over the seed, by the characteristic organization of hyphae, and chlamydospores in each Candida specie.

http://dx.doi.org/10.5772/52383

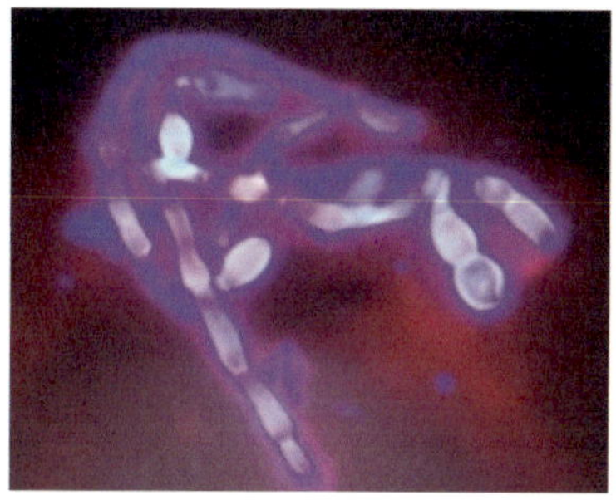

Figure 2. Calcofluor-Evans Blue stain and florescence microscopic view of a corneal smear in a keratomycose in a case patient

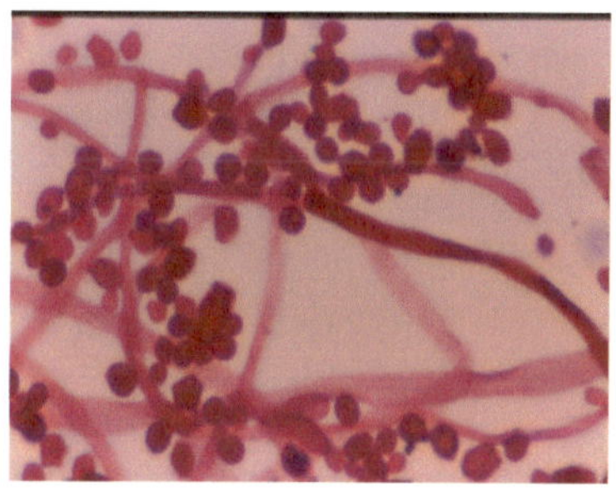

Figure 3. *Candida albicans* pseudomicelium test stained with PAS 1000 X

Recommendations	
1. The sample must be taken before the start of treatment 2. It is nedded the use of 2 drops of topical anesthetic (tetracaine5 mgs/ml) before scraping any corneal lesion.	
Giemsa Cytology	
Polymorphonuclear leukocytes +++ Bacterial or fungal keratitis Polymorphonuclear leukocytes +++, Eosinophils ++ Allergic keratoconjunctivitis Lymphocytes and macrophages +++ Viral or toxic keratitis.	
Mico-organism	Stain
Bacteria and fungus	Gram
Fungus	Periodic-Acid Schiff, calcofluor-Evans Blue
Mycobacteria	Ziehl-Neelsen
Actinomycetes (Actinomyces, Nocardia)	Kinyoun
Parasites (Acanthamoeba)	Giemsa, calcofluor-Evans Blue (Cist).

Table 1. Clinical and laboratory features in bacterial and fungal keratitis

For white filamentous and melanized fungus cultures, it may be observed for its morphology and pigmentation, on surface and reverse of the colony and for its final identification in microcultures for his characteristics conidial forms, prepared with lactophenol blue and direct optical microscopy observation according to the Manual of Clinical Microbiology [14] and Larone [15].

10. Gram positive bacteria and *Mycobacterium*

Coagulase negative *Staphylococcus*. Frequently keratitis associated to coagulase negative *Staphylococcus* are located in the paracentral sites or even near the limbo in patients whom have some systemic immunologic involvement like arthritis or Sjögreen syndrome. The main species isolated are *S hominis, S haemolyticus* and in all cases the bacteria came from conjunctiva flora. In all series consulted *Staphylococcus epidermidis* are the most frequent keratitis bacteria isolated [16].

Staphylococcus aureus. Keratitis caused by this bacterium begin as an epithelial defect, in concomitant conjunctivitis, indiabetic patients or treated with topical steroids patients, beginning as a superficial and stroma, multifocal opacity with few inflammatory cells. After two or three days without antibiotic treatment, a dense infiltrate is observed in the immediate area below the ulcer, and it may progress in indolent form or take a rapid development with a deep and abundant secretion over the corneal surface and conjunctiva. At same time, it can be observed an important cilliary inflammatory reaction close to the ulcer, and conjunctiva vascularization,(Figure 4). In some patients, a sterile ulcer located in the inferior corneal zone (8 to 4 clockaround) are caused by immune reaction to dermonecrotic toxins and staphylolisin generated by *Staphylococcus aureus* blepharitis demonstrated by cultures of both; eye lids superior and inferior (Figure 5).

The corneal smears showed inflammatory cells and Gram positive intracellular or extra-cellular round bacteria (Figure 6). In a diabetic patient, the sample cultures yielded abundant colonies of *Staphylococcus aureus* in cornea and in conjunctiva samples (Figure 7).

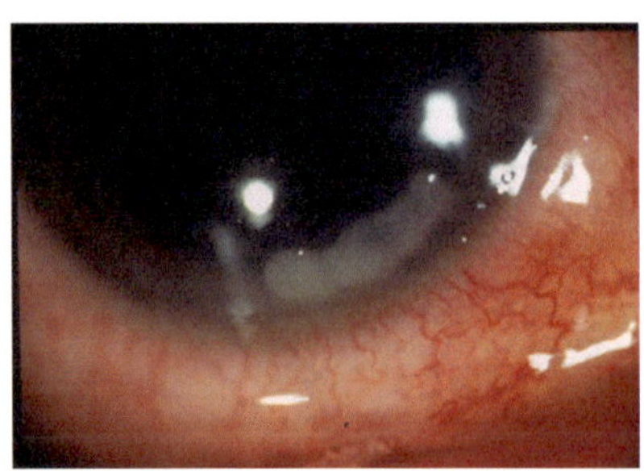

Figure 4. *Staphylococcus aureus* near the limbus keratitis and cilliar reaction.

http://dx.doi.org/10.5772/52383

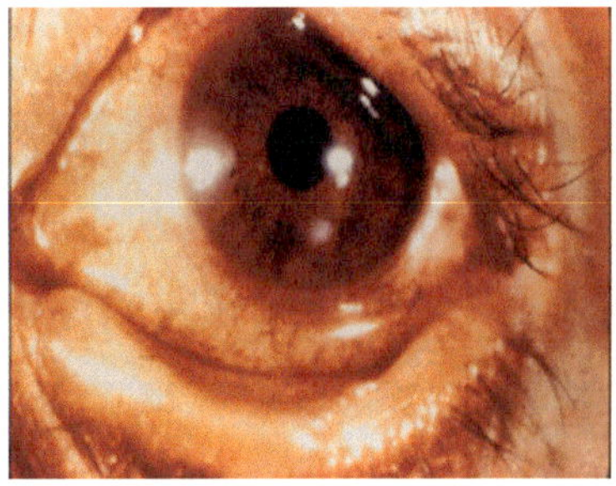

Figure 5. Immune inflammatory reactions in cornea, due to *Staphylococcus aureus* toxins in a patient diagnosed with bacterial blepharitis.

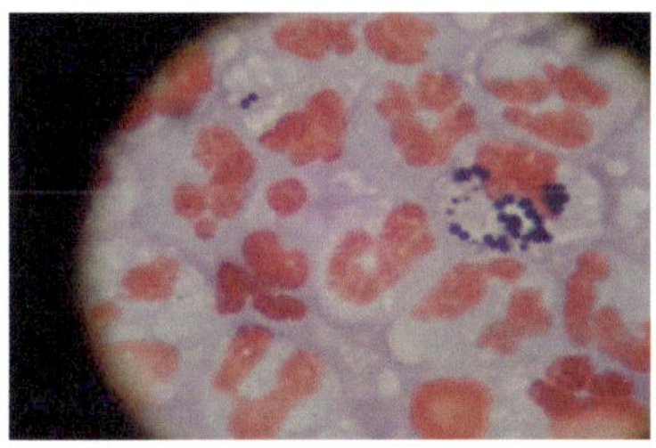

Figure 6. *Staphylococcus* cells ingested by polymorphonuclear leukocytes in a Gram smear of bacterial keratitis. 1000 X

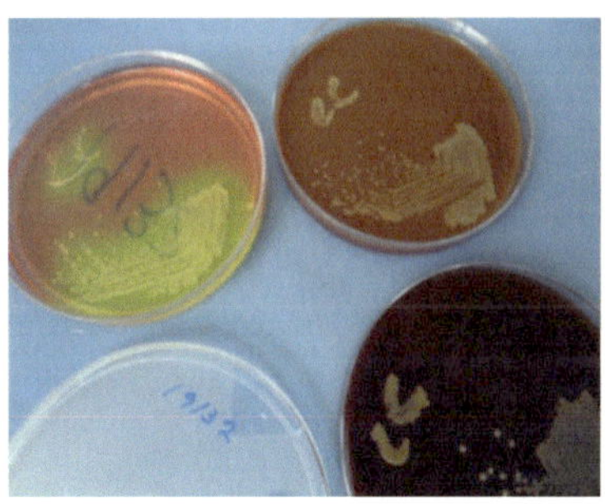

Figure 7. Culture of *Staphylococcus aureus* keratitis showing incorneal C streaks and conjunctiva sample abundant colonies, from a diabetic patient

Streptococcus pneumonia, S viridians and S agalactiae. Formerly named serpinginous ulcer, begins in central cornea with a focal suppurative stromal infiltrate that can reach superficial spread with leading edges, and dense infiltrate below the ulcer (Figure 8), in 70% of the case, hypopyon is observed in some cases occupying 50 % or more in anterior chamber and abundant conjunctiva yellowish secretion, patients refers severe pain. In diabetic patient and treated with topical steroid, the severe inflammatory process that reaches vitreous can cause an inflammatory or infectious endophtalmitis.

In infrequent contaminated post LASIK surgeries, keratitis is originated on streptococcal conjunctivitis developed after the surgery and it is observed like white inflammatory spots in the inter-phase wound and below the corneal flap. (Figure 9)

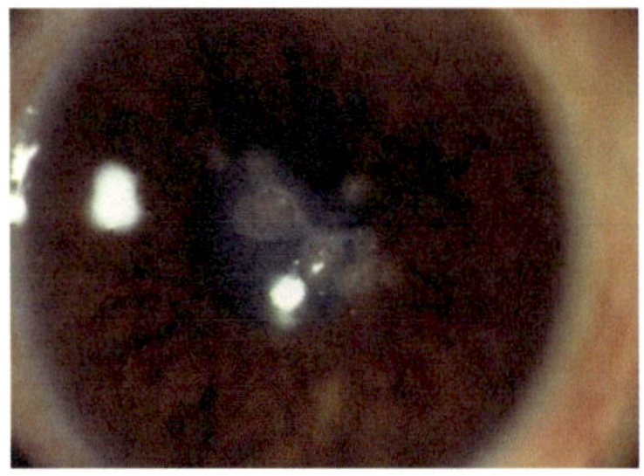

Figure 8. Central, suppurative *Streptoccocus pneumoniae* keratitis in a immuno suppressed female patient.

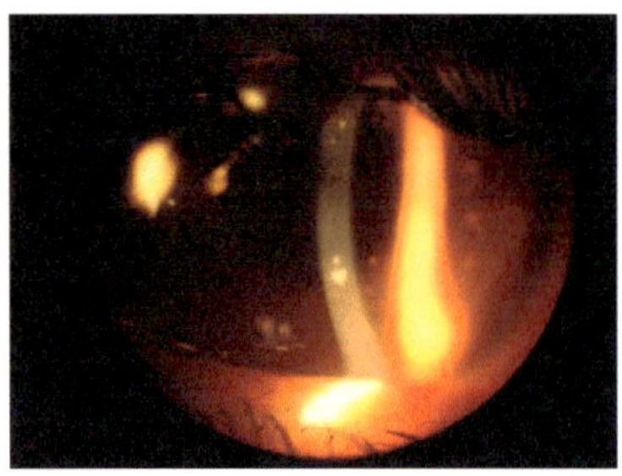

Figure 9. Post LASIK *Streptococcus pneumoniae* keratitis.

In the corneal samples smears, Gram positive *diplococcus* are observed. (Figure 1), and in cultures, *Streptococcus pneumoniae* colonies are obtained(Figure 10), the presumptive identification test for inhibition growth with cooper compound Optoquine is shown in Figure 11

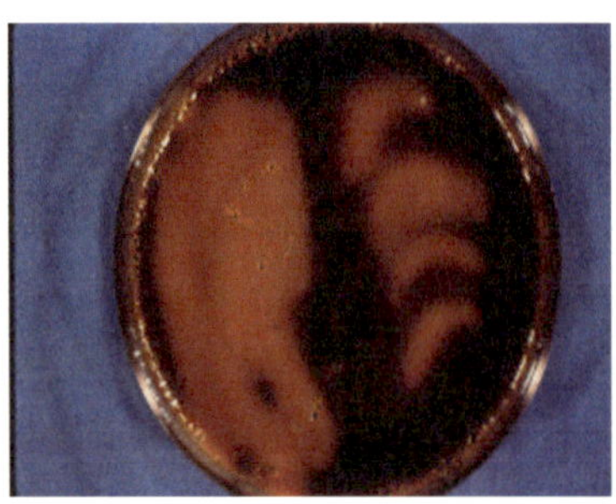

Figure 10. Abundant colonies of *Streptococcus pneumoniae* in conjunctiva and cornea samples from patient of figure 9 (Left).

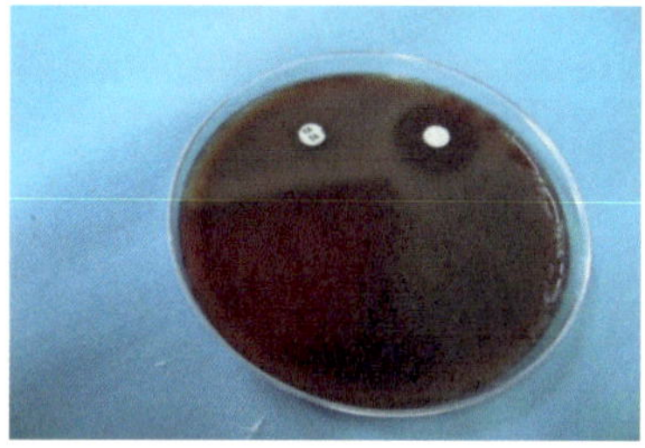

Figure 11. Optoquine inhibition test for *Streptococcus pneumoniae,* and Bacitracine disk without inhibition (Right).

Actinomycetes. Keratitis caused by anaerobic Actinomycetes like Actinomyces israelí, A bovis or aerobic Actinomycetes classified in the genus Nocardia, Actinomadura, Gordonia, Nocardiopsis, Oerskovia, Rhodococcus, Streptomyces, Sacharomonospora, Thermmoactinomyces, Tsukamurella [17], are indolent and with torpid evolution, without response to topical antibiotic like 4a generation quinolone, the traumatic and soil contaminated antecedent are considered in 30%, the infiltrate shows some dense spots in clear cornea and the corneal ulcer is above the infiltrate zone (Figure 12), the smears reveal filamentous Gram positive bacteria (Figure 13) and the culture show yellowish-white colonies in the C strakes of the corneal sample (Figure 14) the medical topical treatment recommended are topical amikacin or sulfadiazine and oral sulfamethoxazole and trimetoprim in regular doses. [18]

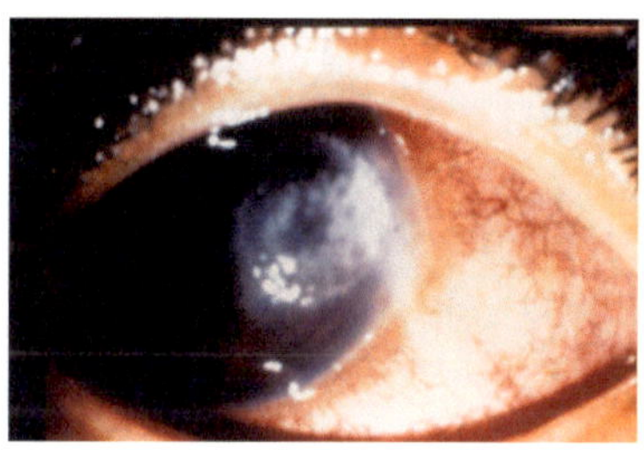

Figure 12. Keratitis due to Nocardia in a traumatic soil contaminated, 5 days of evolution in an adolescent male.

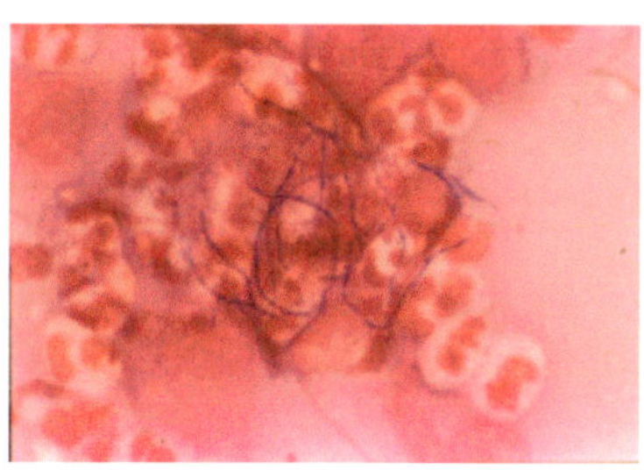

Figure 13. Gram positive filamentous bacteria showing ramifications in the cornea sample (Left).

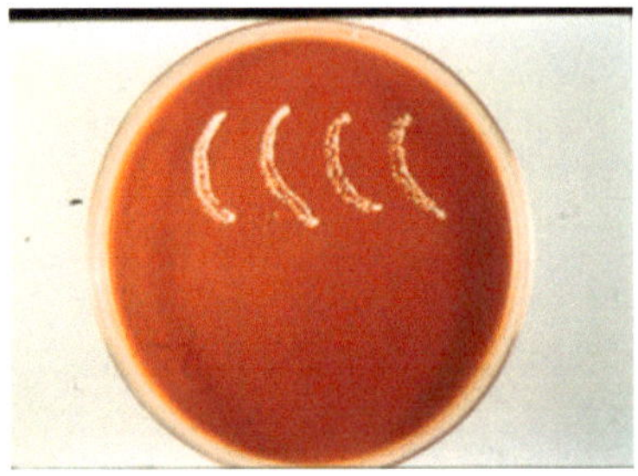

Figure 14. *Nocardia asteroides* cultures from cornea sample of patient in figure 12.

Non tuberculous Mycobacterium:*Mycobacterium chelonae, M intracelulare* are rapidly growing bacteria (7 to 8 days) and are related to low pain or indolent keratitis with torpid evolution, difficulty in diagnosis and with poor results in the treatment. The risky antecedent are corneal erosions or cornea transplant (Figure 15). The topical treatment needs long time and various antibiotics; fourth generation quinolones, amikacyn and clarytromycin. In the smears often it is observed Gram irregular and curved bacilli that in Zihel-Neelsen stain appear in a reddish color (Figure 16), and the cultures grows visible colonies in 7 days. (Figure 17)

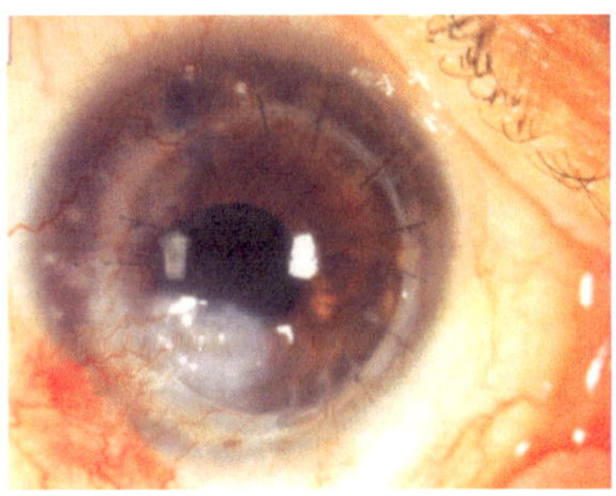

Figure 15. Post-penetrate keratoplasty contaminated with *Mycobacterium chelonae*

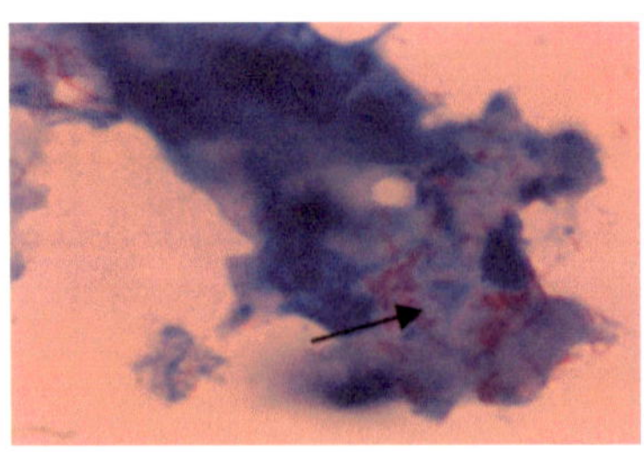

Figure 16. Corneal smear Zihel-Neelsen stained, showing acid-fast bacilli (black arrow) of the patient in figure 12 1000 X (Left).

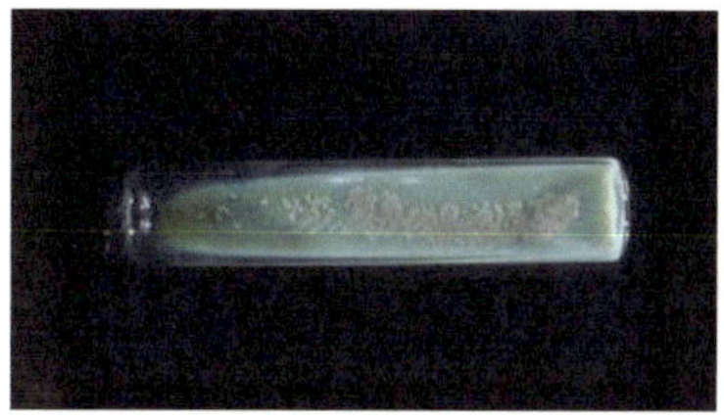

Figure 17. White-yellow colonies of *Mycobacterium chelonae* obtained from the sample of patient in Figure 12.

11. Gram negative bacteria

Pseudomonas aeruginosa: Keratitis caused by *Pseudomonas* that are initiated by the prolonged use of contaminated contact lens, or by traumatic erosion over the corneal epithelium, rapidly progress into cornea stroma and edema in clear cornea zones (Figure 18), these ulcers are painful, and without early antibiotic treatment can progress to endophtalmitis and in some rare cases to severe panophthalmia and vision loss. In the Gram stain of the smear it is observed red small rods (Figure 19), in blood agar white-gray mucous colonies are developed in 18 to 24 hours surrounded by beta hemolytic zone and greenish fluorescein pigment (Figure 20).

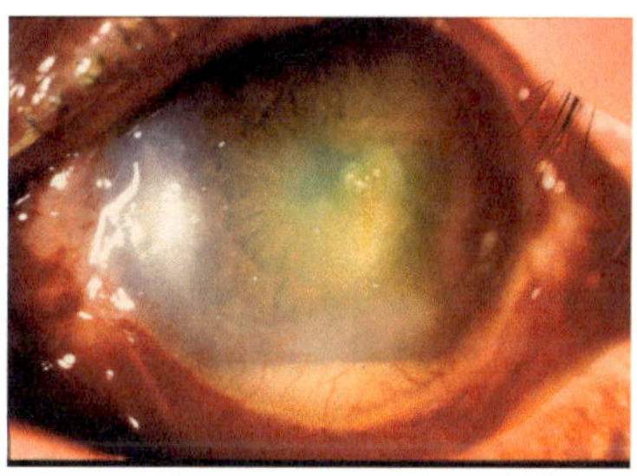

Figure 18. *Pseudomonas,* post-trauma keratitis with hypopyon and corneal vessels in unresponsive case to topic antibiotic treatment.

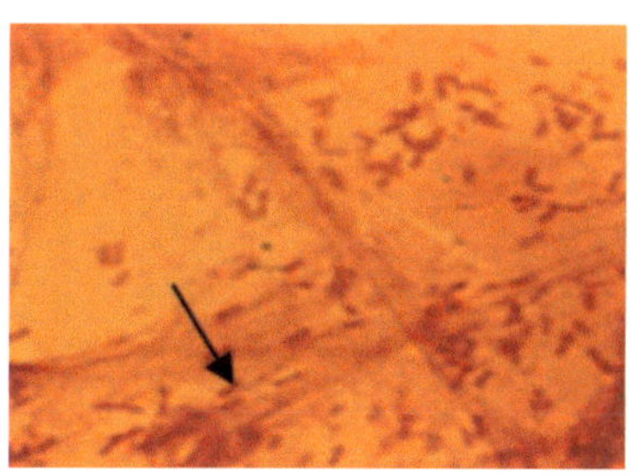

Figure 19. Gram negative rods, (black arrow) in the smear from corneal ulcer from patient in figure 15. 1000 X.

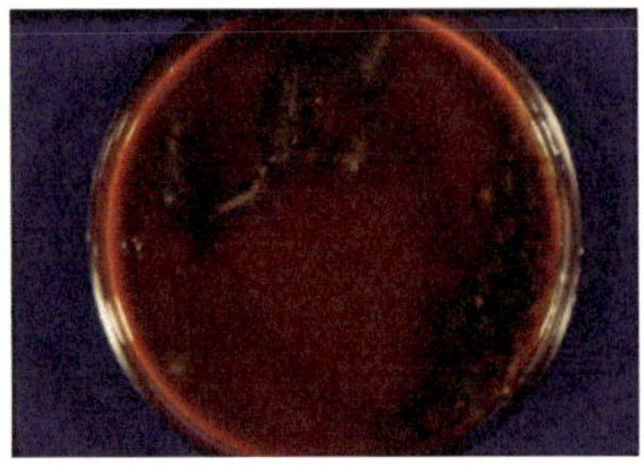

Figure 20. Gray mucous colonies of *Pseudomonas aeruginosa* surrounded by greenish hemolytic zone of fluorescein pigment.

Capnocytophagasputigena.*Capnocytophaga* is a rare keratitis cause, it was described in immuno suppressed patients as risk factor but it was also found in normal young adult patients, (Figure 21). *Capnocytophaga* is normal flora in human and animal (dogs) mouth and the cornea contamination can be by its own patient saliva, in contact lens wearers that use saliva for humectation before putting on his contact lens. In Gram stain smears it appears like negative long rod, (Figure 22) it is a bacterium that grows in 5 to 10% CO2 environment and move away from the site of seed because it is *flagellae* as is showed in cultures. (Figure 23)

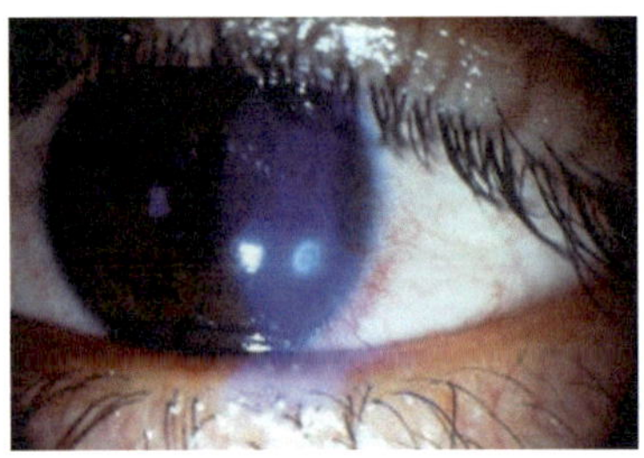

Figure 21. Paracentral, temporal inferior corneal ulceration, caused by *Capnocytophaga sputigena* in a young adult male.

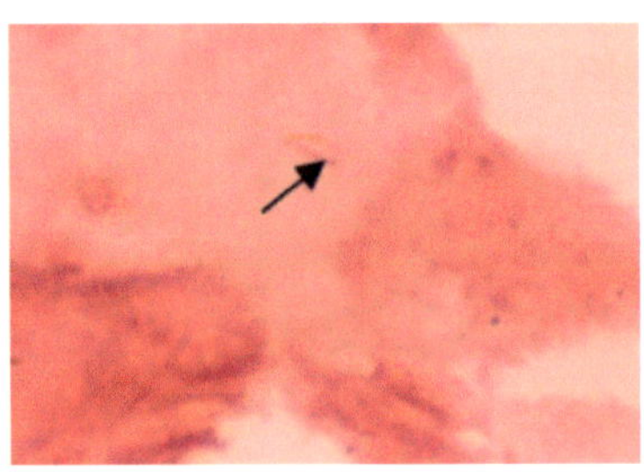

Figure 22. Long and folded Gram negative rod of *Capnocytophaga sputigena* (black arrow) in the secretion keratitis from patient in figure 21

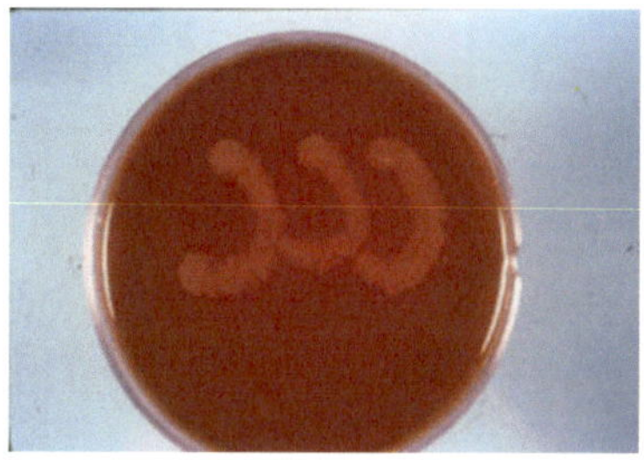

Figure 23. C strikes seeds of *Capnocytophaga sputigena* obtained in the corneal sample culture from patient in figure 21.

Moraxella lacunata. Keratitis related to *Moraxella lacunata* or other *Moraxella* species are observed in patients ofany age, in some cases,the authors [19] describe some immunodeficiency in elderly or malnourished people. Keratitis appear like an abscess or like non severe keratitis, with chronic evolution (Figure 24), in the smears Gram and Giemsa stained appear like broad rods (Figure 25) and in culture the colonies are small and translucent (Figure 26), *Moraxella* is a non fermentative bacteria.

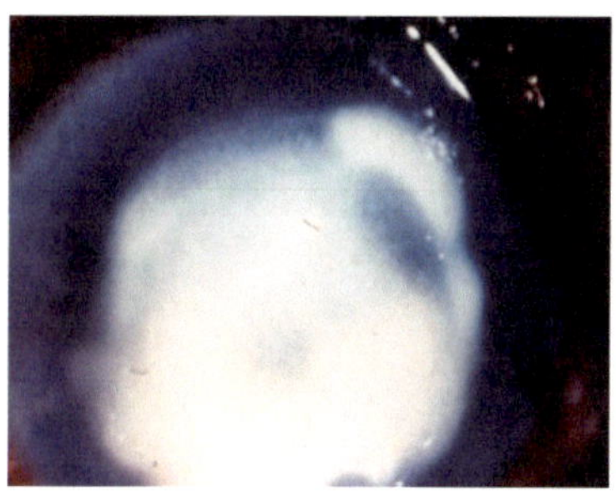

Figure 24. Corneal abscesses in an adult female caused by *Moraxella lacunata.*

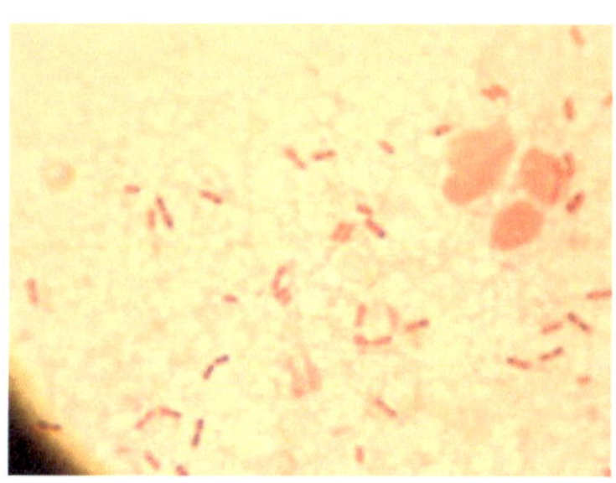

Figure 25. Gram negative broad rods *Moraxella*, from a cornea scraping smear Gram stained. 1000 X.

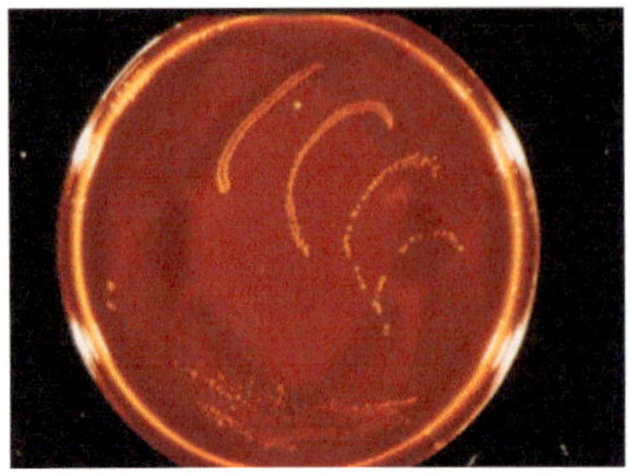

Figure 26. White-yellow colonies, in the C strikes from cornea samples and conjunctiva samples.

Neisseria gonorrhoae, N meningitidis. Keratitis related to *Neisseria* conjunctivitis or meningitis is always severe and painful, it appears in newborns and in young adults involved in sexual activities. The conjunctiva with unilateral presentation is often observed with a very important edema (chemosis) and for this reason, the patient can no open the eye, after the oral or intravenous administration of adequate antibiotic from betalactamic group, the conjunctiva return to normality and the ophthalmologist can explore searching corneal deep ulcers (Figure 27). An early laboratory diagnostic is mandatory by Gram stain on the abundant conjunctiva secretion, always is observed intracellular Gram negative diplococcic in polymorphonuclear leukocytes (Figure 28), in cultures in agar chocolate and CO_2 ambient colonies are small, gray-translucent, oxidase test positive, and by sugar fermentation, semi automated, automated test or latex coaglutination can be specie recognized, and tested for betalactamic antibiotic susceptibility (figure 29).

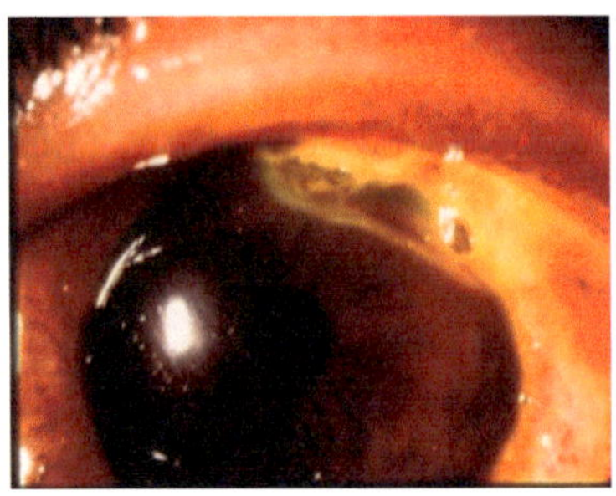

Figure 27. Deep cornea ulceration near the *limbus*, in a male young adult in a case of *Neisseria gonorrhoae* kerato conjunctivitis.

12. Fungal keratitis

Mainly ocular trauma, surgical trauma like corneal transplantation (PKP), Laser in situ keratomieleusis (LASIK) or Photorefractive keratectomy (PRK), use of contaminated contact lens and dry eye originated from tears alterations are the most common precipitating events for fungal keratitis, some of them are caused by opportunistic white filamentous,melanized, or yeast like fungus. Early diagnosis and treatment of these chronic and torpid in clinical evolution infections are important, to achieve a better visual acuity.

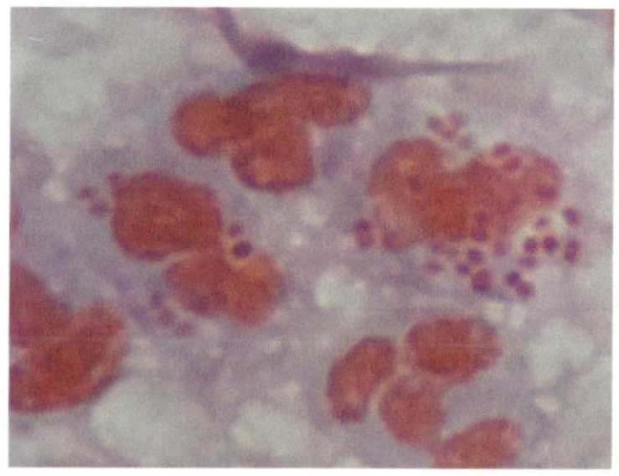

Figure 28. Intracellular in polymorphonuclear leukocyte, Gram negative diplococci observed in conjunctiva secretion in patient from Figure 24 1000X

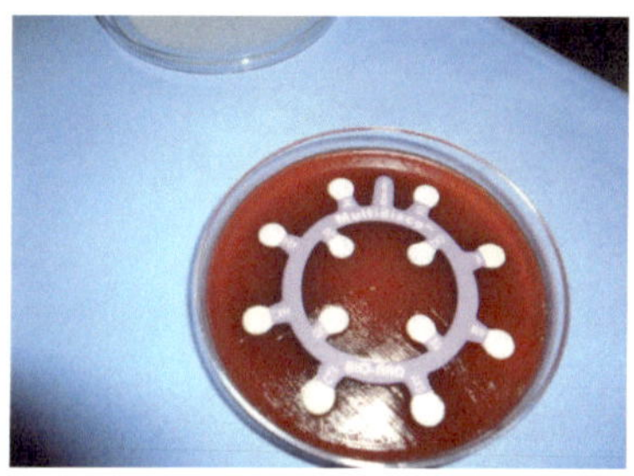

Figure 29. Antibiogram in Mueller-Hinton Blood agar by diffusion disk method (Kirby and Bauer) of *Neisseria gonorrhoeae*

Some of opportunistic fungus are normal flora in the mouth mucous like Candida, others arrive to conjunctiva in the spores forms and do not cause any harmful to conjunctiva or cornea because the normal blink and tear film wash them away [20], the risky factor mentioned above can cause the entrance of the fungi living cells to deep cornea and originate edema and other chronic keratitis with severe clinical manifestations even the ocular loss.

White filamentous Fungi.

Fusarium:*Fusarium solani* are the most frequent cause of keratitis in the series published [21]. In México, 37.2 % fungal keratitis is caused by *F solani, F dimerum, F oxysoporum*, trauma was referred in 35.5 % cases. 75% of cases were observed in males, 38.1% with agricultural activities referred as risk factor, and only 25% in females. In 18 % cases were observed at slit lamp satellite lesions [22], (Figure 30) and 6 % progressed to inflammatory or fungal endophthalmitis, this complication is not frequent in the course of keratitis. [23, 24]

In the laboratory, the diagnosis is made in the scraped sample from the cornea infiltrate as above referred, stained with PAS (Figure 31) or, calcofluor-Evans Blue (Cellfluor) and epifluorescent light microscopy. In the cultures *Fusarium* grows fast, cottony white colonies appear at 48 or 72 hours in Sabouraud-Emmons at 37° C incubation (Figure 32) [23]. In microcultures for identification, round or piriform microconidia and long-curved macroconidia 3 to 4 cells are characteristic for specie identification.

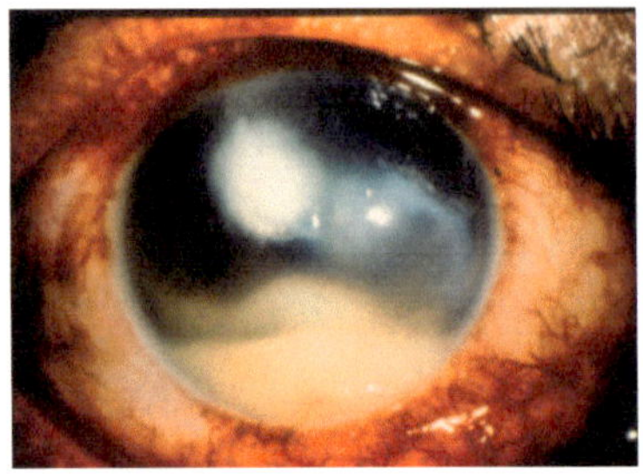

Figure 30. Satellite lesions, hypopyon in anterior and posterior chamber in a *Fusarium* keratitis in 45 year-old male.

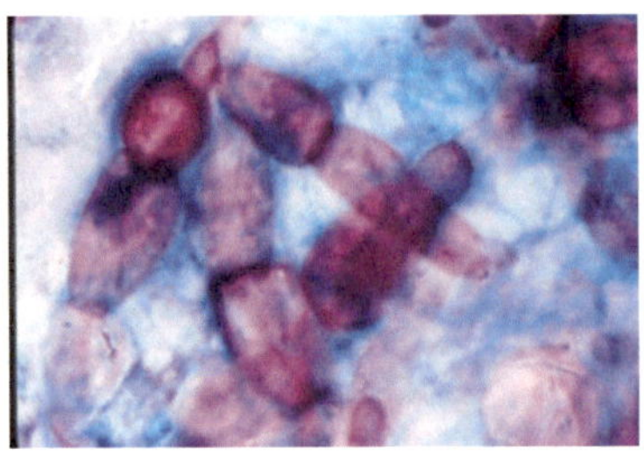

Figure 31. Septate hyphae in corneal scraping smear stained with PAS 1000 X

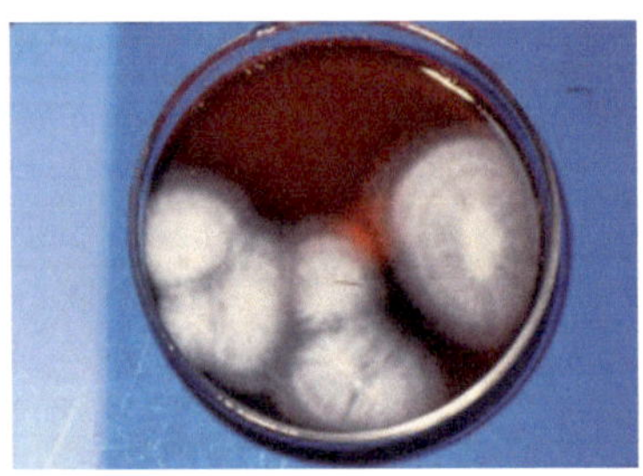

Figure 32. *Fusarium solani* culture from Figure 30 patient

Aspergillus In keratomycose cases *Aspergillus fumigatus, A. nidulans A. flavus, A. niger,* and other species are often isolated, corneal infections are severe and with a poor response to antifungal treatment because *Aspergillus* are intrinsically resistant, in Mexico 10.6 % of fungal keratitis was caused by *Aspergillus* in a serial study including 219 cases; 26% patients involved in agricultural activities, 78.6% males and 21.4 females, 26% cases were eviscerated with the ocular loss (Figure 33) [25].

In Sabouraud-Emmons without cicloeximide media growth white greenish-blue or black *Aspergillus niger* colonies in 3 to 4 incubation 27° C days or in blood agar plates (Figure 34), and in microcultures and cotton blue stain shows the characteristic collumela and conidiophores with phialides uniseriate or biseriate with round or oval conidia growing over them (Figure 35).

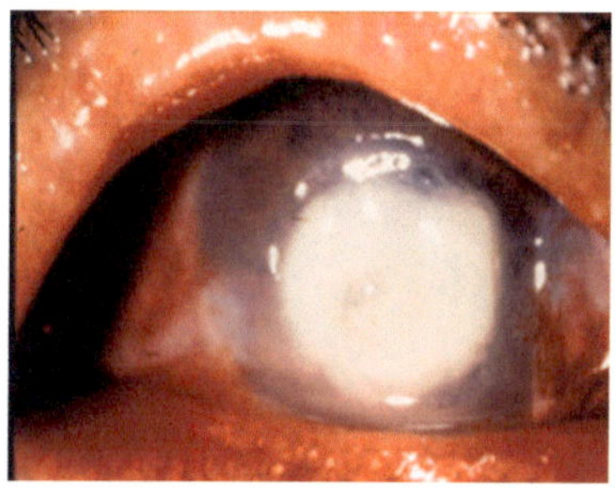

Figure 33. *Aspergillus flavus* keratitis, three weeks after trauma contaminated with organic soil material.

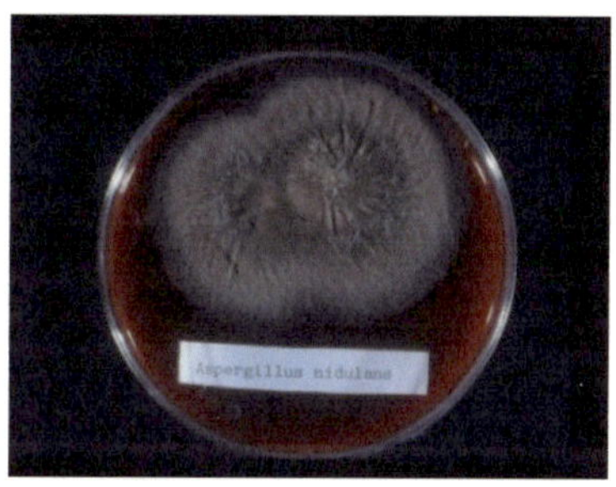

Figure 34. *Aspergillus nidulans* colony from keratomycose patient in Figure 33

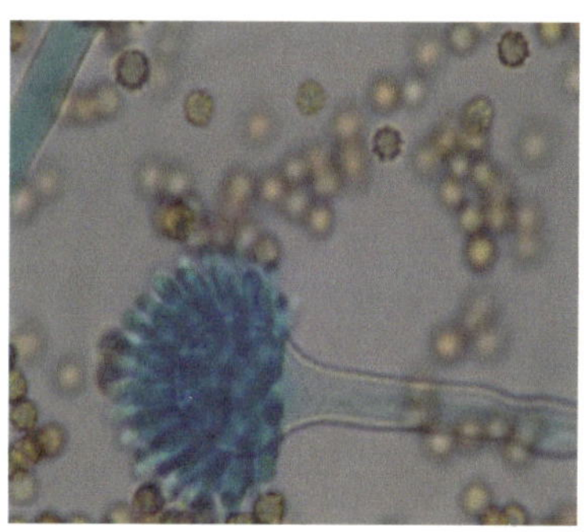

Figure 35. *Aspergillus niger* conidial head, uniseriate phialides and round conidia in lactophenol blue direct microscopic observation from microcultures.

Filamentous Melanized fungus. Many species of opportunistic filamentous melanized (formerly Dematiaceous) fungus related to keratomycoses have been described. *Curvularia, Alternaria, Phialophora, Scyntalydium, Cladosporium, Scedosporium* in India patients serial studies [26]. In Mexico in a serial patients study of 219 cases 19.1% was caused by melanized fungus [25]. Clinical signs and symptoms seems to keratomycoses caused by white filamentous fungus, (Figure 36) in rare cases the corneal scraping samples shows brown fungal cells (Figure 37), and in microcultures the identification are made by its morphological characteristics.

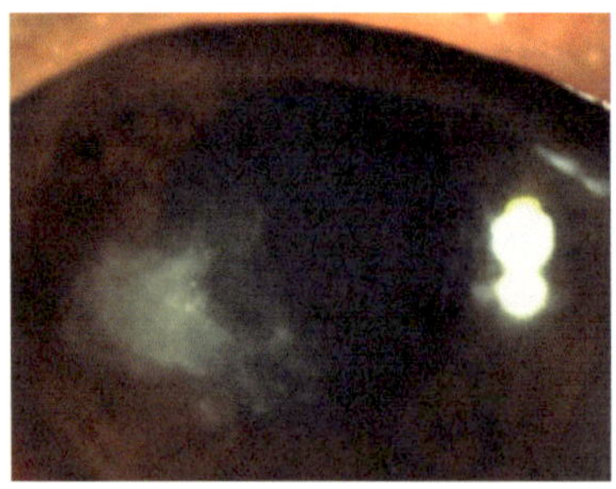

Figure 36. Keratomycose caused by *Curvularia lunata* showing satellite lesions.

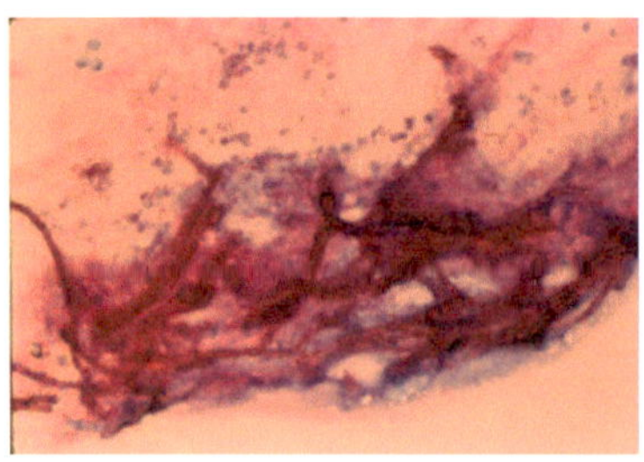

Figure 37. Brown hyphae in cornea smear stained with Schiff periodic acid 400X

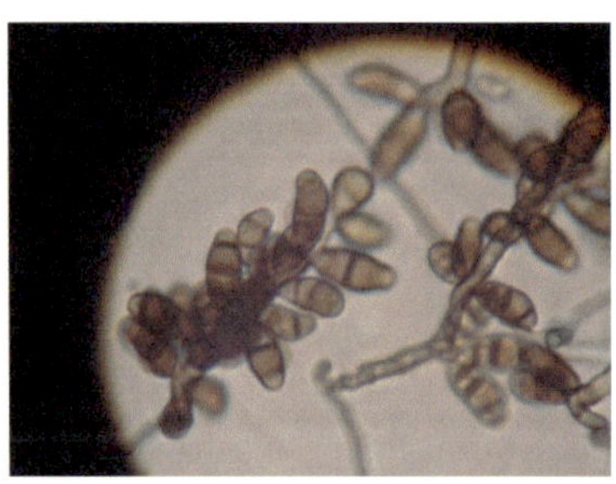

Figure 38. *Curvularia lunata* microcultures from the sample of fungal keratitis in the patient of figure 36

http://dx.doi.org/10.5772/52383

Candida. The yeast fungus *Candida albicans, C parapsilosis, C dubliniensis, C tropicalis,* are often isolated from corneal samples in patient with keratitis with post surgical trauma like in cornea transplant, meantime the patient is topically treated with corticosteroids (Figure 39), or in diabetic type 1 or 2patients. The infiltrate is dense and similar to bacterial keratitis, but without antibiotic treatment response, are indolent and of chronic course, in smears of the corneal secretion can be observed yeast like cells in the PAS stain (Figure 40).

The colonies are obtained in 24 to 48 hours, in blood agar mediums, chocolate agar, Sabouraud-Emmons media, it is suggested to make susceptibility test for Fluconazol and Voriconazole or-amphotericin B as recommended by CLSI (Clinical and Laboratory Standard Institute)

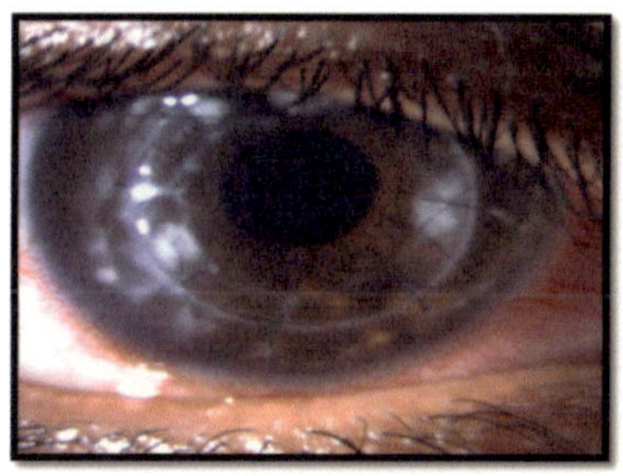

Figure 39. Candida keratomycose in a young male after penetrating keratoplasty for keratoconus

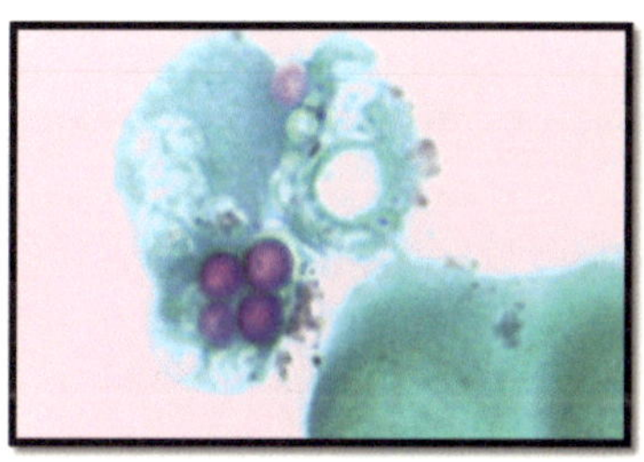

Figure 40. Buddy yeast like cells stained with PAS from corneal smear in patient in Figure 39 1000 X.

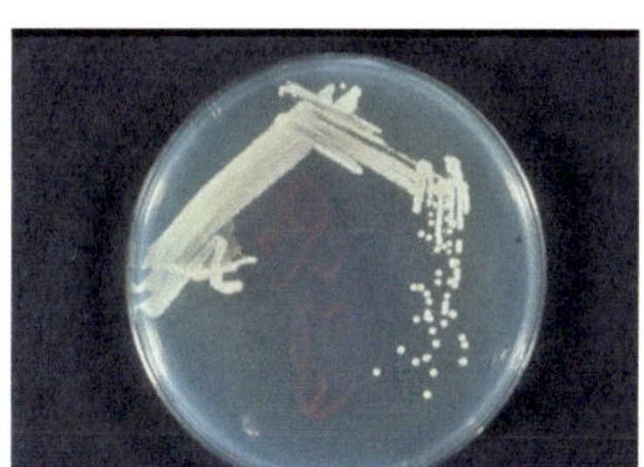

Figure 41. Creamy-white colonies of Candida *tropicalis* in Sabouraud media.

13. Conclusion

Bacterial or fungal corneal inflammation or ulcerations are threatening condition for visual function; the early and accurate diagnosis and specific medical treatment are the gold standard to achieve the best prognosis.

Keratitis caused by Gram negative bacteria and a fungal keratitis clinically seems very similar by clinical signs, the support that the laboratory of microbiology can give for the differentiation between two entities are very important because the medical treatment are made with different drugs, in the other hand keratitis caused by Gram positive bacteria and yeast like fungus, are very similar in inflammatory signs, and in this cases one smear can make the differentiation.

In *Neisseria gonohorroae* keratitis, one delayed or not laboratory confirmation diagnosis is of high risk because the corneal tissue loss is always important and there is risk to lose the whole cornea.

Other options for detection of yeast or filamentous fungi in corneal samples are PCR techniques as suggest Baine using 18S rRNA: 28S rRNA or ITS PCR [27] when the patient has been previously antifungal treated and the corneal smears and cultures are negative for fungal cells search, he suggest PCR as complementary test for traditional cultures as mentioned above. Goldschmidt et al. using High-resolution melting technique [28], detected and differentiated yeast like and filamentous fungi in keratomycose samples in 46 patient in a more simple, specific and cost-efficient test. In 10 negative culture samples they detected 7 cases positive for fungal infections. We have no experience in mycotic keratitis detected by PCR or PCR derived techniques, never the less in one culture proved *Histoplasma capsulatum* scleritis [29].

It is very important for the best prognosis in keratitis cases, to confirm the clinical diagnosis by the laboratory work since the first consultation, for to start immediately the specific medical topical treatment.

For all those reasons the laboratory support in the clinical diagnosis of keratitis is very important in order to achieve a shorter evolution time and to achieve a small scar for the better visual acuity in a patient suffering for a corneal infection.

Acknowledgments

To Miss Elia Portugal for its invaluable help in editorial work.

Author details

Virginia Vanzzini Zago* and Ana Lilia Perez-Balbuena
*Address all correspondence to: vivanzzini@yahoo.com

Laboratory of Microbiology, Hospital Asociación Para Evitar la Ceguera en México "Dr Luis Sánchez Bulnes", México City, Mexico

References

[1] Jones DB. Strategy for the initial management of suspected microbial keratitis. Trans Act. New Orleans Accad. Ophthalmol. Ed. CV. Mosby. St. Louis Mo. 1980: 86-119.

[2] Wilhelmus KR, Liesegang TJ, Osato MS, Jones DB. Laboratory diagnosis of ocular infections.Cumitech. 13A. Washington DC: American Society for Microbiology; 1994.

[3] Wilson DJ, Howes EL. Structural consequences of ocular infection. In Peppose JS, Holland GN, Wilhelmus KR. Ocular Infection and Immunity. Mosby Ed. St. Louis Mo. 1998: 245-251.

[4] Osato M, Normal Ocular Flora in Pepose J, Holland GN, Wilhelmus KR. Ed. Mosby Co St Louis 1998; 191- 199.

[5] Wretlind B, Pavlovskis OR. The role of proteases and exotoxin A in the pathogenicity of Pseudomonasaeruginosa infections. Scand. Infect Dis. Suppl 1981; 29: 13-19.

[6] O'Callaghan RJ, Engel LS, Hobden JA, Callehan MC, Green LC, Hill JM. Pseudomonaskeratitis. The role of an uncharacterized exoprotein, protease IV, in corneal virulence. Invest Ophthalmol Vis. Sci. 1996. 37(4): 534-43.

[7] Wilhelmus KR, Bacterial Keratitis in Pepose JS, Holland GN, Wilhelmus KR. Ocular Infection and Immunity. Edited by Mosby Co St Louis Mo. 1998; 970-103.

[8] Yi X, Wang Y, Yu FS. Corneal epithelial tight junctions and their response tolipopolysaccharides challenge. Invest. Ophthalmol. Vis. Sci. 2000, 41(13); 4093-40100.

[9] Zhao J, Wu XY. Aspergillusfumigtus antigens activate immortalized human corneal epithelial cells via toll-like receptors 2 and 4. Curr Eye Res. 2008; 33(5): 447-454.

[10] Leema G, Kaliamurthy J, Geraldine P, Thomas PA. Keratitis due to aspergillusflavus: clinical profile, molecular identification of fungal strains and detection of aflatoxin production. Mol. Vis. 2010; 16: 843-854.

[11] Jones DB, Liesegang TJ, Robinson N. CUMITEC 13 American Soc. for Microbiology. Washington DC. 1981; 1-27.

[12] WilhelmusK Bacterial Keratitis. In Pepose JS, Holland GN, Wilhelmus KR. Ocular Infections and Immunity. Mosby ed. St. Louis Mo. 1998; 970-1031.

[13] Prophet EB. Laboratory methods in histotechnology. Armed Force Institute of Pathology. Washington DC, 1992.

[14] 14. Murray PR, Jo Baron E, Pfaller MA, Tenover FC, Yolken RH. Manual of clinical Microbiology AMS. 7th. Edition, Washington DC.1998.1161-1242.

[15] Larone DH, Medically important fungi. A guide to identification. ASM press. 4th edition. Washington DC. 2002.

[16] Lichtinger A Yeung SN, Kim P, Amiran MD, Iovieno A, Elbaz U, Ku FK, Wolff R, Rootman DS, Slomovic AR. Shifting trends in bacterial keratitis in Toronto: An 11-

year review. Ophthalmology.2012: May 23.[Epub ahead of print] ISSN 0161-6420/12/ Shttp//dx.doi.org/10.106/j.ophtha.2012.03.031.

[17] Conville PS, Witebsky FG. Nocardia, Rhodococcus, GordoniaActinomadura,Strepotomyces and other aerobic Actinomycetes In Vesalovic J, Carroll KC, Funke G, Jorgensen JH, Landry ML, Warnock. Manual of Clinical Microbiology. 10th Ed. Vol. 1;2011: 443-471.

[18] Sridhar MS, Gopinathan U, Garg P, Sharma S, Rao GN. Ocular Nocardiainfections with special emphasis on the cornea. Surv of Ophtlmol. 2001: 45(5); 361-378.

[19] Das S, Constantinou M, Daniell M, Taylor H. Moraxella keratitis: predisposing factors and clinical review of 95 cases. Br. Jour. Ophthalmol 2006; 90: 1236-1238.

[20] Ando N, Takatori K. Fungal Flora of the Conjunctival Sac. Am Jour Ophthalmol1982; 94(1): 67-74.

[21] Gopinathan U, Garg P, Fernandes M, Sharma S, Athmanathan S. The epidemiologicalfeatures and laboratory results of fungal keratitis. Cornea 2002; 21(6): 555-559.

[22] Perez-Balbuena AL, Vanzzini-Rosano V, Valadez-Virgen JJ, Campos Muller X. Fusarium Keratitis in Mexico. Cornea 2009; 28(6): 626-630.

[23] Dursun D, Fernandez V, Miller D, Alfonso EC. Advanced Fusarium keratitis progressing to endophthalmitis. Cornea 2003: 23(4); 300-303.

[24] Marangon FB, Miller D, Giaconi J, Alfonso EC. In vitro investigation of Voriconazole-susceptibility for keratitis and endophthalmitis fungal pathogens. Am Jour Ophthalmol. 2004; 137:820-825.

[25] Vanzzini VZ. Manzano-Gayoso P, Hernandez-Hernandez F, Gomez-Leal A, Mendez-Tovar LJ, Lopez-Martinez R, Queratomicosisen un centro de atenciónoftalmológica enla Ciudad de México. Rev. IberoamerMicol. 2010; 27(2): 57-61.

[26] Srinivasan M, Gonzalez CA, George C, Cevallos V, Mascareñas JM, Asokan B, Wilkins J, Smolin G, Whitcher JP. Epidemiology and etiological diagnosis of corneal ulcerations inMadurai south India. Br. J. Ophthalmol. 1997; 81(11): 965-971.

[27] Baine PK, Reddy AK, Kodiganti M, Gorli SR, Garg P. Evaluation of three PCR assays for the detection of fungi in patient with mycotic keratitis.. Br J. Ophthalmol 2012.96:911-912.

[28] Goldschmidt P, Degorge S, Benallaoua D, Semoun O, Borsali E, Le Bouter A, Battelier L, Borderie V, Laroche L, Chaumeil C. New strategy for rapid diagnosis andcharacterization of keratomicosis. Ophthalmology 2012; 119: 945-950.

[29] Vanzzini Z. Alcantara-Castro M, Naranjo TR, Support of the laboratory of fungal ocular infections. Int Jour. Inflam.Vol 2012 article ID. 643104doc.10.1155/2012/643104.

Chapter 5

Bacterial Keratitis Infection: A Battle Between Virulence Factors and the Immune Response

Atzin Robles-Contreras, Hector Javier Perez-Cano,
Alejandro Babayan-Sosa and Oscar Baca-Lozada

Additional information is available at the end of the chapter

http://dx.doi.org/10.5772/52264

1. Introduction

1.1. Epidemiology

Microbial keratitis is a potentially serious corneal infection and a major cause of visual impairment worldwide. A conservative estimate of the number of corneal ulcers occurring annually in the developing world alone is 1.5–2 million [1]. The incidence of this condition varies from 11.0 per 100 000 person years in the United States to 799 per 100 000 person years the developing nation of Nepal [2, 3]. Microbial keratitis is thus a significant public health problem, and numerous studies have been performed describing the microbiology of corneal infection. Wide geographical variation exists in the epidemiology of microbial keratitis based on economic and climate factors. To some degree, this variation is explained by economic factors as well as contact-lens wear. A high proportion of bacterial ulcers were reported from centres in developed countries (North America, Australia and Western Europe). In these countries, patients are far less likely to be agricultural workers, and so have a reduced risk of trauma from organic matter, which is known to be a risk factor for fungal infection.

Almost any microorganism can invade the corneal stroma if the normal corneal defense mechanisms are compromised. A wide spectrum of microbial organisms can produce corneal infections and, consequently, the therapeutic strategies adopted for its treatment may be varied. As there is no definite pathognomonic clinical feature, it is difficult to establish the aetiology of corneal ulcer merely on the basis of clinical features. Hence, microbiological evaluation is a must in order to attain a definitive diagnosis and to ensure specific therapy for keratitis.

Regarding bacterial keratitis there are several potential risk factors such as contact lenses, trauma, aqueous tear deficiencies, neurotrophic keratopathy, eyelid alterations or malposition, decreased immunologic defenses, use of topical corticoid medications and surgery [4]. Trauma is a major risk factor for corneal infection in developing countries. In Paraguay, the percentage of cases with preceding trauma was 48%, in Madurai, South India, 65% and 83% in Eastern India [5, 6, 7]. By far the most common cause of trauma to the corneal epithelium and the main risk factor for bacterial keratitis in developed countries is the use of contact lenses, particularly extended-wear contact lenses. Patients with bacterial keratitis, 19-42% are contact lens wearers; incidence of bacterial keratitis secondary to use of extended-wear contact lenses is about 8,000 cases per year. The annual incidence of bacterial keratitis with daily-wear lenses is 3 cases per 10,000 [8].

Traditionally the more common groups responsible for bacterial keratitis are: *Streptococcus sp.*, *Pseudomonas sp.*, *Enterobacteriaceae* (including *Klebsiella*, *Enterobacter*, *Serratia*, and *Proteus*), and *Staphylococcus sp.* Although there is also a wide variation depending on the setting of the series reported. A high percentage of *Staphylococcus sp.* (79%) was recorded in a study from Paraguay, although the reason for this is not clear. Another study found the highest proportion of *Streptococcus sp.* (46.8%), the authors noted that this figure was only 18.5% in 1986 and suggest that the trend might represent a genuine change in the bacterial flora owing to changes in the climate and environment [9]. A study from Bangkok [10] had the highest proportion of *Pseudomonas* infections (55%). Interestingly, this study did not have the highest proportion of contact-lens wearers. Other studies reported far higher proportions of contact-lens wearers—for example, 44% in a study from Taiwan [11] and 50% in a study from Paris [12]. When compared the percentage of contact-lens wearers with the percentage of pseudomonal infections, the Spearman correlation coefficient was not statistically significant. Cohen et al. at Wills Eye Hospital reported a decline in contact lens-related ulcers: during 1991 to 1998, contact-lens wear accounted for 44% of all ulcers, but during 1992 to 1995, it accounted for only 30%. Liesegang reports the following risk factors for development of bacterial keratitis among contact lenses wearers: overnight wear, smoking, male sex, and socioeconomic status. The risk with therapeutic contact lenses is much higher: approximately 52/10,000 per year [13].

Jeng [14] commented on the emerging resistance of bacterial infections to fluoroquinolones. In addition to changes in resistance patterns, studies have also demonstrated changing patterns of causative organisms over time in a given geographical location. Varaprasathan et al [15] reported that the proportion of *Streptococcus pneumoniae* and *Pesudomonas aeruginosa* ulcers in Northern California had decreased over a 50-year period, while that of *Serratia marcescens* had increased over the same period. Sun et al [16] reported a rise in the percentage of Gram positive (+) cocci in North China from 25% in 1991 to 70.8% in 1997, as well as a decrease in Gram negative (-) bacilli from 69% to 23.4% over a similar period. Hsiao et al [17] reported on a 10 year follow up that there was a significant decrease in the percentage of Gram(+) microorganisms over time. The sensitivity of Gram(-) isolates to tested antimicrobials was >97% response for all the reported antibiotics; this was not the case for Gram(+) isolates, in which resistance to the antibiotics was more common, methicillin-resistant organisms accounted for 29.1% of all Gram(+) cultures.

The overview of bacterial keratitis is quite extensive, from the epidemiological point of view is important to consider the wide variety of presentations even within the same regions of a country. Microbiological studies are essential to determine the casuistry of each center in a given time. A common problem throughout the world is the ever increasing resistance to antibiotics including the new fluoroquinolones.

2. Immune response

We have a lot of mechanisms to evade a bacterial infection: physical, chemical, microbiological, and immunological mechanisms. But not all of the mechanisms are described in a bacterial keratitis infection.

2.1. Exterior defense

The eye has several mechanisms to prevent colonization by bacteria, among which are three main types: the mechanics, such as blinking, or that the Tight Junctions present in the corneal epithelial cells, preventing the entry of bacteria into the corneal stroma or other intraocular structures, it is important to mention that certain bacteria are able to penetrate the intact corneal epithelium such as *Corynebacterium diphtheriae, Haemophilus aegyptus, Neisseria sp., Listeria sp.* and *Shigella sp.* [18, 19]; Chemicals, which are the presence of soluble molecules involved in controlling the growth of bacteria, such mechanisms are presence of lactoferrin, lysozyme, antimicrobial peptides, antibodies, etc. [20-21] and finally microbiologic mechanisms, these mechanisms refer the normal microbiota of the ocular surface (*S. epidermidis, S. aureus and Propionibacterium sp.*) [22-26], the microbiota generates substances called bacteriocins, which will be mentioned later in item 3 of this chapter.

2.2. Complement

It was reported in murine models, that anaphylatoxins (C3a, C4a, and C5a) could be generated when the cornea was injured with lipopolysaccharides (LPS), immune complexes, acid, or alkali. Interestingly membrane attack complex (MAC) could only be generated when the cornea was exposed to LPS or immune complexes. Cornea failed to generate MAC when affronted with acid or alkali. The immune response mounted to LPS or immune complex is similar to that generated against infectious agents like Gram(-) bacteria. Indeed the complement system has been shown to play a critical role in protection against *Pseudomonas aeruginosa* infection that causes keratitis [27,28]. Additionally, complement activation is believed to play an important role in ulceration of human cornea induced by Gram(-) bacteria [29].

2.3. Receptors

There are different receptors that recognizes bacteria molecules, these receptors in general are called pattern recognition receptors and exists several types of receptors (TLR, CLR, NLR and RLR). In bacterial keratitis infections are studied in murine and *in vitro* models, the presence, activation and function of TLR. The functions described in TLR activation are cytokine secretion, chemokines secretion, and antimicrobian peptides secretion, recruitment of cells to inflammation site. For example corneal TLR4 expression is increased in *P. aeruginosa* infection and deficiency of this receptor in BALB/c mice resulted in a susceptible rather than resistant phenotype [30], these observations suggest that TLR4 is critical for resistance to *P. aeruginosa* keratitis.

2.4. Effects of receptors activation

2.4.1. Chemokines

In other studies, UV killed *S. aureus* and Pam3Cys (TLR2 synthetic ligand) stimulated the phosphorylation of MAP kinases, JNK, p38 MAPK and ERK, and the blockade of JNK, but not that of p38 or ERK phosphorylation, had an inhibitory effect on IκBα degradation and CXC chemokine production [31]. Furthermore they also found that corneal inflammation was significantly impaired in mice deficient in JNK1 mice compared with control mice, suggesting that JNK has an essential role in TLR2-induced corneal inflammation.

2.4.2. Antimicrobian peptides

Activation with pathogens and TLR agonists of ocular surface epithelial cells by also leads to the production of antimicrobial peptides such as hBD-2 and the cathelicidin LL-37 [32-34]. In an interesting *in vitro* study [35], Maltseva et al., reported that a MyD88 dependent increase in corneal epithelial hBD-2 expression caused by exposure to *P. aeruginosa* supernatant was abrogated by the presence of a contact lens, thus giving new insight into the mechanism by which contact lens wear predisposes to *P. aeruginosa* keratitis.

Additional *in vivo* studies have shown that defensins and LL-37 play an important role in protecting the ocular surface from *P. aeruginosa* infections. In particular, mice deficient in cathelicidin-related antimicrobial peptide (CRAMP), the murine homologue of LL-37, are more susceptible to *P. aeruginosa* keratitis, had significantly delayed bacterial clearance and an increased number of infiltrating neutrophils in the cornea [36]. A similar finding was reported in BALB/c mice following knock down of mBD-2 or mBD-3, but not of mBD-1 or mBD-4, by siRNA [37-38]. Furthermore Wu et al. also found that silencing mBD2, mBD3 or both defensins resulted in a significant upregulation of TLR2, TLR4 and MyD88 but not TLR5 or TLR9 [39].

Kumar et al. [40] observed that pre-treatment with the TLR5 agonist flagellin markedly reduced the severity of subsequent *P. aeruginosa* infection in C57BL/6 mice. This was in part due to induction of corneal expression of the antimicrobial molecules, nitric oxide and CRAMP. They also observed similar results *in vitro*, as flagellin pre-treatment enhanced *P. aeruginosa* induced expression of hBD-2 and LL-37 in human corneal epithelial cells [39]. These observations raise the possibility of utilizing TLR activation as a prophylactic means of preventing an overwhelming inflammatory response and corneal destruction in *P. aeruginosa* keratitis.

2.5. Recruited cells

2.5.1. Polymorphonuclear cells

In animal models as characterized by bacterial invasion of the underlying stroma and intense neutrophil infiltration which results in corneal opacification and potentially loss of vision [41-45]. In an murine model of *S. aureus* keratitis, exposure of corneal epithelium to *S. aureus* increased neutrophil recruitment to the corneal stroma, corneal thickness and corneal haze in normal C57Bl/6 mice, mice deficient TLR4 or TLR9, but not in mice deficient in TLR2 or MyD88, suggesting that *S. aureus*-induced corneal inflammation is mediated by TLR2 and MyD88 [46].

In 2005 Huang et al., reported that silencing TLR9 by siRNA in C57BL/6 mice resulted in less severe inflammation, reduced polymorphonuclear infiltration but consequently increased bacterial load [47]. These data suggested that TLR9 activation is required to adequately eliminate bacteria but that it also contributes to corneal destruction.

2.5.2. T cell populations

Extensive study of the underlying mechanism of the pathogenesis of *P. aeruginosa* keratitis in experimental models has revealed that mice can be divided in two groups based upon their immune response to the pathogen [48]. BALB/c mice are resistant to *P. aeruginosa* infection as they mount a Th2 based response that facilitates recovery and corneal healing. While C57BL/6 mice are susceptible to *P. aeruginosa* infection as they mount a Th1 based immune response leading to corneal perforation. Comparison among these mouse strains provides a unique opportunity to understand the immune response to *P. aeruginosa.*

Exists other type of efectors in the immune response not characterized yet, like the presence of other receptors like NLR or CLR. It is important to mention that the immune response previous described are in animal models or *in vitro* models; a few studies are in patients and we need to study in the future to explain the immunopathogenesis and found new treatments for patients.

3. Virulence factors and mechanisms of bacterial resistance

To understand why bacterial keratitis is often of difficult treatment is necessary to first review the virulence factors and mechanisms of bacterial resistance, this will help us to make decisions about treatment, patient management and contribute to prevent the emergence and development resistant strains.

The treatment for bacterial keratitis consist mainly in antibiotics, so it is necessary to know: bacterial structure, biochemical action, identified important immunogens, and virulence factors. Molecular biology also has had a great participation and that made possible the development of molecular techniques with applications to research to learn more about the bacterial virulence factors and in the diagnosis of pathogens to give a prompt and timely treatment [49].

3.1. Virulence factors

Virulence is a term that comes from the Latin virulent (virus = poison and virulent = poisonous) and that is a property to allows pathogenic bacteria to colonize the host and thus obtain their nutritional requirements, for this it is necessary to evade the defense mechanisms, multiply, establish and cause harm. All this is achieved through the expression of bacterial virulence factors (bacteriocins) that allow microbial adherence, invasion, or both, the harmfulness and pathogenic microorganism determines its virulence o their ability to do harm. Within the virulence factors we can mention the following:

- Adhesins. These substances are membrane receptors involved not only in the cell-cell interactions but also cell-extracellular matrix and cell-trafficking cell. Among the adhesins find bacterial pili, fimbrial proteins, lipoteichoic acids and glycocalyx.
- Invasins. Surface proteins which are responsible for reorganization of actin filaments near the cytoskeleton, thus, when a bacterium comes into contact with the host cell occurs a change in its structure similar to a drop of liquid on a solid surface falls due the reorganization of the cytoskeleton so that it can be incorporated into the cell, once inside the bacteria uses actin to move from one cell to another.
- Impedins. Molecules that help the bacteria evade the host immune response to perpetuate and maintain their infectivity, as examples we can mention the mucinases that using mechanical effects generated by the movement of flagella prevent skidding and disposal, also we can mention proteases that are found mainly in the mucous membranes and destroy the IgA antibodies. In addition exist molecules that help evasion of phagocytosis as coagulase, DNAse, phosphatases, LPS that interfere with complement and finally the production of toxic metabolites to overcome the normal flora.
- Aggressins. Hypothetical substance held to contribute to the virulence of pathogenic bacteria by paralyzing the host defensive mechanisms which, by their chemical nature, can lead to tissue damage, inflammation and shock. Some examples we can cite alpha and beta toxins, lytic enzymes, DNases, lipases, hyaluronidases, kinases, teichoic acid.
- Modulins are bacterial components that promote the production of cytokines among which we can find the lipopolysaccharide of Gram(-), superantigens and murein fragments.

3.2. Bacterial resistance

The principal objective about the study of bacterial virulence factors is the quest from new preventive and therapeutic tools against many infectious diseases. However, there is another condition called bacterial resistance[50].

Antibiotic resistance in bacteria has become a health problem worldwide. The developments of new antibacterial drugs, the indiscriminate and irrational use, besides the evolutionary pressure exerted by therapeutic use have gone masking the increase of the resistance. It appears that the design or discovery of new antibiotics solve the problem, however, also new mechanisms of resistance are difficult to control

Infections caused by multiresistant bacteria, causing extensive morbidity and mortality and the cost per hospitalization and complications is high. The selective pressure plays an important role in the occurrence of resistant strains and is favored by free prescription and formal therapeutic use, the widespread use of antimicrobials in immunocompromised patients, in the intensive care unit, the use of inadequate dose or insufficient duration of antimicrobial therapy and indiscriminate use without establishing a profile sensitivity of isolates. The selective pressure is a process of adaptation and this is not an attribute of individual organisms or nature or life, but it is attributes of a species. In Darwinian terms, the response to the selective pressure is not the individual, not life or nature as a whole but the population itself [51], this means that when a treatment is handled improperly, only susceptible organisms will be destroyed and reduce the bacterial load and hence the infection symptoms, however resistant microorganisms remain in small amounts and gives rise to a new generation of resistant strains (figure 1).

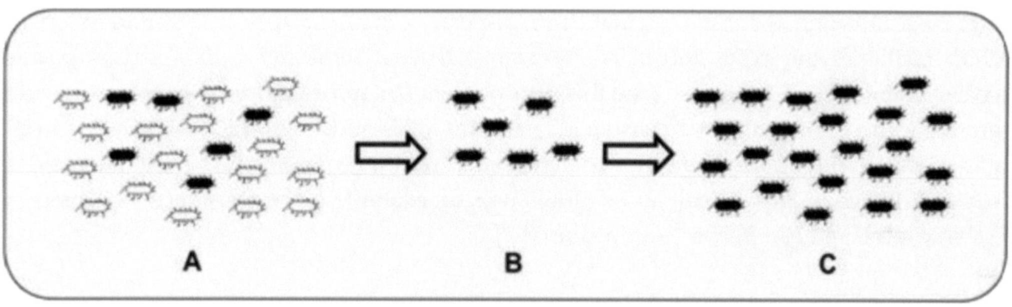

Figure 1. Selective pressure after a treatment with dosage, time or inadequate concentration of the antibiotic. (A) mixture of sensitive and resistant bacteria to an antibiotic (B) Resistant bacteria (C) Proliferation of bacteria resistant proliferation.

The phenotypic expression of bacterial resistance has intrinsic or acquired genetic basis and is mainly expressed by biochemical mechanisms [52]. Briefly describe the two mechanisms of bacterial resistance, the naturally occurring and acquired by the same bacteria.

3.2.1. Natural resistance

Natural resistance is a constant feature of strains of the same bacterial species and is a permanent mechanism determined genetically and furthermore correlated with dose of antibiotic. Some examples of this, we can mention the resistance presented by *Proteus mirabilis* to the tetracyclines and colistin, *P. aeruginosa* to the Benzylpenicillins and trimethoprim-sulfamethoxazole, aerobic Gram(-) bacilli to the clindamycin, *Klebsiella pneumoniae* to the penicillins (ampicillin and amoxicillin), [53].

3.2.2. Acquired resistance

Bacterial species, which by nature is sensitive to an antibiotic, can be genetically modified either by mutation or by acquisition of resistance genes (plasmids, transposons and integrons), these are evolutionary and their frequency depends on the use of antibiotics. An example of mutation of a gene involved in the mechanism of action of an antibiotic is the DNA gyrase involved in DNA replication process of enterobacterias and that a mutation in these genes can confer resistance to quinolones; can also be mutations generated in genes encoding the porins which results in blocking the entrance of the antibiotic into the microorganism. The acquisition of resistance genes can be obtained by transfer from a strain of a species identical or different, mechanisms responsible for these are the plasmids, transposons and integrons [53-54].

The plasmids and transposons are mobile genetic elements which carry resistance genes. The plasmids are fragments of bacterial DNA with variable length; some have the ability to replicate independently of the genetic machinery available to the cell. Other hand transposons are sequences of DNA (double stranded) which can be translocated from chromosome to chromosome or a plasmid to plasmids, thanks to a proper recombination system, this adds to the ability of plasmids to move from one cell to another during conjugation, this allows the acquisition of resistance genes from bacteria of the same species or different species which facilitates the expansion of the resistance strains. Some plasmids and transposons have elements called integrons gene that allows them to capture more exogenous genes determining the development of resistance to several antibiotics (multiple resistance). Antibiotics particularly affected by this mechanism are the beta-lactams, aminoglycosides, tetracyclines, chloramphenicol, and sulfonamide, an example is the resistance presented by *Escherichia coli* and *P. mirabilis* to ampicillin [55].

3.3. Resistance mechanisms

Bacterial resistance both acquired and natural can be approached from the standpoint molecular and biochemical and can be classified into three basic mechanisms of resistance expressed according to the mechanism expressed and the antibiotics mechanism action and may occur simultaneously [55]. The figure 2 shows a schematic representation of the mechanisms of resistance.

- Inactivation of antibiotic by destruction or modification of chemical structure. Is a molecular process characterized by the production of enzymes that carry out this function. For example, enzymes that destroy the chemical structure of an antibiotic against beta-lactamases are characterized by hydrolyzing the beta-lactam nucleus through amide bond cleavage and erythromycin esterase which catalyses the hydrolysis of the lactone ring of the antibiotic, while the enzymes responsible to the modification of the structure we can mention the chloramphenicol acetyl transferase, enzymes that modify aminoglycosides, lincosamides and streptogramins, other enzymes belonging to this group are acetylases, adenilasas and phosphatases [56, 57].

http://dx.doi.org/10.5772/52264

- Altered target site of the antibiotic. Is the modification of bacterial specific sites such as the cell wall, cell membrane, or both 30S and 50S ribosomal subunit. The modification by mutation of GyrA and GyrB genes that coding for topoisomerase II and IV offer bacterial resistance to *S. aureus, S. epidermidis, P. aeruginosa* and *E. coli* to quinolones [57]. Among the ribosomal level changes can include changes in the 30S and 50S subunits which are sites of action of aminoglycosides, macrolides, tetracyclines and lincosamides. Methylation of ribosomal RNA from the 50S subunit confers resistance to *S. aureus* and *S. epidermidis* against tetracycline, chloramphenicol and macrolides. Mutation of the 30S subunit confers resistance to gentamicin, tobramycin and amikacin [55,58].

- Altered permeability barriers. Is due to specific changes in structure of antimicrobial receptors or alterations in the components of the wall or cell membrane and occur changes in the permeability, as well as the loss of the ability of active transport across the cell membrane or the expression of efflux pumps which are activated at the time that the antibiotic is introduced into the bacterial cell [53]. The internalization of hydrophilic compounds is carried out by channels called porins which are filled with water, penetration of the antibacterial in this case depend on the size of the molecule, hydrophobicity and electric charge [55].

- Efflux pumps: On the cell membrane are efflux pumps that carry out the internalization and removal of antimicrobials, a wide variety of these provide antimicrobial resistance both Gram(+) and Gram(-). Active efflux of antibiotics is mediated by transmembrane proteins and the Gram(-) bacteria, involves the membrane components and cytoplasm. These proteins are exported active channels to an antimicrobial agent outside the cell as fast as it comes. These mechanisms confer resistance to tetracycline, quinolones, chloramphenicol, beta lactam antibiotics, antiseptics and disinfectants quaternary ammonium type used for cleaning surfaces [53, 55, 57, 58].

3.4. Biofilm production

In nature, bacteria can grow like planktonic or free-floating, but can also grow colonies embedded in a matrix known as biofilm. Deserves special mention the formation of biofilms, since being a microbial ecosystem composed of one or more microorganisms associated with living or inert surface with functional features and complex structures can be considered a virulence factor and the same time a resistance mechanism. Biofilm formation enables the adhesion to the surface where the bacteria is present and can be one of many causes of chronic infections, for example the chronic infectious keratitis. The structural organization of the bacterial biofilm is composed of polysaccharides, nucleic acids and proteins and all this set is known as extracellular polymeric substances (EPS) and its production is affected by the nutritional quality of the environment in which bacteria develop when the environment is suitable to form biofilms with multiple microcolonies, so the structure that forms is so great that prevents phagocytosis and effects of the immune system against them, for this reason is considered a virulence factor. A very important advantage from the clinical point of view is that biofilms confer resistance to antibiotics such that the dose can be increased thousands of times without causing damage [59]. Two hypotheses to explain the resistance generated by the production of biofilms, the first indicating that occurs a limited penetration of the drug and the bulk is left on the surface such that the antibiotic never reaches its target. The second refers to the physiological limitation and proposes that some microorganisms within the biofilm can exist in a more recalcitrant phenotypic state. Anderl JN et al [60] in a study of *K. pneumoniae* found that the planktonic form was sensitive to ampicillin and reported minimum inhibitory concentration (MIC) of 22µg/mL while the same strain that grew as a biofilm presented a survival of 66% increasing the concentration of ampicillin to 5000µg/mL which corresponds to 2500 times the MIC.

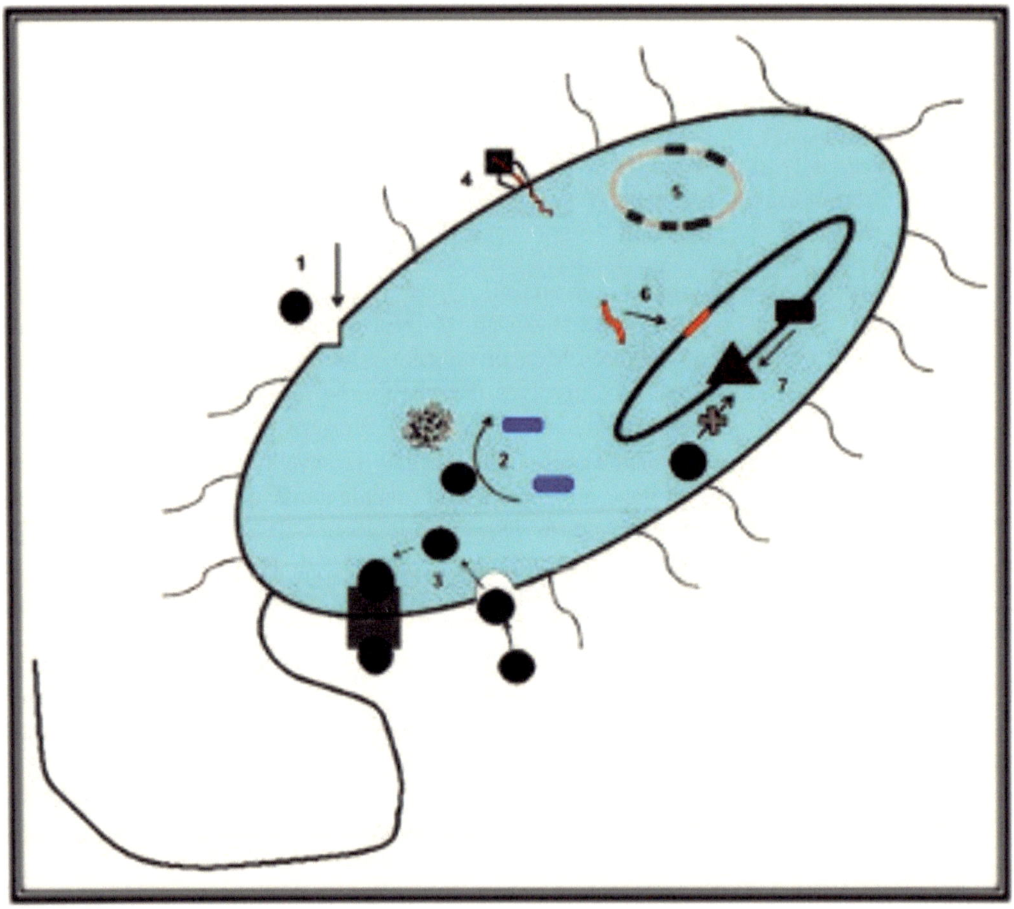

Figure 2. Resistant mechanism (1) Altered target site of the antibiotic and altered permeability barriers (2) Inactivation of antibiotic by destruction or modification of chemical structure (3) Efflux pumps (4) acquisition of resistance genes by fagos (5) Plasmids (6) Transposons and Integrons (7) modification by mutation of topoisomerase.

Having recognized the role of biofilm as responsible of infectious diseases, it is necessary the search for new approaches in both the treatment and prevention. A proposal to counteract this resistance factor is the alteration of the surface to inhibit adhesion. In the area of ophthalmology, for example, chelating agents could be used in contact lens solutions, mainly iron-trapping agent which is necessary for adhesion of the pili of *Pseudomonas sp.* [59, 60].

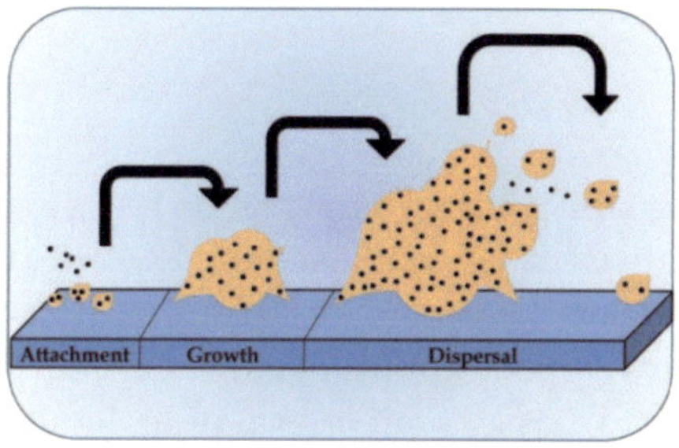

Figure 3. Biofilm production (1) Planktonic bacteria encounter a submerged surface. They begin to produce slimy extracellular polymeric substances (EPS) and to colonize the surface. (2) EPS production allows the emerging biofilm community to develop a complex three-dimensional structure (3) Biofilms can propagate through detachment of small or large clumps of cells that releases individual cells.

4. Clinical characteristics

4.1. Common characteristics

When developing a bacterial corneal ulcer usually appears chemosis and conjunctival injection, eyelid edema, decreased vision, pain, tearing, photophobia, and purulent discharge. Conjunctival reaction is nonspecific, with a predominantly papillary response, is primarily limbal injection. The corneal epithelium and stroma ulcer shows a gray-white infiltrate, may appear necrotic. Infiltration and edema of the cornea can be observed even in areas remote from the ulcer. Appears frequently, an anterior chamber reaction, and in severe cases can be observed fibrin plates on the endothelium and may be a fibrinoid aqueous or hypopyon [61-64].

The hypopyon is produced by the toxic effects of infection on vessels iris and ciliary body, with consequent pouring of fibrin and polymorphonuclear leukocytes. Usually, the hypopyon is sterile as Descemet's membrane is intact. Hypopyon can be seen with any bacterial infection, most frequently in ulcers caused by *S. pneumoniae* and *Pseudomonas sp.;* not forgetting also can occur in viral and fungal ulcers [64-66].

Signs and symptoms of bacterial corneal ulcers vary depending on the virulence of the organism, the previous state of the cornea, the duration of infection, host immune status and prior use of antibiotics and steroids [67-70]. The use of hydrophilic contact lenses can alter the presentation of bacterial ulcers. Infections associated with contact lenses are often multifocal and epithelial and stromal infiltrate is more diffuse. The contact lens wearers presenting with corneal abrasions may have bacterial infections early[71, 72]. Figure 4 are clinical pictures representative in bacterial keratitis.

The aspect sometimes ulcer suggesting the presence of a specific bacterial agent or a group of them. Are indicated below the characteristic signs of infection caused by some agents. However, one must take into account the clinical aspect is never diagnosis, isolation and identification of causative agents is always essential.

4.2. *Staphylococcus sp.*

S. aureus produces coagulase and mannitol fermentation being more aggressive, and *S. epidermidis* does not produce coagulase or ferment mannitol. The latter two are usually opportunistic pathogens that cause infections in compromised corneas, for example, persistent epithelial defects, bullous keratopathy, herpetic epitheliopathy, diabetic epitheliopathy, etcetera. The corneal appearance in *S. aureus*, has a round or oval ulcer, localized, with distinct edges and tends to be deeper, usually accompanied by a creamy white stromal infiltrate and well-defined gray with overlying epithelial defect and can be multifocal. In severe cases, you can get to see hypopyon and endothelial plaque, staphylococcal blepharitis is common [73-75].

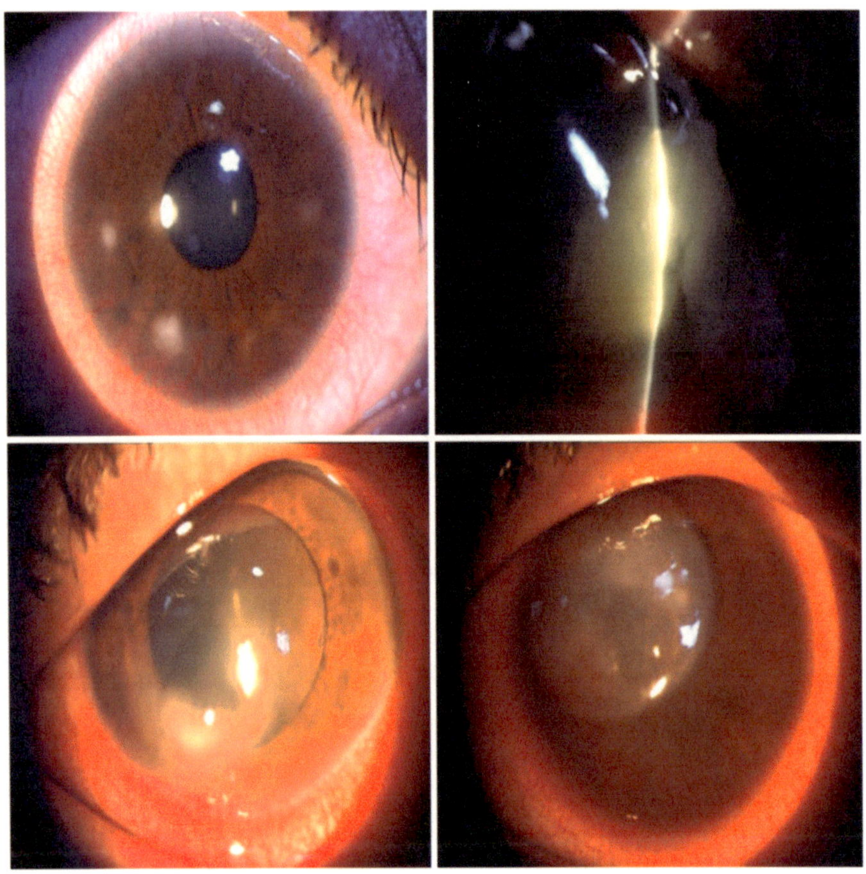

Figure 4. Representative Clinical pictures of patients with Bacterial Keratitis infection..

4.3. *Pseudomonas sp.*

Pseudomonas sp. is a Gram(-) often associated with contact lens use, which adheres to the damaged epithelium and stromal cause rapid invasion, the ulcer has a deep peripheral extension in hours (can reach twice its size in 24 hrs.) peripheral infiltration with diffuse gray, yellow-green discharge, severe reaction and hypopyon in the anterior chamber, which may extend to sclera and cause necrotizing scleritis and/or perforation in 2-5 days. You can also get to see a multifocal pattern that is more associated with use of soft contact lens [67, 76].

4.4. *Streptococcus sp.*

S. pneumoniae isolates in the upper respiratory tract half of the population, their proximity to the eye may explain the frequency of problems associated with it. *Streptococcus sp.* generates hemolysis of erythrocytes, being in full by the *S. pyogenes*, and partially by the alpha hemolytic as *S. viridans* and *S. pneumoniae*. The infection usually arises after corneal trauma and is often associated with chronic dacryocystitis. We present a deep stromal abscess with fibrin deposition, plaque formation, severe anterior chamber reaction, hypopyon, synechiae iridianas, if left untreated can lead to perforation. *S. viridans* has a less aggressive course and is responsible for cristalinean keratopathy, also related to the indiscriminate use of topical anesthetic, use of contact lenses and chemical burns [77-79].

4.5. *Bacillus sp.*

Bacillus cereus are bacilli anaerobic Gram + in soil, water and vegetation. The infection usually occurs within 24 hours after penetrating trauma in the presence of chemosis, severe eyelid edema, proptosis, edema peripheral microcystic with a ring followed by a circumferential corneal abscess may lead to drilling in hours [80-82].

4.6. Less common infectious agents

4.6.1. *Corynebacterium diphtheriae*

Corynebacterium diphtheriae are bacilli Gram + that rarely causes corneal disease but does remark commonly as a cause of pseudomembranous conjunctivitis with preauricular lymphadenopathy resulting in corneal epithelial opacity diffuse stromal necrosis and thinning [83-87].

4.6.2. *Listeria monocytogenes*

Listeria monocytogenes is a facultative anaerobe that causes infection in people who are dedicated to animal care. It is colonizing persistent epithelial defects and keratitis developed a type of necrotizing ulcer-shaped ring with large anterior chamber reaction, fibrinoid exudation and hypopyon [87-89].

4.6.3. Propionibacterium acnes

Propionibacterium acnes are bacilli anaerobic Gram + rod that is part of normal flora, so the infection occurs before a surgical trauma, contact lens use, chronic use of steroids or other associated corneal disease. It takes the form of corneal stromal abscess with intact epithelium [90-93].

5. Conclusions

In order to minimize the effect of bacterial resistance have begun to develop programs among which we mention the use of antibiotics, increased medical education plans in the study of infectious diseases, the use of antimicrobial agents and their prescription based on the evidence, the establishment of surveillance programs to detect the emergence of resistant strains, and improving the quality of antimicrobial susceptibility methods.

In the future it will continue to develop new antibiotic molecules looking to have a better effect. However, we must control a number of factors that facilitate the increase and acceleration of development of resistance, it is necessary to continuously monitor the levels of resistance of each bacterial species and thus able to make a rational antibiotic selection for the benefit of patients and reduce the risk of developing resistance. Simple measures and common sense will remain the main limiting resource for development of bacterial resistance.

Acknowledgements

Fundacion Hospital Nuestra Señora de la Luz. To Ingrid Vanessa Gonzalez-Leon for her support. The authors declare that they have no financial and personal relationships with other people or organizations that could inappropriately influence this work.

Author details

Atzin Robles-Contreras[1], Hector Javier Perez-Cano[1], Alejandro Babayan-Sosa[2] and Oscar Baca-Lozada[2]

1 Biomedical Research Center, "Nuestra Señora de la Luz" Hospital Foundation, Mexico

2 Cornea Department, "Nuestra Señora de la Luz" Hospital Foundation, Mexico

References

[1] Whitcher JP, Srinivasan M & Upadhyay MP. Corneal blindness: a global perspective. Bull World Health Organ 2001; 79:214-21.

[2] Erie JC, Nevitt MP, Hodge DO & Ballard DJ et al. Incidence of ulcerative keratitis in a defined population from 1950 through 1988. Arch Ophthalmol 1993; 111:1665–71.

[3] Upadhyay MP, Karmacharya PC, Koirala S, Shah DN, Shakya S, et al. The Bhaktapur eye study: ocular trauma and antibiotic prophylaxis for the prevention of corneal ulceration in Nepal. BrJOphthalmol 2001;85:388–92.1997; 104:1902–9.

[4] Green M, Apel A & Stapleton F. Risk factors and causative organisms in microbial keratitis. Cornea 2008 Jan; 27:22-7.

[5] Laspina F, Samudio M, Cibils D, Ta CN, Fariña N, et al. Epidemiological characteristics of microbiological results on patients with infectious corneal ulcers: a 13-year survey in Paraguay. Graefes Arch Clin Exp Ophthalmol 2004; 242:204–9.

[6] Srinivasan M, Gonzales CA, George C, et al.. Epidemiology and aetiological diagnosis of corneal ulceration in Madurai, south India. Br J Ophthalmol 1997; 81:965–71.

[7] Basak SK, Basak S, Mohanta A, et al. Epidemiological and microbiological diagnosis of suppurative keratitis in Gangetic West Bengal, eastern India. Indian J Ophthalmol 2005; 53:17–22.

[8] Cohen EJ, Fulton JC, Hoffman CJ, et al. Trends in contact lens-associated corneal ulcers. Cornea 1996; 15:566–70.

[9] Shah A, Sachdev A, Coggon D, et al. Geographic variations in microbial keratitis:an analysis of the peer-reviewed literature. Br J Ophthalmol. 2011; 95:762-7.

[10] Sirikul T, Prabriputaloong T, Smathivat A, et al.. Predisposing factors and aetiologic diagnosis of ulcerative keratitis. Cornea 2008; 27:283–7.

[11] Fong CF, Tseng CH, Hu FR, et al.. Clinical characteristics of microbial keratitis in a university hospital in Taiwan. Am J Ophthalmol 2004;137:329–36

[12] Bourcier T, Thomas F, Borderie V, et al. Bacterial keratitis: predisposing factors, clinical and microbiological review of 300 cases. Br J Ophthalmol 2003;87:834.

[13] Liesegang TJ. Contact lens-related microbial keratitis: Part I: Epidemiology. Cornea 1997;16:125-31.

[14] Jeng BH & McLeod SD. Microbial keratitis. Br J Ophthalmol 2003;87:805–6.

[15] Varaprasathan G, Miller K, Lietman T, et al.. Trends in the aetiology of infectious corneal ulcers at the F.I. Proctor Foundation. Cornea 2004;23:360–4

[16] Sun X, Deng S, Li R, et al. Distribution and shifting trends of bacterial keratitis in north China . Br J Ophthalmol 2004;88:165.

[17] Hsiao CH, Chuang CC, Tan HY,et al. Methicillin-resistant Staphylococcus aureus ocular infection: a 10-year hospital-based study. Ophthalmology. 2012 Mar; 119(3): 522-7.

[18] Yang KS, Lin HC, Ma DH, et al. Ulcerative keratitis caused by Haemophilus influenzae. Cornea. 2006 Jul;25(6):701-4.

[19] Tjia KF, van Putten JP, Pels E, et al. The interaction between Neisseria gonorrhoeae and the human cornea in organ culture. An electron microscopic study. Graefes Arch Clin Exp Ophthalmol. 1988;226(4):341-5.

[20] Zhou L, Zhao SZ, Koh SK, et al. In-depth analysis of the human tear proteome. J Proteomics. 2012; 75(13):3877-85. Epub 2012 May 23.

[21] Zhou L & Beuerman RW. Tear analysis in ocular surface diseases. Prog Retin Eye Res. 2012 Jun 23. [Epub ahead of print].

[22] Keay L, Willcox MD, Sweeney DF, et al. Bacterial populations on 30-night extended wear silicone hydrogel lenses. CLAO J. 2001; 27(1):30-4.

[23] Leitch EC, Harmis NY, Corrigan KM, Willcox MD. Identification and enumeration of staphylococci from the eye during soft contact lens wear. Optom Vis Sci. 1998; 75(4): 258-65.

[24] Leitch EC, Willcox MD. Interactions between the constitutive host defences of tears and Staphylococcus epidermidis. Aust N Z J Ophthalmol. 1997 ;25 Suppl 1:S20-2.

[25] Hart DE, Hosmer M, Georgescu M, et al. Bacterial assay of contact lens wearers. Optom Vis Sci. 1996; 73(3):204-7.

[26] Ramachandran L, Sharma S, Sankaridurg PR, et al., Examination of the conjunctival microbiota after 8 hours of eye closure. CLAO J. 1995; 21(3):195-9.

[27] Cleveland RP, Hazlett LD, Leon MA, Berk RS. Role of complement in murine corneal infection caused by Pseudomonas aeruginosa. Invest Ophthalmol Vis Sci. 1983; 24(2): 237-42.

[28] Hazlett LD & Berk RS. Effect of C3 depletion on experimental Pseudomonas aeruginosa ocular infection: histopathological analysis. Infect Immun. 1984 Mar;43(3): 783-90.

[29] Mondino BJ, Brown SI, Rabin BS, et al. Alternate pathway activation of complement in a Proteus mirabilis ulceration of the cornea. Arch Ophthalmol 96(9): 1659–1661.

[30] Huang X, Du W, McClellan SA, et al. TLR4 is required for host resistance in Pseudomonas aeruginosa keratitis. Invest Ophthalmol Vis Sci. 2006; 47(11):4910-6.

[31] Adhikary G, Sun Y & Pearlman E. C-Jun NH2 terminal kinase (JNK) is an essential mediator of Toll-like receptor 2-induced corneal inflammation. J Leukoc Biol. 2008 Apr;83(4):991-7. Epub 2008 Jan 24.

[32] Kumar A, Zhang J & Yu F-SX. Toll-like receptor 3 agonist poly(I:C)-induced antiviral response in human corneal epithelial cells. Immunology. 2006; 117:11–21.

[33] Kumar A, Yin J, Zhange J, et al. Modulation of corneal epithelial innate immune response to Pseudomonas infection by flagellin pretreatment. Invest Opthalmol Vis Sci. 2007; 48:4664–4670.

[34] McNamara NA, Van R, Tuchin OS, et al. Ocular surface epithelia express mRNA for human beta defensin-2. Exp Eye Res. 1999; 69:483–490.

[35] Maltseva IA, Fleiszig SMJ, et al. Exposure of human corneal epithelial cells to contact lenses in vitro suppresses the upregulation of human β-defensin-2 in response to antigens of Pseudomonas aeruginosa. Exp Eye Res. 2007;85:142–153.

[36] Huang X, Du W, Barrett RP, et al. ST2 is essential for TH2 responsiveness and resistance to Pseudomonas aeruginosa keratitis. Invest Ophthalmol Vis Sci. 2007;48:4626–4633.

[37] Wu X, Gao J & Ren M. Expression profiles and function of Toll-like receptors in human corneal epithelia. Chin Med J. 2007;120:893–897

[38] Wu M, McClellan SA, Barrett RP, et al. Beta-defensin-2 promotes resistance against infection with P. aeruginosa. J Immunol. 2009; 182:1609–16.

[39] Wu M, McClellan SA, Barrett RP, et al. Beta-defensins 2 and 3 together promote resistance to Pseudomonas aeruginosa keratitis. J Immunol. 2009; 183:8054–60.

[40] Kumar A, Hazlett LD & Yu FS. Flagellin suppresses inflammatory response and enhances bacterial clearance in murine model of Pseudomonas keratitis. Infect Immun. 2008; 76:89–96.

[41] Hume EB, Dajcs JJ, Moreau JM, et al. Staphylococcus corneal virulence in a new topical model of infection. Invest. Ophthalmol. Vis. Sci. 2001; 42:2904–2908.

[42] Girgis DO, Sloop GD, Reed JM, et al. A new topical model of Staphylococcus corneal infection in the mouse Invest. Ophthalmol. Vis. Sci. 2003; 44:1591–1597.

[43] Hume EB, Cole N, Khan S, et al. A Staphylococcus aureus mouse keratitis topical infection model: cytokine balance in different strains of mice. Immunol. Cell Biol. 2005; 83:294–300.

[44] Bourcier T, Thomas F, Borderie V, et al. Bacterial keratitis: predisposing factors, clinical and microbiological review of 300 cases. Br. J. Ophthalmol. 2003; 87:834–838.

[45] Sloop GD, Moreau JM, Conerly LL, et al. Acute inflammation of the eyelid and cornea in Staphylococcus keratitis in the rabbit. Invest. Ophthalmol. Vis. Sci. 1999; 40:385–391.

[46] Sun Y, Hise AG, Kalsow CM, et al. Staphylococcus aureus-induced corneal inflammation is dependent on Toll-like receptor 2 and myeloid differentiation factor 88. Infect Immun. 2006; 74:5325–32.

[47] Huang X, Barrett RP, McClellan SA, et al. Silencing Toll-like receptor-9 in Pseudomonas aeruginosa keratitis. Invest Ophthalmol Vis Sci. 2005; 46:4209–4216.

[48] Hazlett LD. Corneal response to Pseudomonas aeruginosa infection. Prog Retin Eye Res. 2004; 23:1–30.

[49] Zepeda CJ. Resistencia de las bacterias a los antibióticos. Revista Médica Hondureña. 1998; 66(2): 88-92.

[50] Henderson B, Poole S & Wilson M. Bacterial modulins: a novel class of virulence factors wich cause host tissue pathology by inducing cytokine synthesis. Microbiol Rev. 1996; 60(2):316-341.

[51] Caponi G. Las poblaciones biológicas como sistemas intencionales. In: Martins, RA, Martins LA, Silva CC & Ferreira JM (eds). Filosofia e história da ciencia no Cone Sul: 3º Encontro. Campinas: AFHIC. 2004;212-217.

[52] Tello A, Austin B & Telfer TC. Selective pressure of antibiotic pollution on bacteria of importance to to public health. Environ Health Perspect. 2011 [Epub ahead of print]

[53] Fernández-Riverón F, López Hernández J, Ponce-Martínez LM et al. Resistencia bacteriana. Rev Cubana Med Milit 2003; 32(1):44-48.

[54] Van Hoek AH, Mevius D, Guerra B, et al. Acquired antibiotic resistance genes: an overview. Front Microbiol. 2011; 2:203.

[55] Giedraitienė A, Vitkauskienė A, Naginienė R, et al. Antibiotic resistance mechanisms of clinically important bacteria. Medicina (kaunas). 2011; 47(3):137-146.

[56] Roberts MC. Enviromental macrolide lincosamide streptogramin and tetracycline resistant bacteria. Front Microbiol. 2011; 2:40:1-8.

[57] Livermore DM. Current epidemiology and growing resistance of gram negative pathogens. Korean J Intern Med. 2012; 27(2):128-142.

[58] Lim KT, Hanifah YA, Yusof M, et al. ermA, ermC, tetM and tetK are essential for erythromycin and tetracycline resistance among methicillin-resistant Staphylococcus aureus strains isolated from a tertiary hospital in Malaysia. Indian J Med Microbiol. 2012; 30(2):203-207.

[59] Nazar CJ. Bacterial Biofilms. Rev. Otorrinolaringol. Cir. Cabeza Cuello 2007; 67: 61-72

[60] Anderl JN, Franklin MJ & Stewart PS. Role of antibiotic penetration limitation in Klebsiella pneumonia biofilm resistance to ampicillin and ciprofloxacin. Antimicrob Agents Chemother. 2000; 44(7):1818-1824.

[61] Mascarenhas J, Srinivasan M, Chen M, et al. Differentiation of etiologic agents of bacterial keratitis from presentation characteristics. Int Ophthalmol. 2012 Jun 30. [Epub ahead of print]

[62] Kerautret J, Raobela L & Colin J. Serious bacterial keratitis: a retrospective clinical and microbiological study. J Fr Ophtalmol. 2006; 29(8):883-8.

[63] Srinivasan M, Mascarenhas J, Rajaraman R, et al. Steroids for Corneal Ulcers Trial Group. The steroids for corneal ulcers trial: study design and baseline characteristics. Arch Ophthalmol. 2012; 130(2):151-7.

[64] Bourcier T, Thomas F, Borderie V, et al. Bacterial keratitis: predisposing factors, clinical and microbiological review of 300 cases. Br J Ophthalmol. 2003; 87(7):834-8.

[65] Weiss K, Ardjomand N & El-Shabrawi Y. Mycotic infections of the eye. Wien Med Wochenschr. 2007; 157(19-20):517-21.

[66] Talukder AK, Halder SK, Sultana Z, et al. Epidemiology and outcome of non viral keratitis. Mymensingh Med J. 2011; 20(3):356-61.

[67] Sy A, Srinivasan M, Mascarenhas J, et al. Pseudomonas aeruginosa keratitis: outcomes and response to corticosteroid treatment. Invest Ophthalmol Vis Sci. 2012; 53(1):267-72.

[68] Lalitha P, Srinivasan M, Manikandan P, et al. Relationship of in vitro susceptibility to moxifloxacin and in vivo clinical outcome in bacterial keratitis. Clin Infect Dis. 2012; 54(10):1381-7.

[69] Srinivasan M, Mascarenhas J, Rajaraman R, et al. Steroids for Corneal Ulcers Trial Group. Corticosteroids for bacterial keratitis: the Steroids for Corneal Ulcers Trial (SCUT). Arch Ophthalmol. 2012; 130(2):143-50.

[70] Blair J, Hodge W, Al-Ghamdi S, et al. Comparison of antibiotic-only and antibiotic-steroid combination treatment in corneal ulcer patients: double-blinded randomized clinical trial. Can J Ophthalmol. 2011; 46(1):40-5.

[71] Guyomarch J, van Nuoï DN, Beral L, et al. Infectious keratitis and cosmetic lenses: a five-case retrospective study. J Fr Ophtalmol. 2010; 33(4):258-62.

[72] Donshik PC, Suchecki JK, Ehlers WH. Peripheral corneal infiltrates associated with contact lens wear. Trans Am Ophthalmol Soc. 1995; 93:49-60; discussion 60-4.

[73] Mascarenhas J, Srinivasan M, Chen M, et al. Differentiation of etiologic agents of bacterial keratitis from presentation characteristics. Int Ophthalmol. 2012 Jun 30. [Epub ahead of print].

[74] de Rojas V, Llovet F, Martínez M, et al. Infectious keratitis in 18,651 laser surface ablation procedures. J Cataract Refract Surg. 2011; 37(10):1822-31.

[75] Suzuki T. A new target for Staphylococcus aureus associated with keratitis. Cornea. 2011; 30 Suppl 1:S34-40.

[76] Stewart RM, Wiehlmann L, Ashelford KE, et al. Genetic characterization indicates that a specific subpopulation of Pseudomonas aeruginosa is associated with keratitis infections. J Clin Microbiol. 2011; 49(3):993-1003.

[77] Galperín GJ, Boscaro G, Tau J, et al. Crystalline keratopathy: an infrequent corneal infection produced by the Streptococcus mitis group. Rev Argent Microbiol. 2011; 43(3):195-7.

[78] Millender TW, Reller LB, Meekins LC, et al. Streptococcal pharyngitis leading to corneal ulceration. Ocul Immunol Inflamm. 2012; 20(2):143-4.

[79] Norcross EW, Sanders ME, Moore QC 3rd, et al. Pathogenesis of A Clinical Ocular Strain of Streptococcus pneumoniae and the Interaction of Pneumolysin with Corneal Cells. J Bacteriol Parasitol. 2011; 2(2):108.

[80] Ramos-Esteban JC, Servat JJ, Tauber S, Bia F. Bacillus megaterium delayed onset lamellar keratitis after LASIK. J Refract Surg. 2006; 22(3):309-12.

[81] Pinna A, Sechi LA, Zanetti S, et al. Bacillus cereus keratitis associated with contact lens wear. Ophthalmology. 2001; 108(10):1830-4.

[82] Choudhuri KK, Sharma S, Garg P, et al. Clinical and microbiological profile of Bacillus keratitis. Cornea. 2000; 19(3):301-6.

[83] Fukumoto A, Sotozono C, Hieda O, Kinoshita S. Infectious keratitis caused by fluoroquinolone-resistant Corynebacterium. Jpn J Ophthalmol. 2011; 55(5):579-80.

[84] Willcox M, Sharma S, Naduvilath TJ, et al. External ocular surface and lens microbiota in contact lens wearers with corneal infiltrates during extended wear of hydrogel lenses. Eye Contact Lens. 2011; 37(2):90-5.

[85] Garg P, Chaurasia S, Vaddavalli PK, et al. Microbial keratitis after LASIK. J Refract Surg. 2010 Mar;26(3):209-16.

[86] Suzuki T, Iihara H, Uno T, et al. Suture related keratitis caused by Corynebacterium macginleyi. J Clin Microbiol. 2007; 45(11):3833-6.

[87] Tay E, Rajan M & Tuft S. Listeria monocytogenes sclerokeratitis: a case report and literature review. Cornea. 2008; 27(8):947-9.

[88] Altaie R, Fahy GT, Cormican M. Failure of Listeria monocytogenes keratitis to respond to topical ofloxacin. Cornea. 2006;25(7):849-50.

[89] Zaidman GW, Coudron P & Piros J. Listeria monocytogenes keratitis. Am J Ophthalmol. 1990; 109(3):334-9.

[90] Ovodenko B, Seedor JA, Ritterband DC, et al. The prevalence and pathogenicity of Propionibacterium acnes keratitis. Cornea. 2009; 28(1):36-9.

[91] Brook I. Ocular infections due to anaerobic bacteria in children. J Pediatr Ophthalmol Strabismus. 2008; 45(2):78-84.

[92] Garg P, Sharma S & Underdahl J. Propionibacterium acnes as a cause of visually significant corneal ulcers. Cornea. 200; 20(4):437-8.

[93] Underdahl JP, Florakis GJ, Braunstein RE, et al. Propionibacterium acnes as a cause of visually significant corneal ulcers. Cornea. 2000 Jul;19(4):451-4.

Chapter 6

Preseptal Cellulitis

Monika Fida, Kocinaj Allma, Abazi Flora and
Arjeta Grezda

Additional information is available at the end of the chapter

http://dx.doi.org/10.5772/52709

1. Introduction

Periorbital infections are typically classified as either preseptal or orbital cellulites and are common in children and adults. One of the major anatomical structures determining the location of disease is the orbital septum, which is a thin membrane originating from the orbital periosteum inserting into the anterior surfaces of the tarsal plates of the eyelids. The septum separates the superficial eyelid from the deeper orbital structures, forming a barrier that prevents infection in the eyelid from extending into the orbit.

2. Definition

Preseptal cellulitis is an inflammation and infection of the eyelid (also of the periorbital soft tissues), anterior to orbital septum, not involving the orbit or other ocular structures, characterized by acute eyelid erythema and edema[1].

This is a common infection and tends to be less severe a disease than orbital cellulitis (known as postseptal cellulitis). It may result from the spread of the upper respiratory tract infections, external eye infections, or eyelid traumas[2].

In preseptal cellulitis, the soft tissues anterior to the orbital septum are affected and the orbital structures posterior to the septum are not infected but may be infected secondarily causing subperiosteal and orbital abscesses. In severe cases,this may also cause cavernous sinus thrombosis or meningitis. Patients with periorbital edema, erythema and increase in local hyperemia but without proptosis, ophthalmoplegia and visual impairment have been defined as having preseptal cellulitis. Patients with proptosis, ophthalmoplegia andvisual impairment have been defined as having orbital cellulitis. Preseptal cellulitis is usually managed medically, whereas orbital cellulitis requires an aggressive treatment and may require surgical intervention [3, 4, 5]. Orbital cellulitis is a serious infection, especially in children, and may result in significant complications including blindness, cavernous sinus thrombosis, meningitis, subdural empyema, and brain abscess.

The correct treatment of the preseptal cellulitis during the antibiotic era makes these complications rare but the correct diagnosis and early treatment are important to prevent the life threatening complications [4,5].

3. Etiology

Preseptal cellulitis, as an eyelid infection, may be caused by inoculation following a trauma or skin infection, from spread of sinuses infection, upper respiratory tract infection, and any infection elsewhere disseminated through the blood.

Also, insect (spider) or animal bites, or a chalazion may be followed by eyelid infection[6].

Nearly two thirds of the cases of cellulitis are reported to be associated with upper respiratory tract infections, with one half of these from sinusitis. The most common microorganisms are Staphylococcus aureus, Staphylococcus epidermidis, Streptococcus species, and anaerobes, known organisms that commonly cause upper respiratory tract infections and external eyelid infections[6]. Cold weather and upper respiratory tract infections are sometimes correlated with increased frequency of sinusitis, resulting in orbital cellulitis having seasonal peaks from late fall to early spring [7, 8].

Streptococcus pneumonia predominates when infection arises from sinuses infection, whereas Staphylococcus aureus and Streptococcus pyogenes often accompany local trauma and may be the most important pathology related toperiocular infection in a developing country.

Haemophilusinfluenzae B is now less common and usually occurs following bacteremic spread from a primary focus such as otitis media or pneumonia. Affected patients may have other foci of bacteremic spread including the meninges[9].

Haemophilusinfluenzae was the most common organism isolated in blood cultures before introduction of the vaccine, resulting with positive blood cultures during upper respiratory tract infections and in subcutaneous aspirates in nearly half of the patients with eyelid trauma or external ocular infections[10].

It has also been reported that total cases per year from all pathogens after the introduction of the Haemophilusinfluenzae vaccine declined as well, suggesting that Haemophilusinfluenzae may have played a facilitative role in the pathogenesis of cellulitis[10].

Periorbital cellulitis has also been reported with smallpox and anthrax[6].

Frequent causes of preseptal cellulitis include Acinetobacter species, Nocardiabrasiliensis, Bacillus anthracis, Pseudomonas aeruginosa, Neisseria gonorrhoeae, Proteus spp, Pasteurellamultocida, Mycobacterium tuberculosis, and Trichophytonspp (the cause of "ringworm"). These pathogens can usually be linked to specific exposures[11-20].

Polymicrobial infections are also common[21, 22, 23].

Decreased immune function, as a side effect after the overuse of antibiotics, penetrating injuries, and diabetes mellitus, are all the factors that favor fungal infections such are aspergillosis or mucormycosis.

Risk factors	Percentage
Conjunctivitis	74.1%
Upper respiratory tract infections	37.4%
Focal lesions on the face or near the orbita	25.2%
Sinusitis	24.5%
Odontogenic infections and dental caries	19.4%
Trauma	10.8%
Allergy	3.6%
Hordeolum	3.6%
Other	6.5%

* Modified from Devrimİ, Kanra G, Kara A, Cengiz AB, Orhan M, Ceyhan M, Seçmeer G. Preseptal and orbital cellulitis: 15-year experience with sulbactam ampicillin treatment. Turk J Pediatr 2008; 50: 214-218.

Table 1. Common risk factors for preseptal cellulitis and orbital cellulitis

Focal lesions on the face or near the orbita	Percentage
Acne	5.8%
Insect bite	5.8%
Herpetic lesions	5.8%
Lesions secondary to trauma	5.8%
Impetigo	5%
Acute dacryocystitis	0.7%

* Modified from Devrimİ, Kanra G, Kara A, Cengiz AB, Orhan M, Ceyhan M, Seçmeer G. Preseptal and orbital cellulitis: 15-year experience with sulbactam ampicillin treatment. Turk J Pediatr 2008; 50: 214-218.

Table 2. Common focal lesions on the face or near the orbita as the risk factors for preseptal cellulitis and orbital cellulitis*

Isolated agent	Percentage
Staphylococcus aureus	43%
Coagulase-negative staphylococcus	26.6%
Streptococcus pneumoniae	10%
Haemophylusinfluenzae type B	6.6%
Streptococcus**	6.6%
Klebsiellapneumonia	3.3%
Pseudomonas aeruginosa	3.3%

* Pus and swab cultures from secretion of conjunctiva

** Other than pneumococci

*** Modified from Devrimİ, Kanra G, Kara A, CengizAB, Orhan M, Ceyhan M, Seçmeer G. Preseptal and orbital cellulitis: 15-year experience with sulbactam ampicillin treatment. Turk J Pediatr 2008; 50: 214-218.

Table 3. Common isolated* microorganisms in cases with orbital and preseptal cellulitis***

The causes of preseptal cellulites are classified as:

- exogenous (trauma, postsurgical)
- endogenous (bacteremia)
- extension from periorbital structures (paranasal sinuses, dental infection, intracranial)
- intraorbital (endophtalmitis, dacryoadenitis).

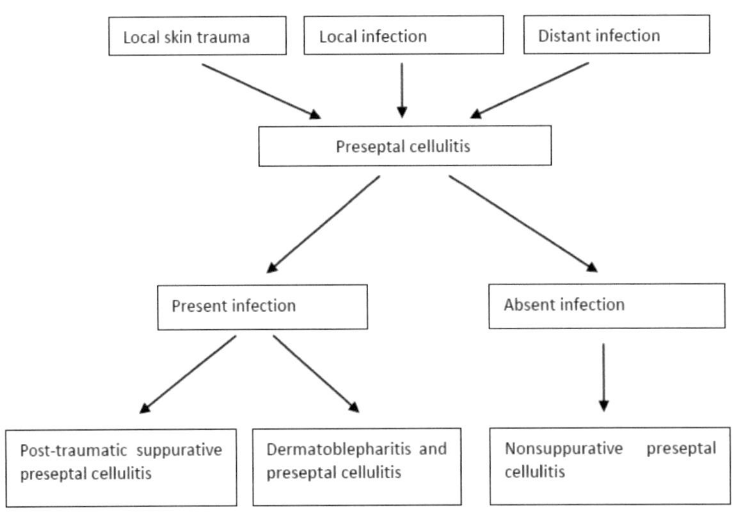

Figure 1. Pathophysiology of preseptal cellulitis

http://dx.doi.org/10.5772/52709

Risk factors [24, 25]

1. Eyelid lesions:
    - Hordeola
    - Chalazia
    - Bug bites
    - Trauma-related lesions
    - Lesions caused by a recent surgical procedure near the eyelids
    - Lesions caused by oral procedures
2. Upper respiratory tract infections (especially sinusitis)
3. Other diseases:
    - Varicella
    - Asthma
    - Nasal polyposis
    - Neutropenia

4. Clinical signs

Patients with preseptal cellulitis clinically complain of eye pain, redness, periorbital lid swelling, and fever. This is a typical clinicalpresentation. Eyelid edema, a violaceous erythema, and inflammation may be severe. Usually the globe is uninvolved; papillary reaction, visual acuity, and ocular motility are not disturbed; pain on eye movement and chemosis are absent. Chemosis may be present in severe cases of preseptal or orbital cellulitis caused by H.influenzae. Focal sinus region tenderness and purulent nasal discharge may be present due to sinus infections. Black eschar within the nasal mucosa indicates a potential fungal infection. Patients diagnosed with preseptal cellulitis have intact extraocular movements and do not have proptoses that differentiate from orbital cellulitis.

Typically, children with Haemophilusinfluenzae cellulites have a history of recent upper respiratory infection and present with high fever, irritability and coryza. A marked leukocytosis may be present but this is evident either in preseptal and orbital cellulites [24, 26, 27].

Preseptal cellulitis: Images show preseptal cellulitis in the second day of inflammation. Marked, isolated, and unilateral periocular inflammation may be noted. The patient presented painless during the eye movement.

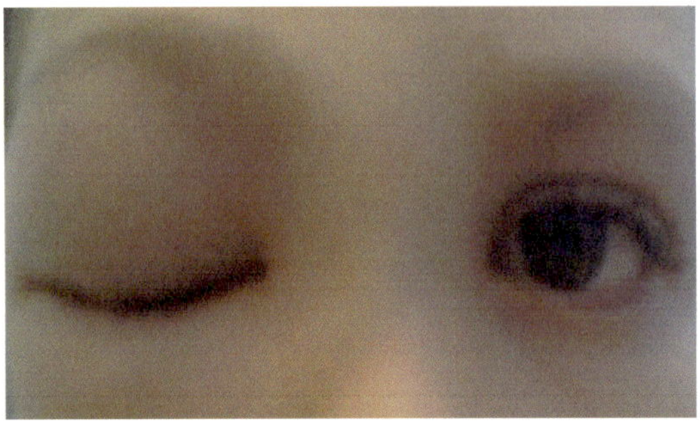

Figure 2.

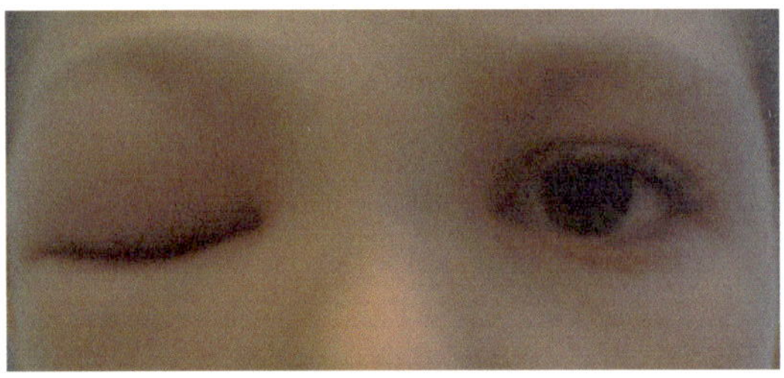

Figure 3.

Same patient with preseptal cellulitis after the treatment: Images show resolved preseptal cellulitis after a whole course of the recommended therapy.

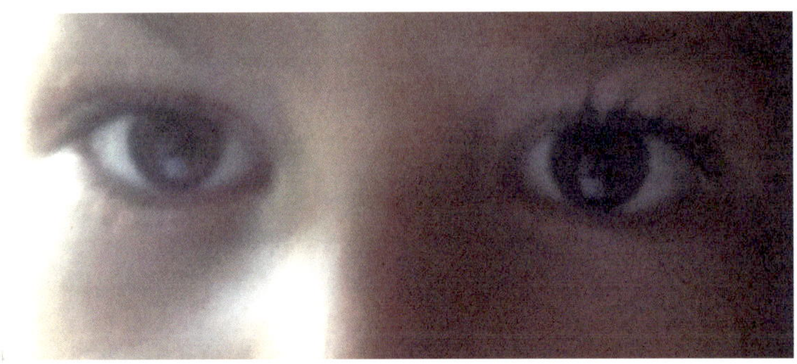

Figure 4.

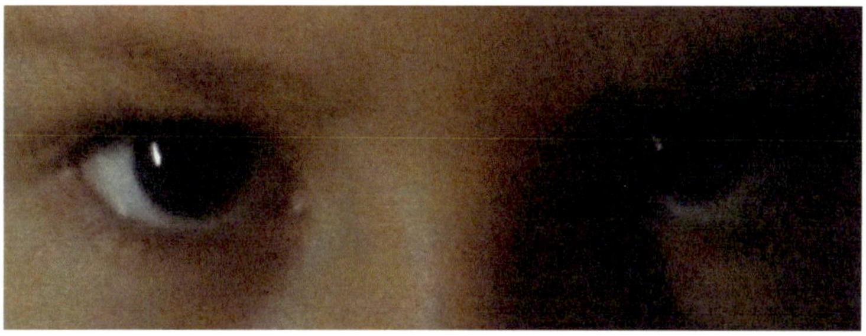

Figure 5.

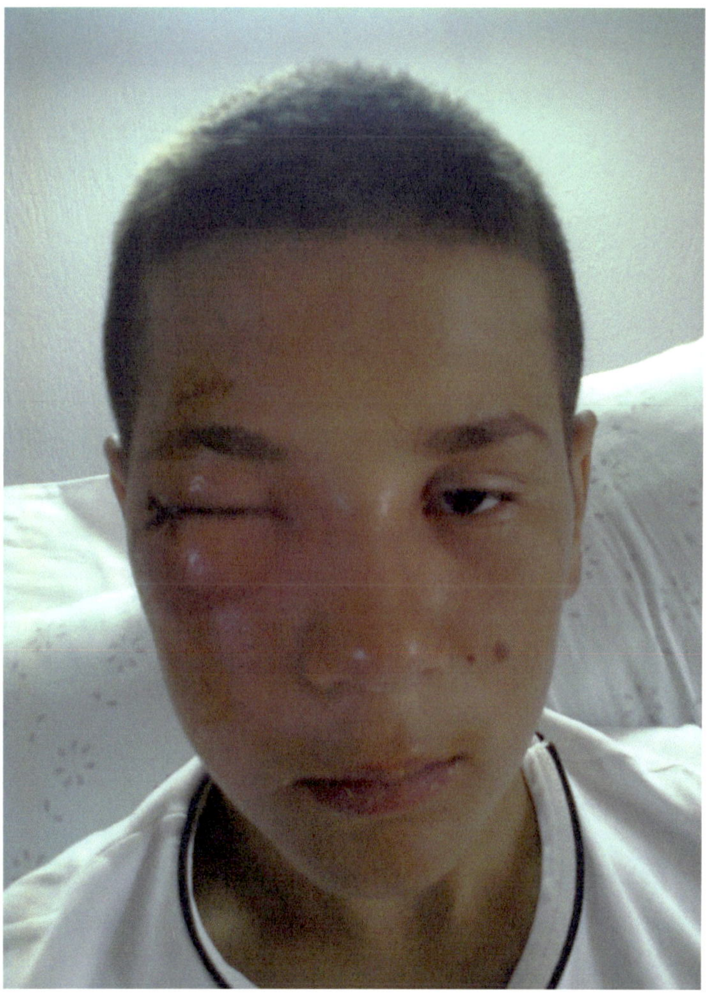

Figure 6.

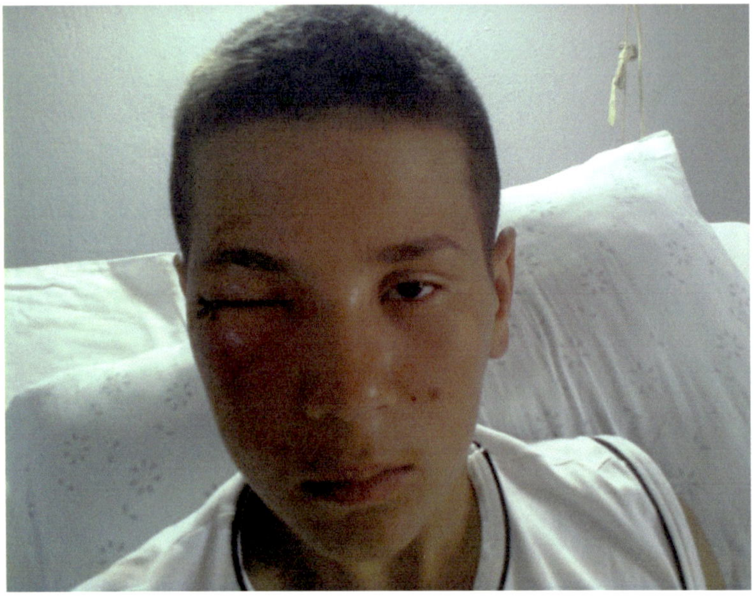

Figure 7.

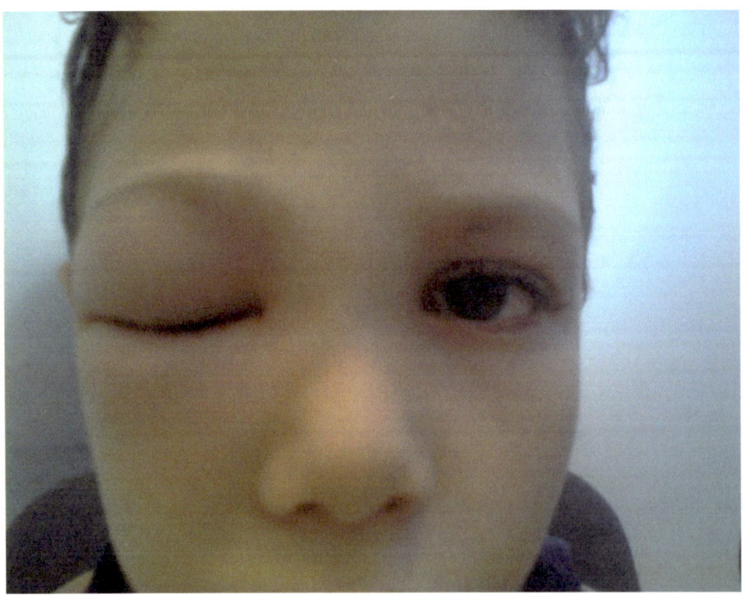

Figure 8.

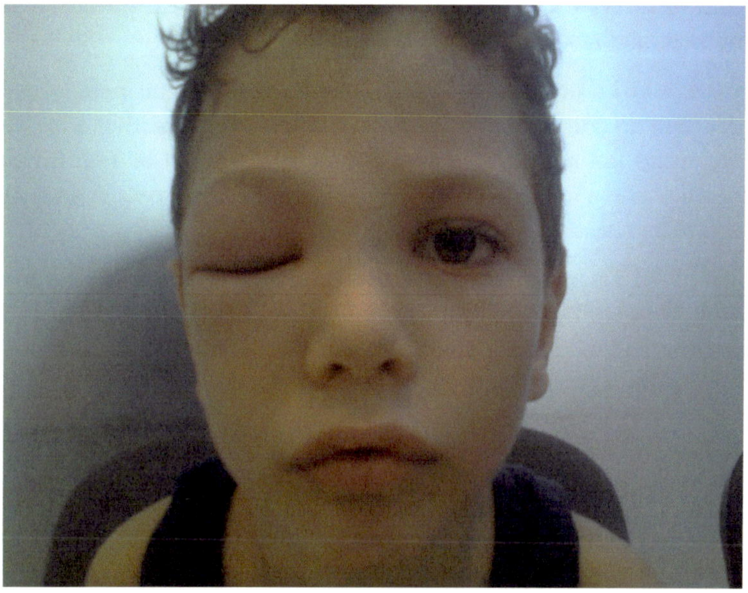

Figure 9.

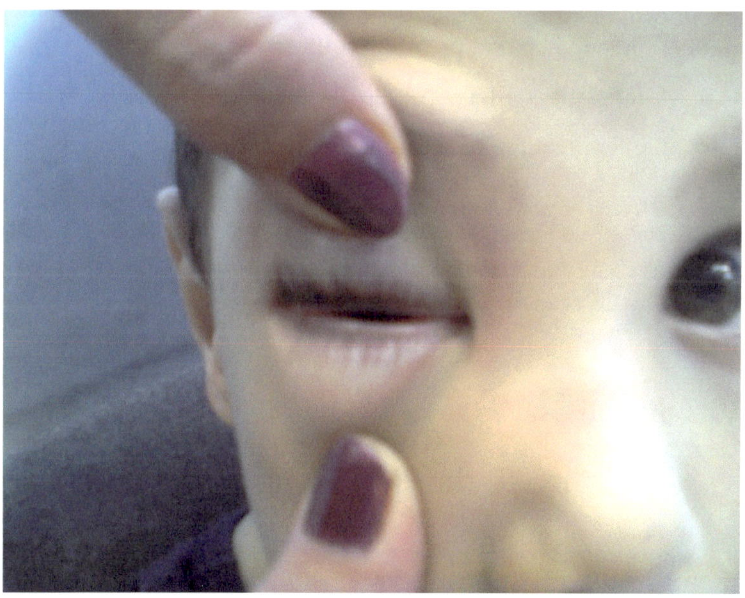

Figure 10.

Diagnosis is usually based upon the clinical findings, microbiological and radiological examination.

Findings on examination include pain on eye movement, afferent pupillary defect, limited extraocular motions, and resistance on retropulsion.

Blood cultures should be obtained as they correlate with orbital pathogens far better in childhood cases than do cultures from the nasopharynx or conjunctiva. Samples of conjunctival discharge, eyelid lesions, and lacrimal sac material should be sent for culture. Blood culture results are positive in less than 10% of cases of preseptal cellulitis, whereas skin culture results tend to be negative.

White blood cell (WBC) counts tend to be elevated and cannot be used to differentiate preseptal cellulitis from orbital cellulitis. Levels of ESR and CRP can help in the differentiation of preseptal and orbital cellulitis. However, it must be kept in mind that all of those high values of routine laboratory results can be seen in preseptal cellulitis.

Biopsy shows edema and polymorphonuclear leukocytes infiltrating tissue planes.

Lumbar puncture may be considered in affected children but not for routine use in the absence of meningitis signs.

Orbital ultrasonography can help in diagnosing orbital inflammation, although it requires experienced observers and specialized equipment.

A computed tomography (CT) scan can delineate the extent of orbital involvement[28].

CT scan findings in preseptal cellulitis include the following:

- Swelling of the eyelid and adjacent preseptal soft tissues
- Obliteration of the fat planes or details of the preseptal soft tissues
- Absence of orbital inflammation

It is quite difficult to distinguish periorbital (preseptal) and orbital cellulitis based just on clinical findings, especially in children. Many of the clinical signs of orbital cellulitis are distinctive, such are proptosis andophthalmoplegia, but the correct diagnosis of orbital cellulitis is best confirmed by CT scan with contrast infusion of the orbit[29, 30, 31, 32].

5. Differential diagnoses

There are several entities to be considered in the differential diagnosis of preseptal cellulitis: [33]

- Rhabdomyosarcoma
- Retinoblastoma
- Orbital pseudotumour (idiopathic orbital inflammation)
- Periocular tinea
- Cellulitis, Orbital

http://dx.doi.org/10.5772/52709

- Conjunctivitis
- Dacryoadenitis
- Dacryocystitis
- Dermatitis, Contact
- Herpes Simplex
- Herpes Zoster
- Hordeolum

6. Staging

A computed tomography (CT) scan can delineate the extent of orbital involvement [28, 31, 32].

The modified Chandler staging system is as follows:

- Stage I - Preseptal cellulitis
- Stage II - Inflammatory orbital edema
- Stage III - Subperiosteal abscess
- Stage IV - Orbital abscess
- Stage V - Cavernous sinus thrombosis

Complications of preseptal cellulitis may be progression to stage II and behind of orbital infections. Preseptal cellulitis in infants and children under the age 5 may be associated with bacteremia, septicemia, and meningitis, and therefore the treatment should start as soon as possible including consultations with a pediatrician. Late complications of preseptal cellulitis include lid abscess, cicatricialectropion, and lid necrosis. Unless appropriately treated, periorbital and orbital cellulitis can result in optic neuritis, opticatrophy, blindness, cavernous sinus thrombosis,superior orbital fissure syndrome, orbital apex syndrome, meningitis, brain abscess, subdural empyema, and even death [34, 35].

7. Treatment

Earlier diagnosis, expeditious treatment, and improved antibiotics have led to a reduction in serious ocular and central nervous system complications in patients with preseptal cellulitis. Treatment involves management of predisposing conditions, antibiotic therapy, and close observation[36]. Starting the antibiotic therapy at all ages should provide coverage for pathogens associated with acute sinusitis (*S. pneumoniae, H. influenzae, M. catarrhalis, S. pyogenes*) as well as anaerobes and *S. aureus*[37, 38].

Preseptal cellulitis treatment is based on oral antibiotics (outpatient treatment) and antiseptic treatment locally provided that a close follow-up can be ensured. Hospitalization is recommended if there is no improvement within 48 hours (or even 24 hours), and parenterally antibiotics (broad-spectrum intravenous antibiotics) are necessary once appropriate cultures have been obtained, undergoing a CT scan to evaluate for orbital cellulitis and its complications. Patients with subtle clinical and/or radiographic findings, suggesting that the orbit is involved, should be treated as a case of orbital cellulitis given the serious complications of this entity.

Also, children younger than one year of age, those who cannot cooperate fully, and patients who are severely ill should generally be admitted to the hospital and managed according to the recommendations.

Teenagers and adults usually respond quickly to appropriate oral antibiotics and there is no need for hospitalization unless orbital involvement cannot be excluded or when the clinical situation is severe.

Initial antibiotic selection is based on the history, clinical findings and laboratory studies, and is almost always empiric and based upon knowledge of the common infecting organisms. Staphylococcus aureus is the most common pathogen in patients with preseptal cellulitis resulting from trauma. The infection usually responds quickly to penicillinase-resistant penicillin. Third-generation cephalosporins or ampicillin have both a broad spectrum coverage including activity against Haemophilusinfluenza, and should be initiated immediately after obtaining the cultures.

Lid abscesses should be drained surgically with the incision and drainage usually performed directly over the abscess, avoiding the damage of the levatoraponeurosis.

In order to avoid contamination of the orbital soft tissue, the orbital septum should not be opened.

One of the following regimens is suggested for empiric oral treatment of preseptal cellulitis: [39]

- Clindamycin (in children: 30 to 40 mg/kg per day in three to four equally divided doses, not to exceed 1.8 grams per day; in adults: 300 mg every eight hours) as monotherapyor
- Trimethoprim-sulfamethoxazole (TMP-SMX; in children: 8 to 12 mg/kg per day of the trimethoprim component divided every 12 hours; in adults: 8 mg/kg per day of the trimethoprim component divided every 8 or 12 hours) plus one of the following:
- Amoxicillin (in children: 80 to 100 mg/kg per day in divided doses every eight hours; in adults: 875 mg orally every 12 hours) or
- Amoxicillin-clavulanic acid (in children: 45 mg/kg per day divided every 12 hours; in adults: 875 mg every 12 hours) or
- Cefpodoxime (in children: 10 mg/kg per day divided every 12 hours, not to exceed 200 mg per dose; in adults: 400 mg every 12 hours) or

- Cefdinir (in children: 7 mg/kg twice daily, maximum daily dose 600 mg; in adults: 300 mg twice daily)

The use of clindamycin alone has shown good efficacy for skin and soft tissue infections caused by staphylococci and streptococci.

One of the combination regimens should be used if the patient has not been immunized against Haemophilusinfluenzae.

Topical antibiotics have no role in the treatment of this infection.

Generally, the treatment is recommend for 7 to 10 days, but if signs of cellulitis persist, treatment should be continued until the eyelid erythema and swelling have resolved or nearly resolved[40, 41].

Recurrent preseptal cellulitis — preseptal cellulitis rarely recurs. When it does, it is usually due to an underlying cause that has not been diagnosed or due to an anatomic abnormality[42, 43].

The presence of subperiosteal or intraorbital abscess is an indication for surgical drainage in addition to antibiotic therapy [44, 45]. Surgical drainage is indicated for complete ophthalmoplegia and/or significant visual impairment (acute optic nerve or retinal compromise) or large well-defined abscesses [46,47,48]. Depending on the patient condition,sinus surgery and sinus endoscopy are recommended,and for patientswith orbital cellulitis, intracranial abscess drainage, orbital surgery or ethmoidectomy.

Author details

Monika Fida[1], Kocinaj Allma[2], Abazi Flora[2] and Arjeta Grezda[1]

1 University Hospital Center "Mother Teresa", Tirana, Albania

2 University Clinical Center of Kosova, Prishtina, Kosovo

References

[1] Botting AM, McIntosh D, Mahadevan M. Paediatric pre- and post-septalperi-orbital infections are different diseases. A retrospective review of 262 cases. Int J PediatrOtorhinolaryngol 2008; 72:377.

[2] Zhang J, Stringer MD. Ophthalmic and facial veins are not valveless. Clin Experiment Ophthalmol 2010; 38:502.

[3] Jain A, Rubin PA. Orbital cellulitis in children.IntOphthalmolClin. 2001;41:71-86.

[4] Ferguson MP, McNab AA. Current treatment and outcome in orbital cellulitis.Aust N Z J Ophthalmol. 1999;27:375-379.

[5] Givner LB. Periorbital versus orbital cellulitis. Pediatr Infect Dis J. 2002;21:1157-1158.

[6] Donahue S, Schwartz G. Preseptal and orbital cellulitis in childhood. A changing microbiologic spectrum. Ophthalmology 1998; 105[10]:1902–6.

[7] Oxford LE, McClay J. Complications of acute sinusitis in children. Otolaryngol Head Neck Surg. 2005;133:32-37.

[8] Jackson K, Baker SR. Clinical implications of orbital cellulitis.Laryngoscope. 1986;96:568-574.

[9] Ambati BK, Ambati J, Azar N, et al. Periorbital and orbital cellulitis before and after the advent of Haemophilusinfluenzae type B vaccination. Ophthalmology 2000; 107:1450.

[10] Artac H, Silahli M, Keles S, Ozdemir M, Reisli I. A rare cause of preseptal cellulitis: anthrax. PediatrDermatol. 2007; 24[3]:330-1.

[11] Miller J. Acinetobacter as a causative agent in preseptal cellulitis. Optometry 2005; 76:176.

[12] Mathews D, Mathews JP, Kwartz J, Inkster C. Preseptal cellulitis caused by Acinetobacterlwoffi. Indian J Ophthalmol 2005; 53:213.

[13] Brannan PA, Kersten RC, Hudak DT, et al. Primary Nocardiabrasiliensis of the eyelid. Am J Ophthalmol 2004; 138:498.

[14] Caça I, Cakmak SS, Unlü K, et al. Cutaneous anthrax on eyelids. Jpn J Ophthalmol 2004; 48:268.

[15] Milstone AM, Ruff AJ, Yeamans C, Higman MA. Pseudomonas aeruginosa pre-septal cellulitis and bacteremia in a pediatric oncology patient. Pediatr Blood Cancer 2005; 45:354.

[16] Raja NS, Singh NN. Bilateral orbital cellulitis due to Neisseria gonorrhoeae and Staphylococcus aureus: a previously unreported case. J Med Microbiol 2005; 54:609.

[17] Sears JM, Gabriel HM, Veith J. Preseptal cellulitis secondary to Proteus species: a case report and review. J Am OptomAssoc 1999; 70:661.

[18] Raina UK, Jain S, Monga S, et al. Tubercular preseptal cellulitis in children: a presenting feature of underlying systemic tuberculosis. Ophthalmology 2004; 111:291.

[19] Velazquez AJ, Goldstein MH, Driebe WT. Preseptal cellulitis caused by trichophyton (ringworm). Cornea 2002; 21:312.

[20] Hutcheson KA, Magbalon M. Periocular abscess and cellulitis from Pasteurellamultocida in a healthy child. Am J Ophthalmol 1999; 128:514.

[21] Brown CL, Graham SM, Griffin MC, et al. Pediatric medial subperiosteal orbital abscess: medical management where possible. Am J Rhinol. 2004;18:321-327.

[22] Harris GJ. Subperiosteal abscess of the orbit. Ophthalmology. 1994;101: 585-595.

[23] Oxford LE, McClay J. Complications of acute sinusitis in children. Otolaryngol Head Neck Surg. 2005;133:32-37.

[24] Chaudhry IA, Shamsi FA, Elzaridi E, Al-Rashed W, Al-Amri A, Arat YO. Inpatient preseptal cellulitis: experience from a tertiary eye care centre. Br J Ophthalmol. 2008; 92[10]:1337-41.

[25] Babar TF, Zaman M, Khan MN, Khan MD. Risk factors of preseptal and orbital cellulitis. J Coll Physicians Surg Pak. Jan 2009; 19[1]:39-42.

[26] Givner LB. Periorbital versus orbital cellulitis. Pediatr Infect Dis J. 2002 Dec; 21[12]: 1157-8.

[27] Murthum K, Pogorelov P, Bergua A. Preseptal cellulitis as a complication of surgical treatment of migraine headaches. KlinMonatsblAugenheilkd. 2009; 226[7]:572-3.

[28] Ho CF, Huang YC, Wang CJ, Chiu CH, Lin TY. Clinical analysis of computed tomography-staged orbital cellulitis in children. J MicrobiolImmunol Infect. 2007; 40[6]: 518-24.

[29] Sobol SE, Marchand J, Tewfik TL, Manoukian JJ, Schloss MD. Orbital complications of sinusitis in children. J Otolaryngol. 2002;31:131-136.

[30] Goldberg F, Berne AS, Oski FA. Differentiation of orbital cellulitis from preseptal cellulitis by computed tomography. Pediatrics. 1978;62:1000-1005.

[31] Sobol SE, Marchand J, Tewfik TL, Manoukian JJ, Schloss MD. Orbital complications of sinusitis in children. J Otolaryngol. 2002;31:131-136.

[32] Starkey CR, Steele RW. Medical management of orbital cellulitis. Pediatr Infect DiseasesJ.2001;20:1002-1005.

[33] Finger Basak SA, Berk DR, Lueder GT, Bayliss SJ. Common features of perioculartinea. Arch Ophthalmol. 2011; 129[3]:306-9.

[34] Israele V, Nelson JD. Periorbital and orbital cellulitis. Pediatr Infect Dis J 1987; 6: 404-410.

[35] Jackson K, Bekar SR. Clinical implications of orbital cellulitis. Laryngoscope 1986; 96: 568-574.

[36] Liu IT, Kao SC, Wang AG, Tsai CC, Liang CK, Hsu WM. Preseptal and orbital cellulitis: a 10-year review of hospitalized patients. J Chin Med Assoc. 2006; 69[9]:415-22.

[37] Garcia GH, Harris GJ. Criteria for nonsurgical management of subperiosteal abscess of the orbit: analysis of outcomes 1988-1998. Ophthalmology. 2000;107:1454-1458.

[38] Kaplan SL, Hulten KG, Gonzalez BE, et al. Three-year surveillance of community-acquired Staphylococcus aureus infections in children. Clin Infect Dis. 2005;40:1785-1791.

[39] Liu C, Bayer A, Cosgrove SE, et al. Clinical practice guidelines by the infectious diseases society of America for the treatment of methicillin-resistant Staphylococcus aureus infections in adults and children. Clin Infect Dis 2011; 52:e18.

[40] Howe L, Jones NS. Guidelines for the management of periorbital cellulitis/abscess. ClinOtolaryngol Allied Sci 2004; 29:725.

[41] Uzcátegui N, Warman R, Smith A, Howard CW. Clinical practice guidelines for the management of orbital cellulitis. J PediatrOphthalmol Strabismus 1998; 35:73.

[42] Sorin A, April MM, Ward RF. Recurrent periorbital cellulitis: an unusual clinical entity. Otolaryngol Head Neck Surg 2006; 134:153.

[43] Karkos PD, Karagama Y, Karkanevatos A, Srinivasan V. Recurrent periorbital cellulitis in a child. A random event or an underlying anatomical abnormality? Int J PediatrOtorhinolaryngol 2004; 68:1529.

[44] Teele DW. Management of the child with a red and swollen eye.Pediatr Infect Dis J. 1983;2:258-262.

[45] Wald ER. Periorbital and orbital infections. In: Long SS, Pickering LK, Prober CG, eds. Principles and Practice of Pediatric Infectious Diseases. 2nd ed. New York, NY: Churchill Livingstone; 2003:508-513.

[46] Wald ER. Periorbital and orbital infections. In: Long SS, Pickering LK, Prober CG, eds.Principles and Practice of Pediatric Infectious Diseases. 2nd ed. New York, NY: Churchill Livingstone; 2003:508-513.

[47] Garcia GH, Harris GJ. Criteria for nonsurgical management of subperiosteal abscess of the orbit: analysis of outcomes 1988-1998. Ophthalmology. 2000;107:1454-1458.

[48] Rahbar R, Robson CD, Petersen RA, et al. Management of orbital subperiosteal abscess in children.Arch Otolaryngol Head Neck Surg. 2001;127:281-286.

Diagnosis and Management of Orbital Cellulitis

Imtiaz A. Chaudhry, Waleed Al-Rashed,
Osama Al-Sheikh and Yonca O. Arat

Additional information is available at the end of the chapter

http://dx.doi.org/10.5772/52719

1. Introduction

Orbital cellulites is an uncommon infectious process in which patient may present with pain, reduced visual acuity, compromised ocular motility and significant proptosis. [1]- [3] In the modern era of relatively early access to the health care facilities, complete loss of vision from orbital cellulitis is rare. In the vast majority of cases, a history of upper respiratory tract infection prior to the onset is very common especially in children. [4], [5] Chandler et al, [6] for simplicity has classified the disease into 5 categories and emphasized the possibility of fatal outcome due to the extension of the abscess to cavernous sinus in the form of thrombosis and intracranial spread. In addition to the loss of vision, orbital cellulitis can be associated with a number of other serious complications that may include intracranial complications in the form of cavernous sinus thrombosis, meningitis, frontal abscess and even death. Historically, since the wide spread use of effective antibiotics, the serious complications of orbital cellulitis have become much less frequent. In the past, loss of vision was a relatively more common outcome of orbital cellulitis. [2] In the recent years, only few case reports of loss of vision following orbital cellulitis has been reported in the literature. For example, Connel et al, [3] reported case of a 69-year-old man who presented with no light perception vision, proptosis and significant ophthalmoplegia. In their case, despite emergent drainage of the abscess and systemic antibiotics, no improvement in vision was noted despite the return of the full ocular motility and disappearance of proptosis. Connel et al, [3] postulated Streptococcal-related ischemic necrosis of the optic nerve as a possible mechanism of loss of vision in their patient. In one of the recent survey of 52 patients treated for orbital cellulitis, over 35% had decreased vision and on their last follow-up, only 4% had decreased visual acuity. [1] Our own experience in treating 218 patients with orbital complications of cellulitis revealed that visual acuity improved in 16.1% and worsened in 6.2%, including 4.3% that sustained complete loss of vision. [8] We attributed the permanent loss of vision to the delay in diagnosis and intervention. Further, there were 9 cases of intracranial orbital abscess extension that required either extended treatment with systemic antibiotics alone or in combination with neurosurgical intervention. [3]

2. Patient presentation

Patients with orbital cellulitis may present with signs of eyelid swelling, conjunctival chemosis, diplopia and proptosis which may not be prominent in cases of preseptal cellulitis. [1], [8], [9] These patients may present with corneal infections resulting from exposure keratopathy due to their inability to close their eyes. Many of these patients come with local symptoms in the form of eyelid edema, redness, chemosis, decreased ocular motility and proptosis (Figure 1). Patients having superficial signs of swelling (preseptal cellulitis) should be differentiated from deeper infection resulting in orbital cellulitis, in which case, signs and symptoms resulting from inflammation may be helpful. [9] In particular, external ophthalmoloplegia, proptosis and decreased visual acuity are associated with orbital cellulitis rather than preseptal cellulitis. [8], [9] Temperature greater than 37.5℃ and leukocytosis resulting in fever may be more prominent feature of the pediatric orbital cellulitis. [4], [5] In children, external ophthalmoplegia and proptosis may be the most common features, while decreased visual acuity and chemosis may be less frequent signs in both the pediatric as well as in the adult patients. In cases of the optic nerve involvement, disc edema or neuritis with rapidly progressing atrophy resulting in blindness may occur. Mechanical pressure on the optic nerve and possibly compression of the central retinal and other feeding arteries results in optic nerve atrophy. [10] Also orbital inflammation itself may spread directly into the substance of the optic nerve causing small necrotic areas or abscesses. [2] Compression of the feeding vessels as well as inflammation may result in the infarction of the optic nerve, infarction of the sclera, choroids as well as the retina. Inflammation may result in septic uveitis, iridocyclitis or choroiditis with a cloudiness of the vitreous, including septic pan ophthalmitis. A less common complication of orbital cellulitis is glaucoma that can cause decreased vision, reduced visual field or even enlarged blind spot on presentation. On occasion, one may not find any fundus abnormalities. Among our patients presenting to a tertiary eye care center in the developing country, presenting signs of 218 patients with orbital cellulitis included, eyelid swelling in 71.5%, proptosis in 68.3%, motility restriction in 59.2%, pain in 52.3%, and decreased visual acuity in 14.2% of cases. [8]

3. Differential diagnosis

Some of the differential diagnosis for patients presenting with orbital cellulitis may include, allergic reaction to topical or systemic medication, edema from hypo-proteinemia due to variety of systemic causes, orbital wall infarction and subperiosteal hematoma due to unrecognized trauma or due to blood coagulation disorders. Differential diagnosis may also include orbital pseudotumor (Figure 2), retinoblastoma, metastatic carcinoma and unilateral or

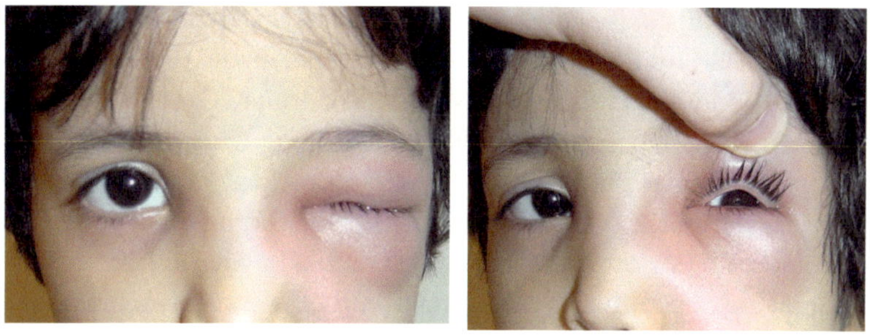

Figure 1. A child with left sided eyelid erythema, swelling and proptosis following a bout of upper respiratory infection.

bilateral exophthalmos secondary to thyroid related orbitopathy. [11] In all cases, careful history, thorough physical examination along with carefully selected imaging studies may help in differentiating orbital cellulitis from other causes of proptosis.

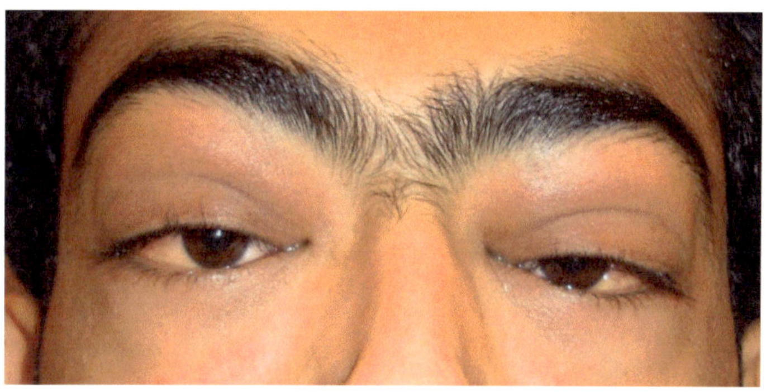

Figure 2. A 25-year-old male with bilateral eyelid swelling, proptosis and painful diplopia was found to have evidence of bilateral orbital pseudotumor and treated with systemic corticosteroids after imaging studies failed to show evidence of any infectious cause of his symptoms.

4. Most common predisposing factors for orbital cellulitis

In the most reported series, the most common predisposing factor for orbital cellulitis is sinus disease, especially in children. [1], [4], [8] Usually, the infection originates from sinusitis. It can originate from face or eyelids after a recent or past trauma, dental abscess or from a distant source by hematogenous spread. [1], [8], [11-13] For simplification purposes, Chandler et al, [6] grouped complication of sinus inflammation into 5 classes. In the group 1, eyelids may be swollen alongwith presence of orbital content edema (preseptal cellulitis). Swelling may reflect impedance of drainage through ethmoidal vessels. Group II reflects evidence of orbital cellulitis in which inflammatory cells diffusely infiltrate orbital tissues. In Group II, the eyelids may be swollen along with conjunctival chemosis as well as some degree of proptosis. Visual loss may be present in Group II patients. Purulent material may be collecting as subperiosteal abscess between the periorbita and the bony walls of the orbit in Group III. These patients may have significant conjunctival chemosis, eyelid edema, along with tenderness in the involved areas with variable degree of proptosis, and decreased ocular motility. The abscess may be anywhere in the vicinity of the orbit. Patients in group IV (orbital abscess), may present with their abscess being inside or outside the muscle cone following untreated orbital cellulitis. These patients may have significantly more pain, proptosis, decreased ocular motility and variable degree of severe visual loss. Patients in group V may present with bilateral eyelid edema along with involvement of third, fifth and sixth cranial nerves which is thought to be due to the extension of the infectious process into the cavernous sinus with formation of thrombosis. These patients may have nausea, vomiting along with signs of nervous system involvement which could also be due to septicemia. Signs of proptosis, eyelid edema, optic neuritis, frozen globe, decreased supra-orbital nerve conduction may be hallmarks of orbital apex syndrome which is thought to be due to the sinusitis in the area of the superior orbital fissure and optic foramen. [14]

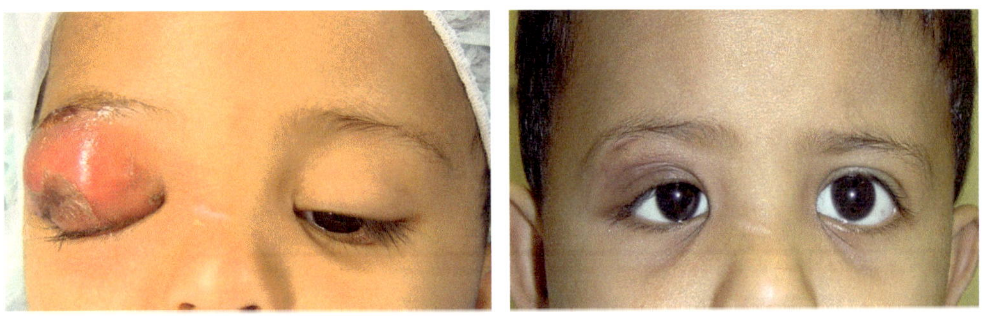

Figure 3. External photographs of a young male child who suffered trauma over his right brow area after which he developed orbital cellulitis and formation of an abscess that required drainage.

Our own experience in treating orbital cellulitis from a developing country confirmed previous observations from the Western countries in which sinusitis has been implicated as the cause of orbital cellulitis in most of the cases. [8] Specifically in children, vast majority of cases with orbital cellulitis had pre-existing sinusitis, and significant number of them had multiple sinuses involved. Our experience revealed that unlike patients from the Western countries, most patients with sinusitis and orbital cellulitis in the developing countries had sought treatment later in the course of their disease. Unlike Western countries, in our patients, prior history of periocular trauma or ocular/ periocular surgery were also very common cause of orbital cellulitis. (Figure 3). [1], [10] Although less common, dacryocystitis, dental infection and endophthalmitis, were also found to be the cause of orbital cellulitis in our patients (Figure 4). [8] Patients with prior history of sinusitis may also develop osteomyelitis and intracranial infection. In these cases, osteomyelitis, commonly involve the frontal bone which is due to a direct extension of frontal infection or septic thrombophlebitis via the valveless sinus of

Breschet. [15] Less common cause of osteomyelitis results from the ethmoidal sinusitis because from this location, infection can rapidly spread through the thin lamina papyracea into the orbit or maxilla, where arterial anastomoses are sufficient to prevent necrosis due to septic thrombosis of a single artery. Although meningitis may be the most common intracranial complication of sinus disease, epidural, subdural and brain parenchymal abscess can also develop. [15]

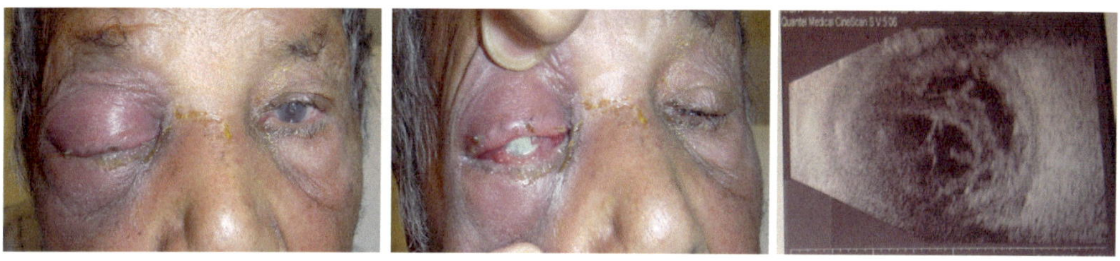

Figure 4. External photograph and U/S of right eye of an 83-years-old male who suffered right eye trauma and then developed panophthalmitis resulting in total loss of his vision.

5. Sources of infection

Usually, orbital cellulitis occurs in the childhood years which has been attributed to the relatively incomplete development of immunity in this age group. [1], [4], [5], [16], [17] In these patients, sinus disease has been found to be the most common predisposing factor. Over 90% of these patients have radiologically confirmed sinusitis, the most common being ethmoidal and maxillary. [1], [8] In the reported series, ethmoidal sinusitis has been demonstrated to be the source of infection in significantly large number of cases. [18], [19]

Ethmoidal sinusitis is usually present with maxillary sinusitis on the same side of the infection. [19], [20] Frontal sinus disease has been frequently identified especially in series in which a large number of adolescents and adults have been studied (Figure 5). [10], [18], [20] Up to 38% of children may have more than one sinus involved and in the adult patients, up to 50% may have underlying sinusitis, while up to 11% may have multiple sinuses involved. [1], [8] Other etiological factors resulting in orbital cellulitis may include dacryocystitis with orbital extension (Figure 6), retained foreign body, panophthalmitis, infected tumor, Herpes Zoster, (Figure 7), and mucormycosis. [8], [21]

As orbital cellulitis has a close relationship with sinus (Figure 5), and upper respiratory disease, a seasonal distribution paralleling that of upper respiratory infections (URI) has been documented with a bi-model seasonal distribution of cases with peak occurring in late winter and early spring season. [1], [8] Bacterial sinusitis can result in orbital cellulitis leading to a subperiosteal abscess from the accumulation of purulent material between the periorbita and the orbital bones. [6], [8], [20] Since the use of modern imaging studies in the form of computed tomography (CT-scan), the concept of subperiosteal abscess has been accepted as a separate

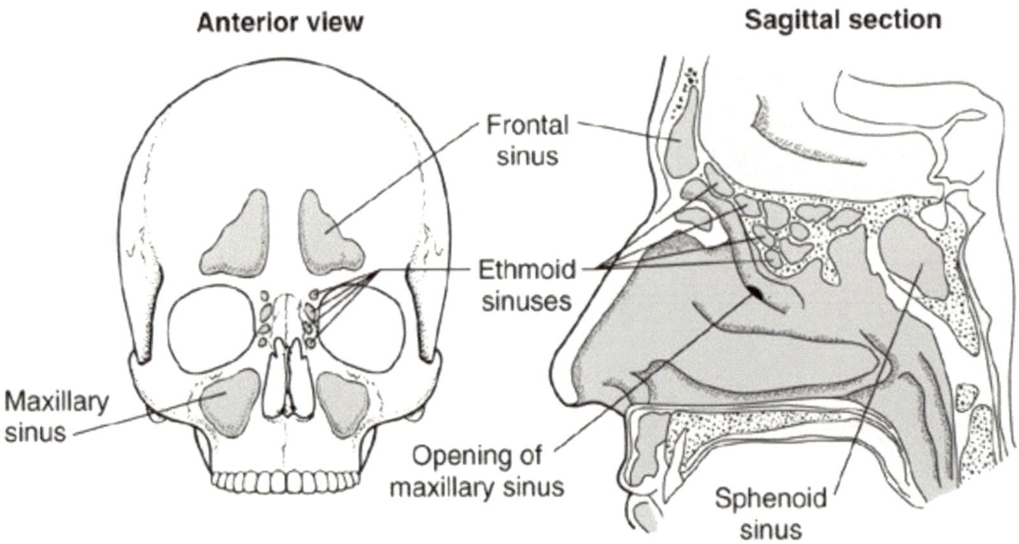

Figure 5. Anterior and sagittal view of the frontal, ehtmoidal, sphenoid and maxillary sinuses and their close relationship with orbital anatomy.

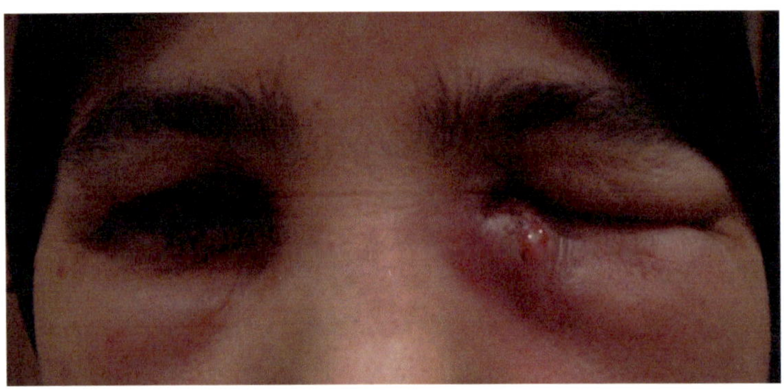

Figure 6. External photograph of a 42-years-old female who presented with left-sided orbital cellulitis and abscess formation due to the acute over chronic dacryocystitis.

entity. [20], [22] Because of the reports of rapidly progressive visual and intracranial complications from subperiosteal abscess, some clinicians argue for the prompt surgical drainage of the abscess and paranasal sinuses when a subperiosteal abscess is first diagnosed by a CT-scan. [15], [20], [22-26] Among our survey of 218 patients who required treatment of their orbital cellulitis, imaging studies revealed that sinus disease was the most cause in 39.4%, trauma in 19.7%, endophthalmitis in 13.3%, (Figure 8), orbital implants in 8.2%, dacryocystitis in 4.6%, retained orbital foreign body in 3.2%, dental infection in 2.7%, and scleral buckle in 2.3%.[8] A history of sinusitis and recent trauma was the cause of orbital cellulitis in 4.1%, and intraocular or orbital tumors were the cause in another 4% of patients.

http://dx.doi.org/10.5772/52719

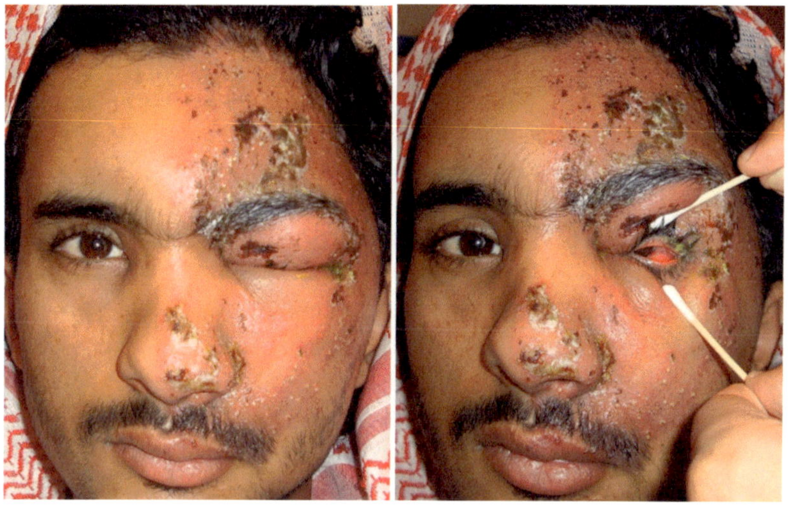

Figure 7. External photograph of a 19-years-old male who presented with 3 day history of left-sided facial erythema, swelling, conjunctival chemosis, proptosis and eruptive skin lesions. A diagnosis of Herpes Zoster Ophthalmicus was made and patient was treated for acute Zoster infection and its complications.

In diabetic and immune-compromised patients one has to rule out fungal infection as the cause of orbital cellulitis, the most common being Mucormycosis and Aspergillosis. While infection with Mucormycosis has no climatic or age restriction, Aspergillosis usually occurs in hot and humid climates in patients older than 20 years of age. Although predisposing factors for Aspergillosis are unclear multiple risk factors for Mucormycosis have been proposed, among them diabetic ketoacidosis is the most common. The course of onset for Mucromycosis infection is rapid (usually 1-7 days) as compared with slow infection due to Aspergillosis which can take a month to a year. Otolaryngologic findings in patients with Mucormycosis may include nasal and palatal necrosis along with paranasal sinusitis. In Aspergillosis, one may find evidence of chronic fibrosis and non-necrotizing granulomatous reaction of the involved structures. In cases of Mucromycosis infections there is evidence of ischemic necrosis along with thrombosed arteries

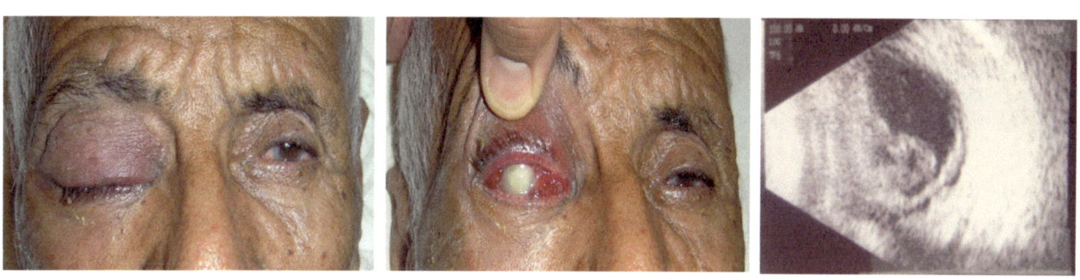

Figure 8. External photographs and U/S of the right eye of a 73-years-old male who developed panophthalmitis after cataract surgery.

6. Epidemiology of orbital cellulitis

Orbital complications of sinusitis have been reported to range anywhere between 0.5 to 3.9%. [1], [17], [27] However, the incidence of abscess formation vary considerably from 0-25% in the reported series. [15] No cases of abscess formation was reported in the published series from the Children's Memorial Hospital in Chicago including 87 patients with orbital cellulitis and from Children's Hospital in Pittsburgh including 104 orbital celulitis cases. [28], [29] On the other hand, a larger study of 6,770 patients from the Hospital for Sick Children in Toronto revealed that 2.3% developed orbital complications; of which 10.7% had abscess formation. [19] Another study reported 20.8% incidence of abscess formation among the 158 patients admitted for orbital cellulitis. There was a 20.8% incidence of abscess formation. [30] Among other series which has reported orbital complications of sinus disease, the incidence of abscess formation had varied from 6.25 to 20 % to as high as 78.6%. [18], [31], [32] One may attribute differences among these studies due to the inclusion criteria, age group and the severity of the complications studied by these authors. The incidence of major complications following sinusitis may be low, however such complications may be associated with considerable morbidity and mortality. [8], [15] According to the published report, in the pre-antibiotic era, orbital cellulitis resulted in death from meningitis in 17% of cases and blindness in 20%. [6] However, in the antibiotic era, incidence of menengitis was reported as 1.9% in patients with orbital cellulitis, despite prompt treatment with systemic antibiotics. [33]

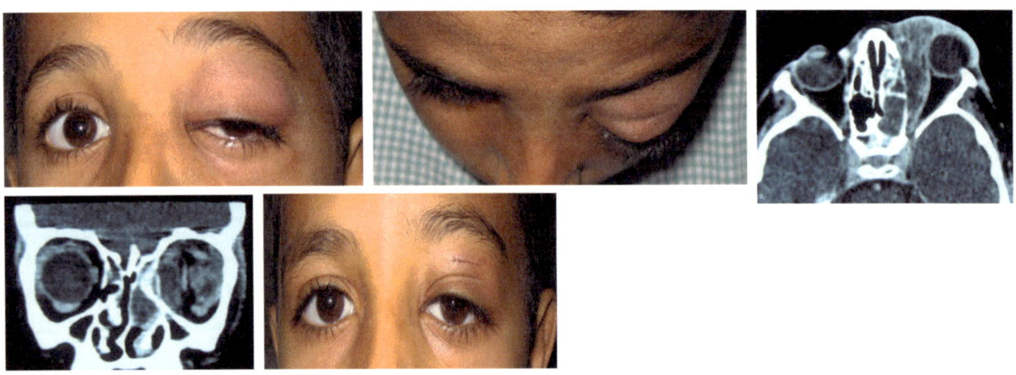

Figure 9. External photographs as well as CT-scan (axial and coronal views) of a 7-year-old boy who presented with upper respiratory infection followed by painful diplopia, left eye proptosis and decreased vision. His symptoms did not improve with a course of systemic antibiotics. This patient required drainage of his orbital abscess which resulted in immediate resolution of his symptoms.

In-spite of systemic antibiotics and surgical intervention, orbital abscesses may have devastating outcome. [15] According to the series in which final visual results have been reported, a significant percentage of patients have been left with non-seeing eyes ranging anywhere from 7.1% to as high as 23.6%. [10] Visual loss in these cases have been attributed to optic atrophy, central retinal artery occlusion, or exposure keratopathy with corneal ulcer formation. [8], [10], [19] Some of the other hypothesized mechanisms of vision loss are septic optic neuritis, embolic or thrombotic lesions in the vascular supply of the optic nerve, choroid or retina. It has been postulated that delayed medical and surgical intervention may produce unacceptable visual outcome. [19], [20], [22]- [25] Among our 218 patients with diagnosis of orbital cellulitis, there were 116 cases of radiologically confirmed subperiosteal abscess, (Figure 9), 87% of them required drainage, and the remaining 13% were observed closely until their resolution while those patients were being treated with systemic antibiotics. [8] Thirty-nine eyes (17.8%) had endophthalmitis causing orbital cellulitis which required evisceration (9.6%) or enucleation (8.2%). Seven orbits required exenteration and 6 infected orbital implants had to be removed. Six patients had dacryocystitis that required a dacryocystorhinostomy to treat orbital cellulitis in addition to the administration of systemic antibiotics. [8]

7. Investigative studies

On orbital ultrasonography (U/S), abscess may show low internal reflectivity and therefore, U/S can be useful as a screening office procedure for patients suspected of having orbital abscess. [8], [27] Computed tomography scan may be necessary to assess the evidence of sinusitis and orbital processes. On CT-scan, orbital abscess may appear as localized, generally homogenous elevation of the periorbita adjacent to an opacified sinus, (Figure 9). On imaging studies, there may be evidence of inflammatory or infective changes in the sinus areas as well as orbital structures. In children, more patients may have subperiosteal abscess as compared to the adult group at the time of their initial presentation. [4] In the series reported by Ferguson and McNab, [1] among children, 29% had inflammatory changes only, while 62% had evidence of a subperiosteal abscess, only 9% had orbital abscesses, compared with 72%, 5% and 22%, respectively, in their adult group. Computed tomography scan may influence the initial therapeutic plan by demonstrating the size and location of the abscess and the specific sinuses involved, features that may be necessary in the approach of surgical drainage. [8], [20], [27] Experience however have shown that the CT-scan characteristics of the subperiosteal collection may not always be predictive of the clinical course. For example, in reports from the patients who recovered with systemic antibiotics alone, findings were similar to the findings in patients who underwent surgical drainage. [22] The imaging studies have shown that the size of an orbital abscess may increase over the first few days of intravenous antibiotics regardless of the bacteriological response to the treatment in these patients. [22] In some patients, the identification of an orbital abscess may be a diagnostic challenge. The reliability of some of the imaging modalities such as CT-scan in demonstrating some orbital abscesses has been questioned. For example from a series of 25 cases of orbital infection, all 15 orbital abscesses were satisfactorily demonstrated only when the CT-scan examination included coronal sections. [34] According to this study, one-third of abscesses would have been missed if coronal sections had not been performed. Magnetic resonance imaging studies have been found to be necessary in some cases where CT-scan have not satisfactorily addressed clinician's concerns.

The development of an orbital abscess does not correlate specifically with visual acuity, proptosis, chemosis, or any other signs. [15], [27] Therefore diagnostic procedures are essential in evaluating the patient with orbital cellulitis and possible abscess or retained orbital foreign bodies. Although sinus X-ray may demonstrate an air-fluid level when present in an abscess cavity, gas-free abscesses may not be readily visible. [15] Ultrasound may detect an abscess of the anterior orbit or the medial wall with 90% accuracy, [25] although an acute abscess may be poorly delineated. Currently, the investigative procedure of choice to diagnose an orbital infection is the CT-scan, although MRI can be utilized when there is a contra-indications for CT-scan. [8], [27], [35] By CT-scan, orbital walls, extraocular muscles, optic nerve, intraconal area and adipose tissue can be seen clearly. An orbital abscess can be seen as a homogenous, a ring-like, or a heterogenous mass. In these studies, the site of origin, orbital or subperiosteal, and extent of abscess are readily visible. [8], [22] When administered, contrast-media can enhance the surrounding wall of an abscess. Computed tomography scan will not differentiate between preseptal cellulitis and eyelid edema but will differentiate between preseptal and orbital cellulitis. [15] Beside foreign bodies, sinus disease and intracranial complications may also be visible on the CT-scan. [8] Our experience has shown that CT-scan may be the most comprehensive source of information about orbital infections and the most sensitive means of monitoring resolving orbital or intracranial lesions. [8], [27] Computed tomography scan is indicated in all patients with periorbital inflammation in whom proptosis, ophthalmoplegia, or a decrease in visual acuity develop, in whom a foreign body or an abscess is suspected, severe eyelid edema prevents an adequate examination, or surgery is contemplated. [8], [15], [20], [22], [35] In our study of the 218 patients with orbital cellulitis, diagnosis was made clinically and confirmed by CT-scans or U/S in 90.4% and 36.2% orbits, respectively. [8] Orbital abscesses were identified in 53.2% of orbits. In all cases of orbital cellulitis, there was evidence of inflammatory or infective changes of the orbital structures. Abscess location was found to be medial in 35%, superior in 33%, intraconal in 13%, superomedial in 6%, inferomedial in 6% and lateral in 2% of orbits. [8]

8. Bacteriology of orbital infection

In the reported series, the bacteriology of orbital abscesses has received little attention. In series in which the contents of the abscess cavity have been cultured, a wide range of organisms have been reported. [8], [36] Most commonly reported bacterial species from the abscesses of the orbit and periorbital area include Staphylococcus aureus, Staphylococcus epidermidis, Streptococci, Diphtheroids, Haemophilus influenzae, Escherichia Coli, multiple species of aerobes and anaerobes. There was no growth in up to 25% of abscesses. [15], [17] Microbiological results from Ferguson and McNab, [1] series varied, with differences in the rate of testing between the pediatric age group and the older age group. In their series, some forms of cultures were performed in 93% of their patients. Fifty percent of their patiens had blood cultures none of which yielded positive results. According to their study, cultures taken from abscesses were more likely to yield positive results. The authors noted that there was no correlation between cultures taken from conjunctival swab and the etiological organisms recovered from the abscesses of those patients with positive cultures. In their study, Staphylococcus aureus was the most common micro-organism recovered. In their pediatric age group various species of Streptococcus predominated. Among their pediatric patients, 4 patients had anaerobic Streptococcus isolates, two had mixed anaerobes and one had Clostridium bifermentans. In Ferguson and McNab's, [1] series, orbital cellulitis due to anaerobes was much less common in adults, with only one case of mixed anaerobes identified. In their series, only 5 adults and 4 pediatric patients had multiple organisms isolated from the abscesses. No pathogenic organisms were isolated from their 6 adult and 15 pediatric patients in whom the cultures were performed. [1] Although in the past, H influenza was a major pathogenic bacteria responsible for orbital cellulitis in the pediatric age group, [8], [15] in the series reported by Ferguson and McNab,[1] no cases of H. influenza were identified in the pediatric age group and only one case was found in an adult patient. This observation has been attributed to the general immunization of children with H. influenza type B vaccine since the early 1990s. [1], [27] Schramm et al,[5] reported 32 cases of orbital abscesses, the predominant microorganisms being Staphylococci, Streptococci and Bacteroids species.

The role of anaerobes, not usually considered pathogens in the sinus disease is unclear, although considerable number of cultures in adult patients have yielded anaerobes. [8], [20], [23] In general, patients during their first decade of life may have infection caused by a single aerobic pathogen which may be responsive to the medical therapy alone. On the other hand, patients older than 15 years of age may have complex infections caused by multiple aerobic and anaerobic organisms that may be slow to clear despite medical and surgical intervention. [23] The virulence of pathogens and responsiveness to anti-microbial agents appear to be age-related. [20], [37] With enlarging of the size of the sinus cavities, the ostia gets narrow creating optimal condition for anaerobic bacterial growth. As the person ages, there is a trend towards appearance of more complex infections. In mixed infections, aerobes utilize oxygen which encourage growth of more anaerobic microorganisms. On the other hand anaerobes produce B-Lactamase which makes antibiotics less effective. Harris, [20] reviewed microbiology results of 37 patients with orbital abscesses in which one-third were younger than 9 years, 58% were culture negative and the rest had single aerobic pathogen. From his series, 16 patients between ages 9-14 years showed transition towards more complex infections. Among these, 9 patients which were older than 15 years had positive cultures despite being on systemic antibiotics for 3 days. In Harris's, [20] study, older group had more often polymicrobial infections and anaerobes were found in all cases. According to our study the most common microorganisms isolated from the drained abscesses were the most common microorganisms isolated from the drained abscesses were Staphylococci and Streptococci species; less common organisms included Propionibacterium acnes, Haemophilus influenzae, Bacillus, and fungi. [8]

9. Medical management

Medical management depends on the patient's appearance, ability to take oral medications, compliance and clinical progression of the disease. Patients presenting with signs and symptoms of eyelid edema, diplopia, reduced visual acuity, abnormal light reflexes, ophthalmoplegia and proptosis need admission (Figure 10). Further, if a patient appears toxic and eye exam is difficult to be completely performed, along with signs of CNS involvement as evident by lethargy, vomiting, seizures, headache or cranial nerve deficit, admission is needed for further evaluation and proper treatment. Intravenous antibiotics are usually started once the diagnosis of orbital cellulitis is suspected, broad-spectrum antibiotics that cover most gram positive and gram negative bacteria are considered initially. The recommendations for antibiotics are usually based on the microorganisms most frequently suspected from abscesses; Staphylococcus aureus, Staphylococcus epidermidis, Streptococci, and Hemophilus species. [15] Empiric antibiotics should cover methicillin-resistant Staph.aureus if suspected. [38], [39] One should suspect mixed infections including aerobic and anaerobic species in the abscesses. [20] Warm compresses over the involved area may help to improve the softening of the tissues to bring in more blood circulation in the area where blood supply is already abundant. If no improvement occurs in 24-48 hours of systemic antibiotics, one may consider Infectious Disease, Ear, Nose and Throat and/or Neurosurgery consultations. [27]

Historically, cultures from the conjunctiva, nose and throat are usually not representative of the pathogens cultured from the abscesses and blood cultures may frequently be negative and are not usually helpful. [15] Most patients in the reported series, had received a combination of a third-generation cephalosporin and flucloxacillin. [1], [8] According to those reports, most patients had received oral antibiotics on discharge for varying periods of time. [40] For example, all patients in the Ferguson and McNab's [1], series had received intravenous antibiotic treatment during their admission and most of these patients had received multidrug therapy with up to 5 different antibiotics at some point. In these cases treatment regimens were empirically based and instituted prior to the identification of responsible organisms. [1] In our experience, most of our patients also had multiple antibiotic regimens administered during their stay in the hospital and most of them were discharged on at least one antibiotic therapy. [8] In our study of 218 patients having orbital cellulitis and abscess, all patients received systemic antibiotic treatment, and in all patients, treatment regimens were empirically based and were instituted before the identification of any responsible organisms. [8] In our study, the most common antibiotic regimen included cephalosporins in 90%, and aminoglycosides in 66% with a combination of other antibiotics. These antibiotics included flucloxacillin in 15%, vancomycin in 13%, ampicillin in 6%, metronidazole in 4%, and penicillin in 3% of patients. In our study, most patients received oral antibiotics on their discharge for varying periods, ranging from 3 days to 3 weeks. [8]

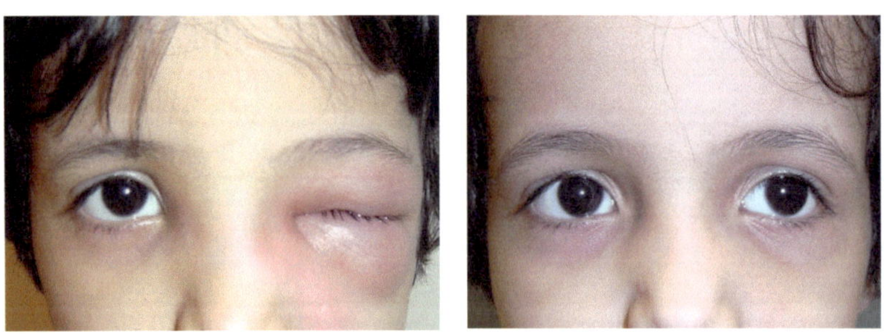

Figure 10. Patient from Figure 1 after medical treatment of her left-sided orbital cellulitis.

From the reported series, patient age has been identified as a factor in the bacteriology and the response of these patients to treatment for their orbital abscesses. [16], [17], [20] In general, children aged <9 years have been found to have simpler, more responsive infections, primarily caused by single aerobic pathogen. Older children and adults have been found to harbor more complex infections caused by multiple aerobic and anaerobic organisms, resistant to both medical and surgical treatment. [20] In addition to starting systemic antibiotics, emergent drainage of the orbital abscesses may be necessary in patients with compromised vision regardless of patient age. Urgent drainage (within 24 hour of presentation) has been recommended for large abscesses, for extensive superior or inferior orbital abscesses, for patients with central nervous system complications and for infections following dental work in which anaerobes might be expected. [20] These patients require surgical option if improvement does not occur as expected. In these patients, careful monitoring of the clinical course is mandatory and comparison of serial CT-scan may be necessary as an adjunct to clinical judgment. In Harris's series 27 of 29 patients which were younger than 9 years old recovered with antibiotic treatment alone with a good clinical outcome. [20] He described "sliding scale" of risk associated with increasing age and argued that patients in the older age group who present with orbital process should undergo prompt sinus surgery even before orbital or intracranial abscesses develop. Once sinus infection in older children or adults has extended into the orbit as an abscess, urgent drainage may include the orbit along with the infected sinuses. [20] Computed tomography scan may not be accurate in assessing clinical course in some of these patients. In a review of 37 cases of orbital abscesses, Harris, found that subperiosteal material could not be predicted from the size or relative radiodensity of the collections from the CT-scans. [22] Initial scans were not as predictive of the clinical course. In fact the serial scans showed enlargement of abscesses during the first few days of systemic antibiotic therapy regardless of the final outcome of the response to treatment. He concluded that expansion of orbital abscess on the serial CT-scans during the initial treatment may not be equated to failure of the infection to respond to the medical management in the form of antibiotics alone. [22]

10. Surgical intervention

From their vast experience with the management of orbital abscesses, Garcia and Harris [23], concluded that surgical therapy for orbital abscesses may be contemplated based on several factors, including the sinuses involved, the presumed pathogens, the anticipated bacterial response to administered antibiotic, visual status, the size and location of the orbital abscess and potential intracranial complications. They recommended emergency drainage of the orbital abscesses and sinuses of patients of any age whose optic nerve or retinal function is compromised. Urgent drainage for large abscesses, in cases of extensive superior or inferior abscesses that might not quickly resolve despite clearance of sinusitis by medical treatment has been recommended, (Figure 11). In cases of intracranial complications at the time of presentation and in frontal sinusitis, in which the risk of intracranial extension is increased, and when complex infections that include anaerobes are suspected, urgent drainage of an abscess is recommended. [23] Again, expectant approach has been recommended for patients younger than 9 years of age in whom simple infections may be suspected. Surgical option may still be exercised if clinical improvement does not occur in a timely manner and if relative afferent pupillary defect develops at any time. Further, surgical option should be considered in cases of fever not abating within 36 hours of systemic antibiotic treatment suggesting that the infection may not be responding to the choice of antibiotics being administered. Surgery should also be considered when there has been deterioration of vision despite 48 hours of appropriate antibiotic therapy and no improvement despite 72 hours of such treatment. Usually, CT-scan improvement should be expected to lag behind the clinical picture. In fact, the CT findings may worsen during the first few days of hospitalization despite successful treatment with antibiotics alone. [23]

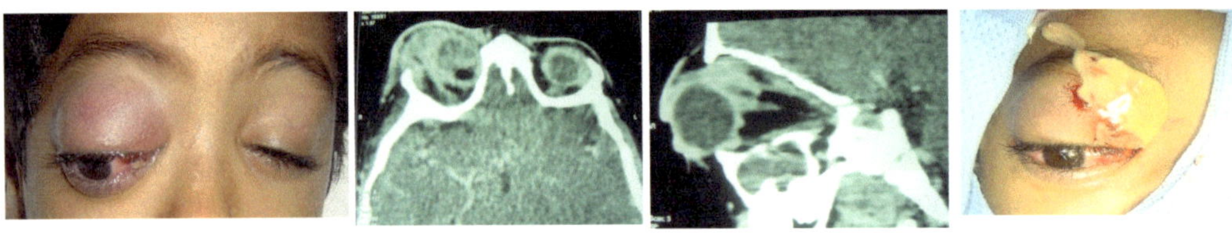

Figure 11. External photograph of an 8-year-old boy who required drainage of his right orbital abscess after failing 3 days of by systemic antibiotic treatment. CT-scan (axial and saggital cuts) showed an evidence of maxillary sinusitis and an abscess formation in the superior orbit.

In majority of the cases, surgical intervention is indicated for significant underlying sinus disease, orbital or subperiosteal abscess, or both in the children, (Figure 11). [1], [5], [8], [17] For older patients, sinus surgery remains the most common surgical intervention. Recent literature suggests that the volume of subperiosteal abscess seems to be the most important criterion in determining medical versus surgical management; the volumes of abscesses needing surgery appears to be larger than the volumes of abscesses not needing surgery. In general, volumes of <1,250 mm may not need surgical intervention. [41], [42] There may be an argument regarding early drainage of an orbital abscess to prevent complications whereas early surgical intervention has the possibility of seeding the infection. [20] For practical purposes, Harris, has outlined a useful approach in the management of an orbital abscess. [20] He emphasizes on the emergent drainage for patients of any age whose visual function may be compromised. Also for the patients in whom a large orbital abscess causes discomfort, presence of superior or inferior orbital abscess, evidence of intracranial extension, involvement of frontal sinuses, and a known dental source of the infection in patients older than 9 years, urgent drainage usually within 24 hours has been recommended. [20] Wait and see approach may be indicated for patients younger than 9 years of age having medial subperiosteal abscess of modest size, for patients having no visual compromise and in those having no intracranial or frontal sinus involvement. In these patients, careful evaluation and close monitoring of their optic nerve function and the level of consciousness and mental state are necessary. When indicated, one may consider making an incision approximately 2-inch down to the periosteum at the inner quadrant of the orbit to drain these orbital abscesses. [27] Patients with suspected fungal orbital cellulitis (especially Mucormycosis), need to be treated with intravenous

Amphotericin B and predisposing factors such as diabetes, acidosis and other medical conditions need to be addressed. Wide excision along with debridement of the necrotic tissue is desired. If necessary, a drain may be inserted and tissues may not need to be sutured and may be left for granulation. One may consider removal of drain when no further drainage occurs. In some cases, endoscopic approach may be utilized and has been found to be effective for the treatment subperiosteal abscess as a result of sinus infection. Some of the advantages of endoscopic surgical drainage may be the avoidance of external ethmoidectomy and associated external facial scar and an early drainage of the affected sinuses and subperosteal abscess at the same time. [27], [43] In our study [8], among the 116 radiologically confirmed orbital abscesses, 87% required drainage, and the remaining 13% required close observation until their resolution while on systemic antibiotics. Thirty-nine eyes (17.8%) had endophthalmitis causing orbital cellulitis and required evisceration or enucleation. Seven orbits required exenteration and 6 infected orbital implants had to be removed. Other 6 patients had dacryocystitis that required a dacryocystorhinostomy to treat orbital cellulitis in addition to the administration of systemic antibiotics. Combined endoscopic sinus surgery with transnasal orbital abscess drainage was carried out in some of our patients with sinusitis and orbital abscess, especially in the medial orbit. [8]

11. Complications of orbital cellulitis

Although less common, major complications related to orbital cellulitis and abscess can occur. Even after the successful treatment of such infections, permanent visual loss or loss of function of the vital structures may remain. Ferguson [1] reported no visual function loss among their patients after resolution of their infections. Only one of their patients from the pediatric age group had proptosis on follow-up; one had ophthalmoplegia and one had recollection of the abscess. One of their adult patients developed presumed meningitis and another adult patient required enucleation. In rare circumstances, the microorganism may cause necrotizing eyelid disease often referred as necrotizing fasciitis. [3], [44]- [46] This may progress to systemic manifestations including the potentially fatal toxic streptococcus syndrome, characterized by multi-organ failure. [44], [46] These complications can occur in the absence of antecedent health problems or history of trauma. [3], [45], [46] The virulence of this organism is related to the production of M proteins and exotoxins A and B. [47] These proteins act as super-antigens in vitro and mediate tissue necrosis by causing massive release of cytokines such as tumor necrosis factor and interleukins.

12. Visual loss in orbital cellulitis

Permanent loss of vision has been noted as a complication of orbital infection and up to one fifth of patients with orbital inflammation had blindness in the pre-antibiotic era. [2] Now, although permanent loss of vision resulting from orbital inflammation is unusual it can still occur, (Figure 12). [8], [25], [26] Patt [26] reported 38 patients with orbital cellulitis and resultant permanent vision loss one of which progressed to no light perception vision. Loss of vision with orbital inflammation may result from optic neuritis as a reaction to adjacent or nearby infection, ischemia due to thrombophlebitis along valveless orbital veins, or compressive/pressure ischemia possibly resulting in central artery/occlusion, (Figure 12). [22], [26] Permanent irreversible visual loss may occur in cases with orbital and subperiosteal abscess despite early intervention. In a survey of 46 cases with confirmed diagnosis of orbital and subperiosteal abscess in which visual results were reported, permanent loss of vision occurred in 15% of the cases. [48] Blindness was attributed to the central retinal artery occlusion in 4, optic atrophy in 2 of hese patients. Permanent visual loss in orbital cellulitis probably has a vascular cause, whereas partial vision loss that respond to antibiotic therapy and drainage procedures may be due to inflammatory infiltrates or presence of compressive optic neuropathy. [21] It is believed that the confinement of the optic nerve in the orbital apex area and within its bony canal along with its proximity to the posterior ethmoid and sphenoid sinuses may further highlight the importance of the these factors in the exacerbation of posterior orbital celluliltis. Physcians need to be aware that patients with sinusitis and associated orbital cellulitis may be at risk for developing severe vision deficit requiring timely intervention. In a review of 148 patients with orbital abscess from 13 series reported by Hornblass [15], 3 patients had evidence of no light perception vision.

Clinical examination by itself may not exactly delineate the nature of orbital inflammatory processes, clinicians may have to rely on imaging studies to select potential surgical candidates. Despite availability of modern CT-Scan and MRI studies, the physician stil needs to rely on the clinical progression of the inflammation based on vision, pupillary fuction, and assessment of ocular motility. Patt and Manning [26], reported 4 patients with vision loss due to orbital cellulitis and in each of these cases had CT-scan readings of "no definite abscess" contributing to the delay in diagnosis of orbital abscess, with a resultant delay in surgical drainage.

Ethmoidal sinuses are separated from the orbital cavity by the lamina papyracea and anterior and posterior ethmoidal foramina serve as additional connections that may allow infection to gain access from ethmoidal air cells to the orbital cavity, (Figure 5). Periorbita in this area is loosely attached to bone and may be elevated by a purulent collection, resulting in subperiosteal abscess. Acute visual loss due to sinusitis may either be secondary to complications of orbital cellulitis or may be seen as a part of orbital apex syndrome. orbital cellulitis or as a part of the orbital apex syndrome. [27] Two cases of acute visual loss have been reported by El-Sayed and Muhaimeid [49], as a complication of orbital cellulitis due to sinusitis. One of these patients had dramatic improvement in vision from hand motion to normal vision after systemic antibiotic treatment of pansinusitis and associated orbital cellulitis. The second patient, (a 10-year old girl), achieved normal visual acuity from no light perception after only surgical intervention by exploration of sphenoid and ethmoid sinuses along-with intravenous antibiotic administration. Three cases of sphenoethmoiditis with minimal signs of orbital inflammation causing permanent loss of vision have been reported by Slavin and Glaser. [48] These authors suggested the use of term "posterior orbital cellulitis" for such cases and defined it as a clinical syndrome in which early severe visual loss overshadows or precedes accompanying inflammatory orbital signs. Acute blindness may also result from orbital infarction syndrome.

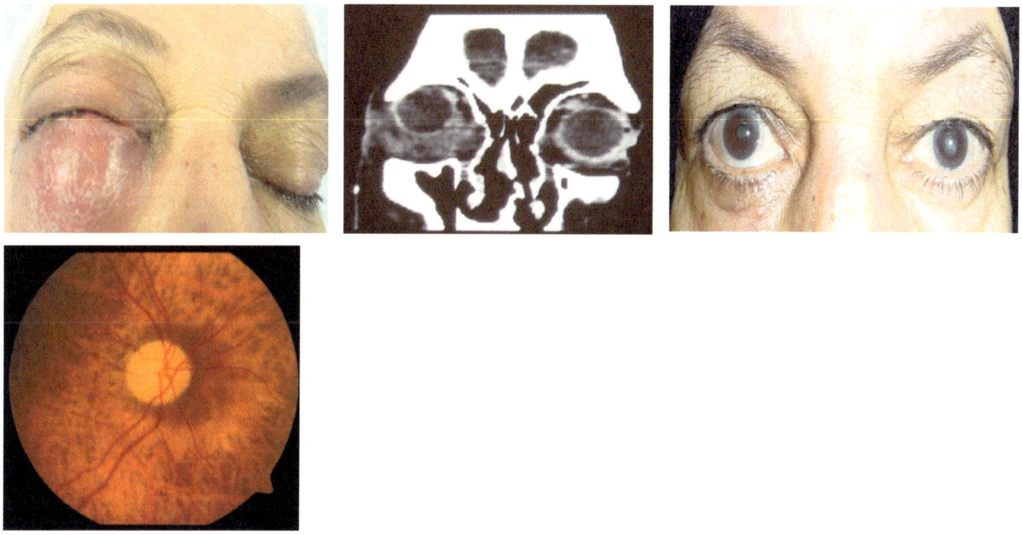

Figure 12. External photographs, CT-scan (coronal view) and right eye fundus photograph of a 70-year-old female who presented late in the course of her right-sided orbital cellulitis/abscess which required surgical drainage. She had complete loss of vision in the right eye which was attributed to central retinal artery occlusion due to orbital infectious process. Fundus photo reveals evidence of a pale optic nerve.

Orbital infarction syndrome is a disorder that may take place secondary to different mechanisms which may include acute perfusion failure like common carotid artery occlusion, systemic vasculitis such as giant-cell arteritis, or as a result of orbital cellulitis with vasculitis such as Mucormycosis. In some of these cases, vision loss can be permanent due to retinal or optic nerve damag. [50] According to our experience in a developing country, most patients with sinusitis and orbital abscess presented late in the course of their disease. [8] Most patients with refractory or complicated subperiosteal abscesses have been older children or adults. In one of the largest studies reported, among the 159 patients with orbital complications of sinusitis, 4 had permanent blindness. [26] All 4 had surgically confirmed subperiosteal abscess, and all were older than 15 years of age. In another study, among the 13 patients with intracranial abscess extension from sinusitis or orbital abscesses, 2 patients were 9 to 14 years of age and 11 were older than 15 years of age. [7] In our study of orbital cellulitis, visual acuity improved in 16.1% and worsened in 6.2%, including 4.3% that sustained complete loss of vision. We attributed the permanent loss of vision to the delay in diagnosis and intervention. [8]

13. Intracranial extension of orbital abscess

In the pre-antibiotic era, Birch-Hirschfeld reported that 19% of 275 cases of orbital cellultis reported in the studies from 1907-1930 died mostly due to the intracranial complications of orbital cellulitis. [2] More recently, Hartstein et al, [51], reported case-studies of 3 patients who were found to have pansinusitis which progressed to subperiosteal abscess of the orbit and subsequent intracranial extension. All 3 patients had been treated with systemic antibiotics and surgical drainage of the orbital abscesses as well as sinuses. Two of the 3 patients required surgical drainage of their intracranial abscesses.

In our series of 218 patients with orbital cellulitis, there were 9 cases of intracranial extension of orbital abscesses that required either extended treatment with systemic antibiotics alone or in combination with neurosurgical intervention. [8] Nineteen cases of intracranial abscesses due to mid-face infection had been reported by Maniglia et al, [7] anaerobic organisms were the most common cause of their abscesses. Most of these intracranial complications were due to the nasal, sinus and orbital disease while cavernous sinus thrombosis occurred in only one of these patients. Intracranial abscesses were mostly located in frontal lobe, epidural or subdural. Handler et al [52], recommend surgical drainage for those with deterioration of ocular motility and vision. Ethmoidal sinusitis was overwhelming predisposing cause in their study of orbital cellulitis and intracranial spread occurred in 6 of their 65 patients with orbital cellulitis. Sinus infections appear to be more common cause of intracranial abscess, the most common being frontal sinus, followed by ethmoid and maxillary sinuses. While the superior ophthalmic vein drains into the cavernous sinus, the inferior ophthalmic vein may drain either into the cavernous sinus through the superior orbital fissure or into the pterigoid plexus through the inferior orbital fissure (Figure 13). [15]

In the past, intracranial abscess formation had a poor prognosis with a significant mortality rate. The valveless veins interconnect the orbit with sinuses, eyelids and the cavernous sinus, (Figure 13). Since intracranial abscess may be a life-threatening complication of orbital processes, it may require aggressive intervention by multidisciplinary team. Undesirable complications of intracranial abscess may result from cavernous sinus thrombosis as well as intracranial rupture of the abscess. Patient with intracranial abscess may be asymptomatic or present with nausea, vomiting, seizures and change of their mental status. [27] Among other signs, neurological signs of intracranial abscess may include fever or altered mental status. The classic neurological presentation of intracranial abscess seen in adults may be typical, while in children these symptoms may be minimal or even absent, (Figure 14). [27] Cavernous sinus thrombosis may represent the most severe form of orbital cellulitis. The condition may be suspected clinically by the presence of bilateral orbital process along with ophthalmoplegia and loss of vision. [53], [54] Repeat imaging studies may be necessary when there is evidence of neurologic deficit, to rule out presence of epidural or subdural empyema, brain abscess, or cavernous sinus thrombosis. [55]- [57] In such cases, successful management of orbital and/or intracranial abscesses may require timely recognition of the infectious process, administration of systemic antibiotics, serial head and orbital imaging studies, early surgical management of orbit disease and often the intracranial process, (Figure 14). Computed tomography scan of the orbit and sinuses with fine cuts is the recommended imaging study of choice. [8], [51], [57] Magnetic resonance imaging studies with fat suppression has been found to be useful for visualizing the intracranial abscesses in suspected cases. The cause of most of the intracranial infectious complications of sinusitis are polymicrobial organisms, with anaerobes being the most common pathogens. [38], [51]- [54] Although no specific species or combination of bacterial microorganisms is

http://dx.doi.org/10.5772/52719

found to be predominant; Streptococcus, Staphylococcus, Bacteriodes, and Fusobacterium species are frequently encountered. Hartstein et al. reported 3 cases of intracranial abscess all of which had evidence of polymicrobial infection with no predominance of any one particular organism. [51] Initial treatment of such patients requires broad-spectrum antibiotics including beta-lactamase resistant antibiotics that have good anaerobic coverage, as well as good central nervous system penetration. [20], [23], [27], [51] Routine follow-up imaging studies may be indicated based on the clinical examination. Proper management of these patients may require a multidisciplinary team that includes an orbital surgeon, otolaryngologists, neurosurgeon, and an infectious disease specialist.

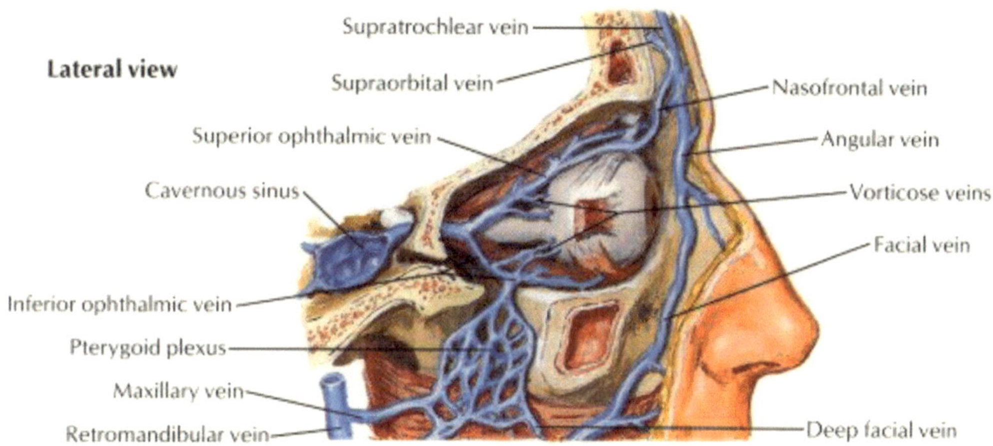

Figure 13. Lateral view of the schematic drawing showing extensive venous drainage of the facial structures along with orbital veins and their direct connections with cavernous sinus.

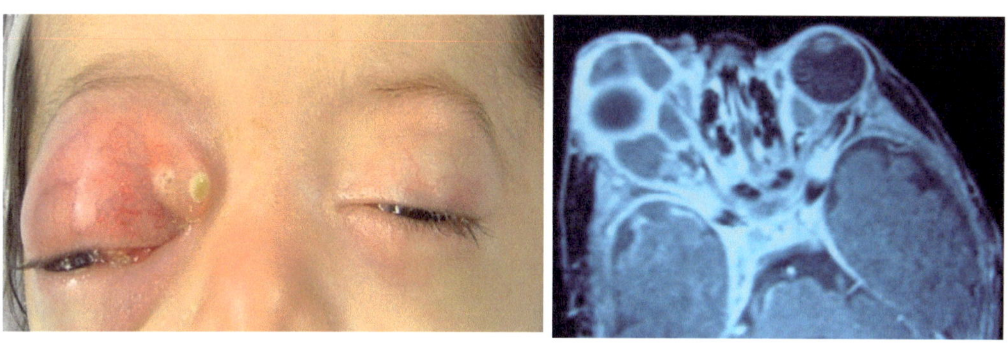

Figure 14. External photograph and MRI (axial view) of the orbits and brain of an infant with bilateral orbital cellulitis/abscesses and its extension to the brain requiring broad-spectrum systemic antibiotics along with drainage of right orbital abscess.

Author details

Imtiaz A. Chaudhry[1], Waleed Al-Rashed[2], Osama Al-Sheikh[3] and Yonca O. Arat[4]

1 Houston Oculoplastics Associates, Memorial Herman Medical Plaza, Texas Medical Center, Houston, Texas, USA

2 Al Imam Mohammad Ibn Saud Islamic University, Faculty of Medicine, Riyadh, Saudi Arabia, Saudi Arabia

3 Oculoplastic and Orbit Division, King Khaled Eye Specialist Hospital, Riyadh, Saudi Arabia

4 Department of Ophthalmology, University of Wisconsin-Madison, Wisconsin, USA

References

[1] Ferguson MP, McNab AA. Current treatment and outcome in orbital cellulitis. Aust N.Z. J Ophthalmol. 1999; 27: 375-9.

[2] Duke-Elder S, MacFaul PA. The ocular adnexa: part 2. Lacrimal orbital and para orbital diseases. In: Duke-Elder S, ed. System of Ophthalmology. Vol. 13. London: Henry Kimpton; 1974:859–89.

[3] Connel B, Kamal Z, McNab AA. Fulminant orbital cellulits with complete loss of vision. Clin Exp Ophthalmol 2001; 29: 260-1.

[4] Meara DJ. Sinonasal disease and orbital cellulitis in children. Oral Maxillofac Surg Clin North Am. 2012;24:487-96.

[5] Bedwell J, Bauman NM. Management of pediatric orbital cellulitis and abscess. Curr Opin Otolaryngol Head Neck Surg. 2011;19:467-73.

[6] Chandler JR, Langenbrunner DJ, Stevens ER. The pathogenesis of orbital complications in acute sinusitis. Laryngoscope. 1970;80:1414 –28.

[7] Maniglia AJ, Goodwin WJ, Arnold JE, Gonz E. Intracranial abscess secondary to nasal, sinus and orbital infections in adults and children. Arch Otolaryngol Head Neck Surg 1989; 115: 1424-9.

[8] Chaudhry IA, Shamsi FA, Elzaridi E, Al-Rashed W. Al-Amri AM, Al-Anezi F, Arat YO, Holck DEE. Outcome of treated orbital cellulitis from a tertiary eye care center in the Middle East. Ophthalmology 2007;114:345-54.

[9] Chaudhry IA, Shamsi FA, Elzaridi E, Al-Rashed W, Al-Amri A, Arat YO. Inpatient preseptal cellulitis: experience from a tertiary eye care centre Br. J. Ophthalmol. 2008;92;1337-41.

[10] Jarrett WH, Gutman FA. Ocular complications of infection in the paranasal sinuses. Arch Ophthalmol, 1969; 81: 683-8.

[11] Fezza J, Chaudhry IA, Kwon YH, Grannum E, Sinard J, Wolfley DE. Orbital melanoma presenting as orbital cellulities: A clinicopathologic report. Ophthal Plastic Reconstr Surg 1998;14:286-9.

[12] Chaudhry IA, Shamsi FA, Morales J. Orbital cellulitis following implantation of aqueous drainage devices for glaucoma. Eur J Ophthalmol, 2007;17:136-140.

[13] Chaudhry IA. Herpes Zoster Presenting with Orbital Cellulitis, Proptosis, and Ophthalmoplegia Middle East J Ophthalmol. 2006;13:167-9.

[14] Krouschnabel EF. Orbital apex syndrome due to sinus infection. The Laryngoscope, 1974: 84: 353-71.

[15] Hornblass A, Herschorn BJ, Stern K, Grimes C. Orbital abscess. Surv Ophthalmol. 1984; 29: 169-78.

[16] Hauser, A and Fogarasi, S. Periorbital and Orbital Cellulitis. Pediatrics in Review. 2010;31:242-9.

[17] Seltz LB, Smith J, Durairaj VD, Enzenauer R, Todd J. Microbiology and antibiotic management of orbital cellulitis. Pediatrics. 2011;127:566-72.

[18] Morgan PR, Morrison WV. Complications of frontal and ethmoid sinusitis. The Laryngoscope, 1980; 90: 661-6.

[19] Fearon B, Edmonds B, Bird R. Orbital-facial complication of sinusitis in children. The Laryngoscope, 1979; 86: 947-53.

[20] Harris GJ. Subperiosteal abscess of the orbit: age as a factor in the bacteriology and response to treatment. Ophthalmology, 1994; 101: 585-95.

[21] Coşkun M, Ilhan Ö, Keskin U, Ayintap E, Tuzcu E, Semiz H, Öksüz H. Central retinal artery occlusion secondary to orbital cellulitis and abscess following dacryocystitis. Eur J Ophthalmol. 2011;21:649-52.

[22] Harris GJ. Subperiosteal abscess of the orbit: computed tomography and the clinical course. Ophth Plast Reconstr Surg. 1996; 12: 1-8.

[23] Garcia GJ, Harris GJ. Criteria from nonsurgical management of subperiosteal abscess of the orbit: analysis of outcomes 1988-1998. Ophthalmology 2000; 107: 1454-8.

[24] Harris GJ. Subperiosteal abscess of the orbit: older children and adults require aggressive treatment: Editorial. Ophth Plast Reconstr Surg. 2001; 17: 395-7.

[25] Schramm VL, Myres EN, Kennerdell JS. Orbital complications of acute sinusitis: Evaluation, management and outcome. ORL Digest. 1979; 86: 221-30.

[26] Patt BS, Manning SC. Blindness resulting from orbital complications of sinusitis. Otolaryngol. Head Neck Surg 1991; 104: 789-95.

[27] Chaudhry IA, Al-Rashed W, Arat YO. The hot orbit: Orbital cellulitis. Middle East Afr J Ophthalmol 2012;19:34-42.

[28] Gellady AM, Shulman ST, Ayoub EM. Periorbital and orbital cellulitis in Children. Pediatrics, 1978; 61: 272-7.

[29] Watters EC, Waller PH. Acute orbital cellulitis. Arch Ophthalmol 1976; 94: 785.

[30] Weiss A, Friendly D, Eglin K. Bacterial periorbital and orbital cellulitis in childhood. Ophthalmology, 1983; 90: 195-204.

[31] Welsh LW, Welsh JJ. Orbital complications of sinus disease. The Laryngoscope, 1974; 84: 848-56.

[32] Giletto JB, Scherr SA, Mikaelian DO. Orbital complications of acute sinusitis in children. Trans Pa Acad Ophthalmol Otolaryngol, 1980; 34: 60.

[33] Smith AT, Spencer JT. Orbital complications resulting from lesions of sinuses, Ann Otology, Rhinology, and Laryngdology, 1948; 57: 5.

[34] Langham – Brown JJ, Rhys-Williams S. Computed tomography of acute orbital infection: the importance of coronal sections. Clin Radiol. 1989; 40: 471-4.

[35] Hilal SK. Computed tomography of the orbit. Ophthalmology, 1979; 86: 864-9.

[36] Bagheri A, Tavakoli M, Aletaha M, Salour H, Ghaderpanah M. Orbital and preseptal cellulitis: a 10-year survey of hospitalized patients in a tertiary eye hospital in Iran. Int Ophthalmol. 2012;32:361-7.

[37] Donahue SP, Schwartz G. Preseptal and orbital cellulitis in childhood: A changing microbiologic spectrum. Ophthalmology, 1998: 105: 585-95.

[38] Mathias MT, Horsley MB, Mawn LA, Laquis SJ, Cahill KV, Foster J, Amato MM, Durairaj VD. Atypical presentations of orbital cellulitis caused by methicillin-resistant Staphylococcus aureus. Ophthalmology. 2012;119:1238-43.

[39] Kobayashi D, Givner LB, Yeatts RP, Anthony EY, Shetty AK. Infantile orbital cellulitis secondary to community-associated methicillin-resistant Staphylococcus aureus. J AAPOS. 2011;15:208-10.

[40] Emmett Hurley P, Harris GJ. Subperiosteal abscess of the orbit: duration of intravenous antibiotic therapy in nonsurgical cases. Ophthal Plast Reconstr Surg. 2012;28:22-6.

[41] Todman MS, Enzer YR. Medical management versus surgical intervention of pediatric orbital cellulitis: the importance of subperiosteal abscess volume as a new criterion. Ophthal Plast Reconstr Surg. 2011;27:255-9.

[42] Gavriel H, Yeheskeli E, Aviram E, Yehoshua L, Eviatar E. Dimension of subperiosteal orbital abscess as an indication for surgical management in children. Otolaryngol Head Neck Surg. 2011;145:823-7.

[43] Bhargava D, Saukhla D, Ganesan A, Chand P. Endoscopic sinus surgery fro orbital subperiosteal abscess secondaryto sinusitis. Rhinology 2001; 39: 151-5.

[44] Ingraham HJ, Ryan ME, Burns JT. Streptococcal preseptal cellulitis complicated by the toxic streptococcus syndrome. Ophthalmology 1994; 102: 1223-6.

[45] Shayegani A, MacFarlane D. Kazim M. Streptococcal gangrene of the eyelids and orbit. Am J Ophthalmol 1995; 120: 784-92.

[46] Marshall DH, Jordan DR, Gilberg SM. Periocular necrotizing fasciitis: a review of five cases. Ophthalmology 1996; 104: 1857-62.

[47] Meyer MA. Streptococcal toxic shock syndrome complicating preseptal cellulitis. Am J Ophthalmol 1996; 123: 841-3.

[48] Slavin ML, Glaser J. Acute severe irreversible visual loss with sphenoethmoiditis - 'posterior' orbital cellulitis. Arch Ophthalmol. 1987; 105: 345-8.

[49] El-Sayed Y, Al-Muhaimeid H. Acute visual loss in association with sinusitis. J Laryng Otol. 1993; 107:840-2.

[50] Borruat FX, Bogousslavasky J, Uffer S, Klainguti G, Schatz NJ. Orbital infarction syndrome. Ophthalmology, 1993; 100:562-8.

[51] Hartstein ME, Steinvurzel MD, Choen CP. Intracranial abscess as a complication of subperiosteal abscess of the orbit. Ophth plast Reconstr Surg. 2001; 17: 398-403.

[52] Handler LC, Davey IC, Hill JC, Lauryssen C. The acute orbit: differentiation of orbital cellulitis from subperiosteal abscess by computerized tomography. Neuroradiology, 1991; 33: 15-18.

[53] Giannoni CM, Stewart MG, Alford EL. Intracranial complications of sinusitis. Laryngoscope 1997; 107: 863-7.

[54] Brook I. Bacteriology of intracranial abscess in children. J Neurosurg 1981; 54: 484-8.

[55] Weber AL, Mikuli D. Inflammatory disorders of the periorbital sinuses and their complications. Radiol Clin North Am 1987; 25: 615-30.

[56] Towbin R, Han B, Kaufmann R, Burke M. Postseptal cellulitis: CT in diagnosis and management. Radiology 1986; 158: 735-7.

[57] Harr DL, Quencer RM, Abrams GW. Computed tomography and ultrasound in the evaluation of orbital infection and pseudotumor. Radiology 1982; 152: 395.

[58] Brook I, Frazier EH. Microbiology of subperiosteal orbital abscess and associated maxillary sinusitis. Laryngoscope 1996; 106: 1010-3.

Chapter 8

Nontuberculous Mycobacterial Keratitis

Ana Lilia Pérez-Balbuena,
David Arturo Ancona-Lezama,
Lorena Gutiérrez-Sánchez and
Virginia Vanzzini-Zago

Additional information is available at the end of the chapter

http://dx.doi.org/10.5772/45964

1. Introduction

Mycobacterium species that are considered typical are the tuberculosis species such as *M.tuberculosis, M.bovis, M.africarium* and *M.leprae*. These species have only human or animal reservoirs and are not transmitted by water. In contrast, the species Non-Tuberculosis or "atypical", naturally are ubiquitous in soil and water and have been found as normal flora of skin, sputum, and gastric contents. These bacteria are resistant to common, disinfectants, chlorine, formaldehyde and glutaraldehyde.

NTM can cause infections on all adnexal and ocular tissues including the cornea, iris, lens, retina, choroid and optic nerve. Most NTM infections are caused by *M.chelonae* and *M. fortuitum*, that as we will discuss later, belong to the rapid growers group.

In this chapter, we will focus on keratitis caused by atypical mycobacterium, since a great number of recent clinical reports of NTM ocular infections are of keratitis. In common general ophthalmology procedures like refractive surgery, for example laser in situ keratomileusis (LASIK), Laser epithelial keratomileusis (LASEK), photorefractive keratectomy (PRK), and other specialized procedures such as penetrating keratoplasty (PKP), a transgression to natural barriers occurs, this constitutes a risk factor for infection by these organisms. In addition, LASIK is one of the most commonly performed procedures in ophthalmology practice.

Several factors may contribute to the development of mycobacterial keratitis following LASIK, making it difficult to determine the true origin of the infection in most cases. This procedure is often performed utilizing aseptic, but non sterile techniques. *Mycobacterium chelonei, M. abscessus, M. fortuitum, M. szulgai,* and *M. mucogenicum* have been reported as the result of improper asepsis.

Atypical Mycobacteria corneal infections are rare, but devastating complications. Although rare, are a diagnostic and therapeutic challenge. Mycobacterium have been involved in several isolated cases as well as in outbreaks.[4-12]

2. Microbiological and laboratory profile

Mycobacterium species that are considered typical are the tuberculosis specie; *M.tuberculosis.* Many species enclosed in genus *Mycobacteriaceae* are true human pathogens as *Mycobacterium tuberculosis* complex, that include *M tuberculosis, M bovis,* non pathogenic *M bovis* BCG, *M africanum, M caprae, M microti,* and *M pinnipedii* are characterized by different phenotypes and mammalian host ranges, displays the most extreme genetic homogeneity with 0.01 to 0.03% nucleotides variation only. Growth rate in this group is 6 to 12 weeks. *M leprae* is the only non cultivable in vitro specie and has some genetic variations in relation to *M tuberculosis complex*.

The only genus of the *Mycobacteriaceae* family is the *Mycobacterium*, the *Mycobacteriaceae* belongs to the order *Actinomycetales*. Mycobacteria is an unusual ocular pathogen that has the following characteristics: intracellular bacilli, slow growing organisms, obligate aerobic, non-motile, non-capsulated, non-sporing, present a large amounts of lipids and true waxes in their cell walls, and are considered gram-positive and acid-fast.

Other places where NTM have been isolated are: contaminated tap water, saline solutions, disinfectant solutions, and hemodialyzers. Mycobacteria influences a number of ocular structures, including the cornea,iris, lens,retina, choroid and optic nerve.

Clinical manifestations of the typical mycobacteria are : lupus vulgaris on eyelid, phlyctenule, scleritis, lacrimal gland involvement, orbital periostitis, granulomatous panuveitis, secondary glaucoma and cataract, chorioretinal plaque or nodule, nerve palsies.

The incidence of tuberculosis has increased due to the growth in homelessness, the upsurge of intravenous drug abuse, neglect of tuberculosis programs, acquired immunodeficiency syndrome.

Runyon classified nontuberculous mycobacteria into four groups, described in [Table 1]. Runyon Classification of tuberculous and non-tuberculous *Mycobacterium* is based, on the growth rate, and pigment production. Groups I to III are slow growers that require approximately 2 to 3 or more weeks to form visible colonies in culture at 27°C. Group IV organisms are rapid growers, forming non-pigmented colonies in culture in one week.[1,14,15]

Out of the more than 130 actually validated species of non-tuberculousmycobacteria, 60 are slowly growingmycobacteria, that shows in solid culture media growth rates of 2 to 4 weeks, the most clinically significance and most frequently in isolated human samples are *M avium, M intracellulare, M kansasii, M marinum, M xenopi, M malmoense and M ulcerans.* In the

http://dx.doi.org/10.5772/45964

rapidly growing mycobacteria group with 7 -10 days of growing rate on solid culture media, there are three major clinically important species responsible for 80% of diseases in humans *M chelonae, M abscessus* and *M fortuitum,* that are too frequently located in tap water and have been related with sepsis in bone marrow transplant, post-traumatic, surgical ocular and other surgical wound infections.

SlowGrowers			**Rapid Growers**
Group I	**Group II**	**Group III**	**Group IV**
(photochromogens) 6-12 weeks	*(scotochromogens)* 2-4 weeks	*(nonchromogens)* 2-4 weeks	*(nonchromogens)* 7-10 days
M. marinum	M. scrofulaceum	M. avium	M. fortuitum group
M. kansasii	M. szulgai	M. intracellulare	*M. fortuitum*
M. simiae	M. gordonae	M. haemophilum	*M. peregrinum*
M. asiaticum	M. xenopi	M. paratuberculosis	*M. mucogenicum*
	M. flavescens	M. gastri	*M. Senegalese*
		M. malmoense	*M. septicum*
		M. nonchromogenicum	*M. mageritense*
		M. terrae	M. chelonae-abscessus group
		M. triviale	*M. chelonae*
			M. abscessus
			M. immunogenum
			M. smegmatis group
			M. smegmatis
			M. goodii
			M. wolinskyi

Problem statement: To describe the experience in México (Asociación Para Evitar La Ceguera I.A.P. "Hospital Dr. Luis Sánchez Bulnes" [APEC]) in the management of keratitis caused by nontuberculous mycobacteria.

Application area: Cornea and Refractive Service and Mycrobiology Service

Research course: To describe of atypical *Mycobacterium* keratitiscases diagnosed and attended in the Cornea Service of our Hospital in the last 10 years.

Methods: This is a descriptive retrospective case series of five patients treated in our service.

Table 1. Runyon's Classification of Nontuberculous Mycobacterium

3. Laboratory diagnosis and bacteriology

In ophthalmological infections traumatic or post-surgical in origin, are frequently involved in non-tuberculous or atypical fast growing *Mycobacteria,* the species *M. chelonae, M. chelonae /abscesus, M. fortuitum* have been isolated in many cases. These rapidly growing *Mycobacteria* share the cellular characteristics of *Mycobacterium* genus,like mycolic acids esters in its cell wall, long straight or curved rods with irregular Gram staining [Figure 1], and specific red-magenta staining characteristic with Ziehl-Neelsen or Kinyoun cold techniques.[Figure 2] They are aerobic and capable of growing in 5 -10% CO_2 atmosphere and in blood agar media.[Figure 3] In addition, these microorganisms are arylsulfatase positive, catalase positive and niacin negative. [Figure 4]

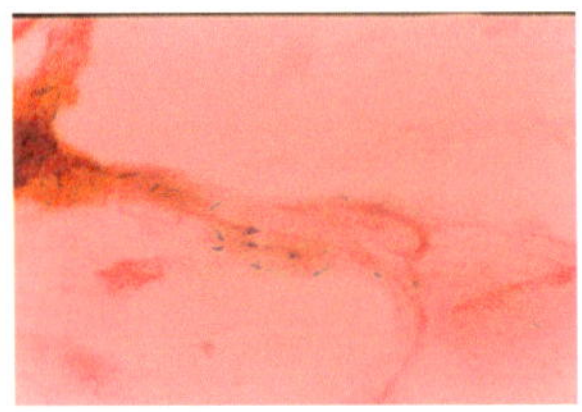

Figure 1. Gram positive and irregular stain and forms of *Mycobacterium chelonae*

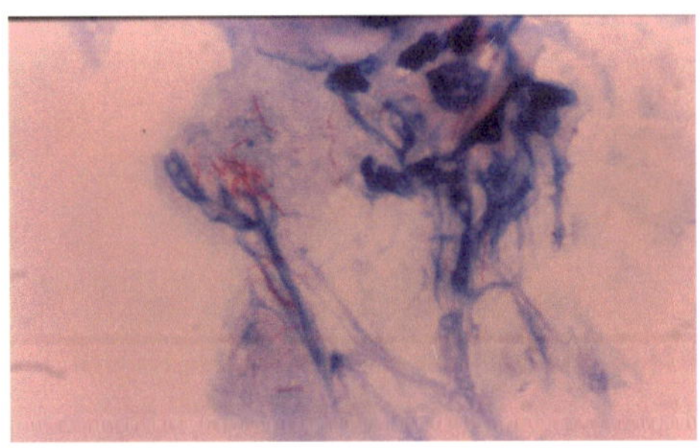

Figure 2. Red-magenta rods of *M. chelonae* in a corneal smear of patient with keratitis.

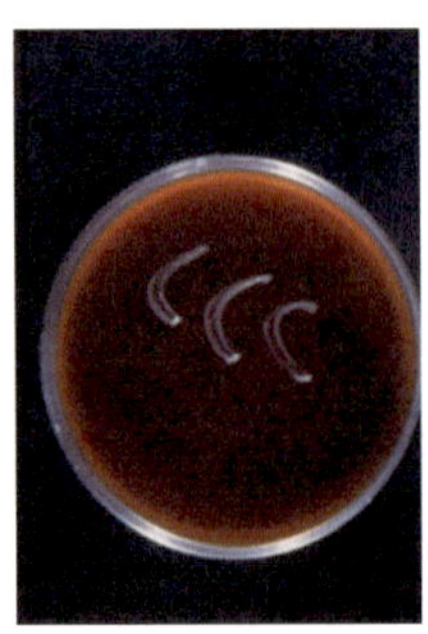

Figure 3. Colonies of *M. chelonae* in agar blood with Brain Heart Infusion (BHI) agar base after 7 days of incubation at 27ºC and 5% CO_2 atmosphere.

http://dx.doi.org/10.5772/45964

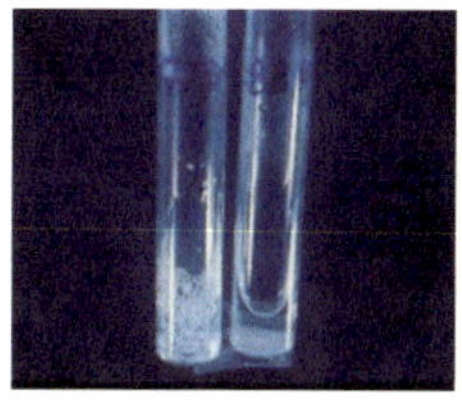

Figure 4. Catalase 65°C positive test (O_2 bubbles) for *Mycobacterium chelonae*.

To identify the microorganism, its phenotypic characteristics were used, such as pigmentation of colonies growing in the darkness (presented in Table 1) on Lowenstein-Jensen media.

The most common species of rapidly growing *Mycobacteria* belong to group IV of Runyon's classification, also known as colorless or nonchromatogens.[Figure 5]

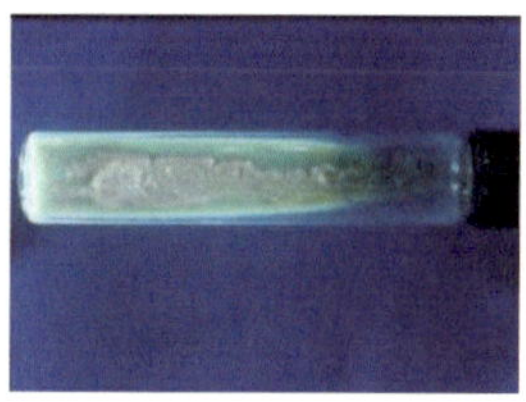

Figure 5. *Mycobacterium chelonae* colonies in Lowenstein-Jensen medium after 7 days of incubation at 27°C.

For genotypic characterization, the 16Sr RNA gene sequencing, high performance liquid chromatography and polymerase chain reaction has been used.

4. Clinical features

Nontuberculous Mycobacteria can cause infections of all adnexal and ocular tissues. Most atypical Mycobacteria infections are caused by *M. chelonae*, and *M. fortuitum*.

Dacryocystitis and Canaliculitis: Present as epiphora and erythematous swelling in the medial canthal area, purulent material can be expressed with massage of the lacrimal sac.

Orbital Infections: Present with a gradual development of periorbital edema, without a significant proptosis and a superficial skin lesion may be present. The visual acuity will depend on the involvement of the optic nerve. [18,19]

Conjuntivitis and Scleritis: Present as conjunctival or as scleral injection and tenderness accompanied with chronic redness, irritation, discharge and pain. Sometimes, marked scleral thinning may develop. Scleral abscesses manifest late in the course of the disease as subconjunctival nodules. [20,21]

Endoftalmitis: Present with severe pain, decreased vision, and redness and discharge, may exist hypopyon, and variable amounts of granulomatous keratitic precipitates. Moderate vitreous inflammation is present in most cases.

Keratitis: The greatest number of recent clinical reports of nontuberculous Mycobacteria ocular infections are of keratitis, as seen in our hospital (Asociación Para Evitar La Ceguera en México "Dr. Luis Sánchez Bulnes" I.A.P. [APEC]). Keratitis most commonly follows trauma or surgery and has been associated with penetrating keratoplasty and refractive surgery.

Nontuberculous Mycobacteria keratitis is characterized by a delayed onset of symptoms that range typically from 1 to 3 weeks following the exposing event. There is decreased vision and an indolent course and some cases various degrees of pain, ranging from indolent to severe.

Presenting symptoms can include any of the following: pain, redness, photophobia, decreased vision, foreign body sensation and/or mild irritation. Presenting clinical signs include infiltrates in the corneal interface that can either be multiple white granular opacities <0.5mm in diameter with well defined borders or radiating projections, or a single white round lesion (0.1-2 mm in diameter) which may progress to satellite lesions. These infiltrates spread subsequently into the corneal stroma posteriorly and anteriorly and can result in perforation though the flap to surface. [Table 2].A hypopyon is often found in untreated or poorly treated cases. [25,26]

Lazar and colleagues first described the presence of a "cracked windshield" appearance to the cornea around the edge of the central area of ulceration and infiltrate, seen transiently early in the course of the infection. [25,27,28] This sign consist of radiating lines from the central infiltrate in the middle third of the corneal stroma. It is important to mention that NTM keratitis has also been noted in the abscence of epithelial defect with deep stromal keratitis. The corneal infiltrate may show irregular margins.

Signs	Symptoms
Single or multiple white granular opacities with well	Pain (mild)
defined borders or radiating projections	Redness
Satellite infiltrates	Photophobia
Hypopyon	Tearing
Mild or absent anterior chamber reaction	Foreign body sensation
"Cracked windshield" appearance	Decreased visual acuity

Table 2. Signs and symptoms of keratitis caused by mycobacterias

5. Predisposing factors

Nontuberculous Mycobacteria are opportunistic pathogens that require an alteration in the ocular barriers to produce infection. In nearly all reports, a previous history of minor to severe trauma is the common denominator.Men and women are equally affected among NTM keratitis patients who have had LASIK, in contrast to a 70% male preponderance among patients who have not had LASIK, the result of a higher prevalence of trauma in males. [Table 3] [5,29]

Risk factors associated with NTM keratitis
Trauma
Surgical trauma
Refractive surgeries
Laser in situ keratomileusis (LASIK)
Laser epithelial keratomileusis (LASEK)
Corneal transplantation
Radial keratotomy
Photorefractive keratectomy (PRK)
Penetrating keratoplasty (PKP)
Other ophthalmologic surgeries
Extracapsular cataract extraction
Small incision corneal cataract surgery
Suture removal
Contact lens wear
Corticosteroid use
Improper aseptic technique or sterilization of surgical instrumentation

Table 3. Risk factors for the development of nontuberculous mycobacterial keratitis.

Post-LASIK NTM keratitis: Laser in situ keratomileusis (LASIK) is the most commonly performed refractive surgical procedure, since it offers rapid visual rehabilitation, decreased stromal scarring, less postoperative pain, and the ability to treat a wider range of refractive disorders. LASIK preserves the integrity of Bowman's membrane and the overlying epithelium, thus decreasing the risk for microbial keratitis. Several studies have reported an incidence of bacterial infection following LASIK procedures varying between 0% to 1.5%. [29,31,32] Solomon et. al published the first survey that provides information about post-LASIK infectious keratitis. The most common organisms cultured were nontuberculous mycobacteria (48%) and staphylococci (33%).. These findings are consistent with Chang's research, where he found that nearly 47% of infectious keratitis cases after LASIK appear to be caused by NTM; 32% being caused by *Mycobacterium chelonei* alone. In contrast to the acute or subacute onset of symptoms generally seen postoperatively in bacterial and fungal keratitis, rapid growing atypical mycobacteria may present with a slower onset of clinical disease, from 3 to 14 weeks (3.5 weeks in average) after the procedure. It is important to keep in mind that this is not a rule, and more rapidly growing NTM such as the *Mycobacterium chelonae-abscessus* group may present as soon as 10 days posterior to the refractive surgery. [1,33,34]

Innoculation of NTM to the flap-stromal interface probably takes place at the time of surgery, therefore, it is infrequent to find an epithelial defect, being present in less than half of cases. Corneal infiltrates appear to be entirely within the lamellar flap or at the flap interface and may be either multiple, tiny, white, granular opacities less than 0.5mm in diameter or a single white lesion ranging between 0.1-0.2mm in diameter. Anterior extension of infiltrate with ulceration or anterior perforation of the corneal flap or posterior extension into the stroma is a rare finding and is usually associated with a delay in diagnosis and the beginning of therapy. Anterior chamber reaction is not a common finding, occurring in only 20% of cases.[1,29]

6. Differential diagnosis

NTM keratitis can often be mistaken with other bacterial infections that cause nonsuppurative keratitis. Several authors suggest to keep in mind other causative organisms that may present, in the course of disease, similar clinical features such as fungal keratitis, infectious crystalline keratopathy, Nocardia keratitis, herpes simplex virus, and rarely Acanthamoeba keratitis. In our experience at APEC, the principal differential diagnosis must be made between fungal and Nocardia keratitis.

Fungal keratitis: Often preceded by history of trauma involving plants or foreign bodies. Like NTM, mycotic keratitis may worsen with the use of topical corticosteroids. These keratitis often do not respond to topical antibiotics, as seen with NTM keratitis. Multiple corneal fungal abscesses may emulate the multifocal presentation of NTM keratitis. Sabouraud's agar is essential for the identification of the causative fungus. [Figure 6]

Infectious Crystalline Keratopathy (ICK): "Cracked windshield" corneal appearance may be also seen in this keratitis caused most commonly by Streptococcus species, but unlike this entity, NTM keratitis presents with this sign transiently early in the course. Gorovoy et al first described Infectious crystalline keratopathy in 1984, describing it as a unique corneal infection characterized by and indolent, progressive course: a paucity of inflammation; and

http://dx.doi.org/10.5772/45964

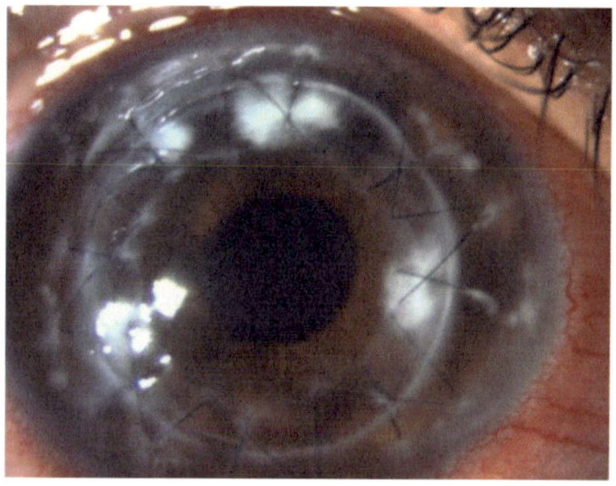

Figure 6. Candida keratitis after penetrating keratoplasty for keratoconus.

the formation of sharply demarcated, gray-white, branching, round, stellate, or needle-like opacities in the corneal stroma. Although the duration of the relatively recalcitrant course of the infectious crystalline keratopathy may mimic NTM keratitis, the crystalline appearance persists in ICK but is transient in NTM keratitis. Among post-LASIK patients, crystalline NTM keratitis occurs rarely (less than 10%).

Nocardiaasteroides infection: should also be considered, since it is an acid-fast microorganism capable of producing bacterial keratitis. The best way to differentiate Nocardia infection from NTM keratitis is with a Gram stain. Nocardia keratitis is more fulminant than NTM keratitis.[Figure 7]

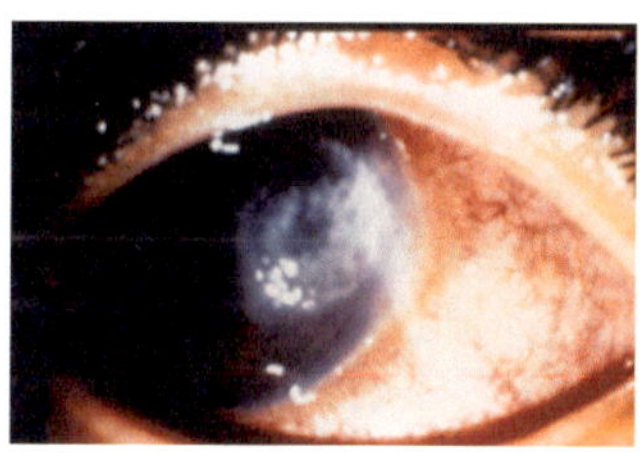

Figure 7. Nocardial keratitis as a differential diagnosis of NTM keratitis.

Deep lamellar keratitis can be confused with post-LASIK NTM keratitis. It usually presents within the first 7 days post-LASIK, and unlike NTM keratitis, it clears with topical corticosteroids. If the wrong diagnosis is made, the improper use of such medications contribute to the delay in diagnosis of post-LASIK NTM keratitis.

Acanthamoeba keratitis generally presents with out-of-proportion pain in comparison to the clinical findings. It is common to see ring ulcers in Acanthamoeba keratitis. This agent responds, unlike NTM, to topical biguanides and diamidines, and topical corticosteroids may be of some benefit.

Herpetic keratitis. In necrotizing stromal keratitis, herpetic keratitis can cause dense white stromal infiltrates that may be confused with NTM keratitis. Special features that are more typically found in herpetic keratitis are decreased corneal sensation and previous or concomitant history of herpes labialis lesions. NTM keratitis may simulate a non-suppurative herpetic keratitis, especially in cases caused by Mycobacterium marinum. There may also be a dendritic or geographic epithelial defect with minimal stromal infiltration, misleading the clinician and prompting treatment with antivirals. This can lead to the development of a severe, wide corneal infiltrate.

7. Our experience

Keratitis caused by atypical *Mycobacteria* is characterized by an indolent course and poor response to antibiotics. The diagnosis requires a high index of suspicion and their treatment is usually very difficult. The early diagnosis of nontuberculous mycobacterial keratitis following LASIK is not easy, because the overlying, noninvolved stroma hinders the collection of sufficient material for culture. In addition, such organisms are only detectable by culture in special media, such as Lowenstein-Jensen, and special stains like Ziehl-Neelsen, which may not be included among routine cultures in the microbiology service.

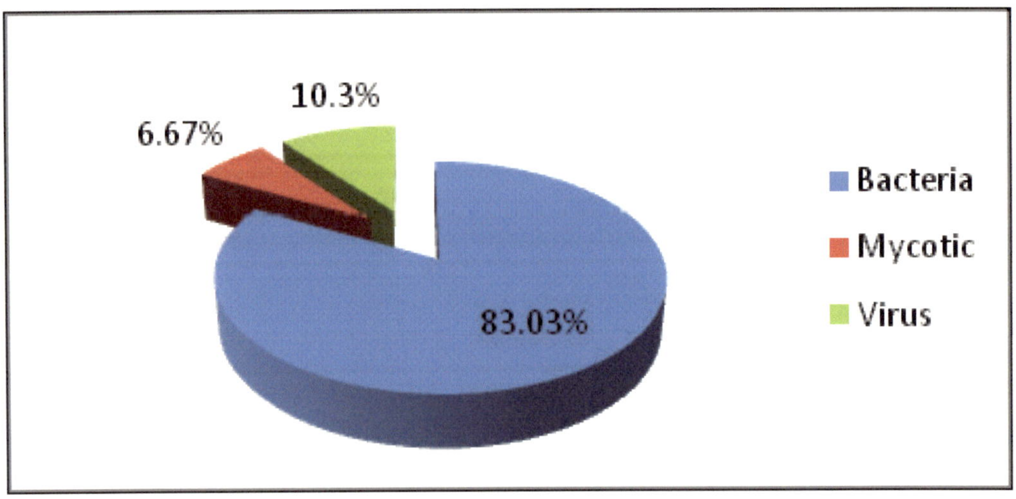

Table 4. Profile of microorganisms causing infectious keratitis; 2025 cases, during 10 years (2000-2010). Data of Asociación Para Evitar La Ceguera en México "Dr. Luis Sánchez Bulnes" I.A.P.

In our hospital, our service found an incidence of 2025 cases of infectious keratitis in the last 10 years (2000-2010). We found that 83.03% corresponded to infections caused by bacteria, 6.67% mycotic, and 10.3% originated by virus. [Table 4] Out of this percentage of bacterial keratitis, we report a frequency of 73.57% caused by gram positive, 9.22% caused by gram negative and 0.24% originated by nontuberculous mycobacteria. [Table 5]

http://dx.doi.org/10.5772/45964

In 100% of cases, the causative agent was *Mycobacterium chelonae*, correlating with the reported in literature.

Several authors reported an incidence between 0% and 1.5% of mycobacterial keratitis post-LASIK, our results (0.24%) correlate with these values. [29,31,32]

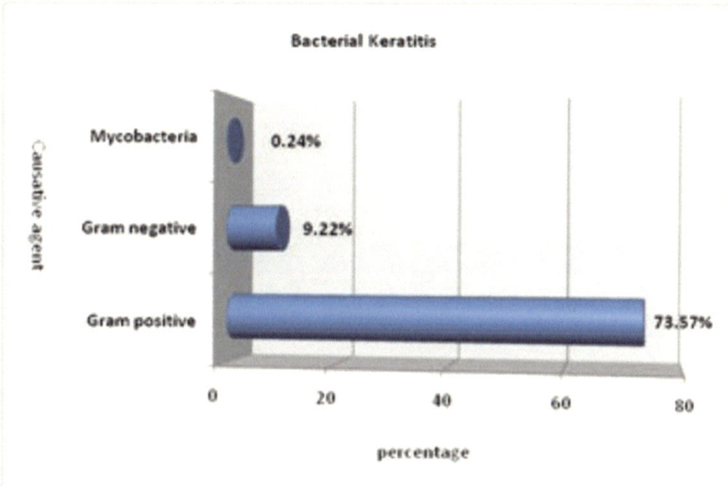

Table 5. The spectrum of bacterial agents causing keratitis. Data of Asociación Para Evitar La Ceguera en México "Dr. Luis Sánchez Bulnes" I.A.P

Almost all our cases (4 out of 6) of nontuberculous mycobacterial keratitis had as common background, a previous history of surgical trauma, specifically speaking of LASIK and PKP. We report one case of a contact lens user. A clinical summary of all cases reported in APEC to date, has been compiled in [Table 6,7]

The average age in our patients was of 36.6 years with a range from 12 to 58 years.

The average time that took from the onset of symptoms to the stabishment of correct diagnosis in patients that underwent previous surgical therapy was 4.25 weeks, which results similar to the average of weeks reported in literature (3.5 weeks). [1,33,34]

In our hospital 15,028 LASIK surgeries were performed from 2001-2011. We report in our service a total of 4 cases ok infectious keratitis following a LASIK procedure, which resembles an incidence of 1 infection every 3,757 procedures (0.026%). 2 cases (50%) correspond to post-LASIK keratitis caused by *Mycobacterium chelonae, a*nd the remaining 2 cases (50%) by gram positive bacteria (*Streptococcus pneumoniae*). These findings correlate with the reported by Solomon et al. (year 2003)of 1 infection for every 2919 procedures (0.034%), Donnenfeld et al. (year 2005) who reported an incidence of 1 in every 2131 (0.04%) LASIK procedures and LLovet et al. (year 2010) with an incidence of 1 in every 2841 cases (0.035%). The study also mentions that 65.5% (76 cases) of the infections reported, presented in the first week postoperatively. 6.03% (7 cases) presented in the second week, 14.65% (17 cases) presented between the second and fourth week and lastly 13.79% (16 cases) presented after 1 month. 2 of our cases, the ones caused by *Streptococcus pneumoniae,* presented in the first week postoperatively. 1 nontuberculous mycobacterial case presented between the second and fourth week (3 weeks), and lastly the remaining NTM keratitis case presented presented after 1 month (7 weeks). Speaking of ethiological factors, Solomon et al. reported that the most common microorganisms involved in post-LASIK keratitis are mycobacteria (48%) and coccus (33%), we found similar data in our retrospective analysis; Mycobacterial keratitis 50% and Streptococcus 50%.[30,39,40]

Case	Age/Sex	Eye	Delay in diagnosis	History	Infiltrates /localization	Initial VA	Previous Eye therapy	Causative organism	Medical therapy
1	57/F	OS	7 weeks	Unilateral redness, photophobia and tearing 6 weeks after bilateral LASIK associated with flap ulcer.	A central epithelial defect measuring 5.0 x 3.0 mm associated with stromal infiltrates involving area of flap. Hypopyon of 1mm.	*CF 50cm*	*Multitreated with Moxifloxacin, Dexamethasone Natamycin and Aciclovir*	*M. chelonae*	Amikacin 3.3% Gatifloxacin 0.3% Topical Rifampin Clarithromycin PO BID
2	58/M	OS	3 weeks	DM. Uneventful bilateral PKP as treatment for keratoglobus. 14 years later unilateral corneal trauma with graft dehiscense and endothelial rejection. Second graft evolved with redness, photophobia, pain and diminished VA, 3 weeks later.	Paracentral lesion 3.0 x 2.0 mm at the graft-host junction, infiltrate with irregular edges, satellite lesion.	*CF 2m*	*Multitreated with Neomycin, Polymixin and Dexamethasone phosphate*	*M. chelonae*	Amikacin 3.3% Gatifloxacin 0.3% Clarithromycin PO BID Fluorometholone
3	27/M	OS	4 weeks	PKP for herpetic leucoma, 4 months later presented with loose suture and ulcer at the site.	Ulcer in graft-host junction.	CF 1m	Multitreated with Prednisolone, Ciprofloxacin, Vancomycin, Fluorometholone	*M. chelonae*	Gatifloxacin 0.3% Ciprofloxacin PO BID Lubricant eye drops
4	43/F	OS	6 weeks	Redness, photophobia and tearing. Contact lens user.	Paracentral infiltrate with satellite lesion.	CF 2m	Multitreated with Vancomycin, Tobramycin, Ofloxacin	*M. chelonae*	Amikacin c/3hrs. Gatifloxacin 0.3% Clarithromycin PO BID
5	23/M	OD	3 weeks	Bilateral LASIK. post surgery unilateral hyperemia, photophobia and tearing.	3.5 mm intralamellar central infiltrate	20/100	Multitreated with Ofloxacin, Vancomycin, Moxifloxacin	*M. chelonae*	Amikacin c/3hrs. Gatifloxacin 0.3% Clarithromycin PO BID

F=female, M=male, CF=count fingers, OS=left eye, OD=right eye, PO=per oral, BID=twice daily, DM=Diabetes Mellitus, VA= visual acuity, PKP=penetrating keratoplasty, LASIK=laser in situ keratomileusis

Table 6. Nontuberculousmycobacterialkeratitis in patients of Asociación Para Evitar La Ceguera en México "Dr. Luis Sánchez Bulnes" I.A.P.

Velotta reported that nearly 90% of NTM keratitis after LASIK cases are unilateral, all of our cases presented in just one eye.

Infectious keratitis after penetrating keratoplasty (PKP) is not a frequent complication with an incidence ranging from 1.8% to 11.0%; however, this infection has a high risk of loss of corneal clarity. In our present analysis, the remaining 2 patients that underwent surgical procedures, developed nontuberculous mycobacterial keratitis posterior to penetrating keratoplasty. Both cases were promptly diagnosed after onset of symptoms, resulting in satisfactory outcomes and good final visual acuity [Table 7] [Figure 8,9]

Case	Surgical Treatment	Follow up	Outcome	Final Visual Acuity	Refraction
1	Flap amputation + scraping + irrigation with gatifloxacin 0.3% First PKP (*with recurrence*) Second PKP + Ahmed valve implant + ECCE & IOL	30 months	resolved	*20/70*	*+8.00=-4.00x140°*
2	None	18 months	resolved	*20/30*	*Contact lens +3.50 D*
3	None	10 months	resolved	20/30	*Contact lens* 8.30 Power -7.00, Diameter 9.6
4	None	3 months	resolved	20/20	-4:00=-3:00 X180°
5	None	3 months	resolved	20/60	-2.00=-1.00x45°

PKP=penetrating keratoplasty, ECCE=extracapsular, IOL=intraocular lens.

Table 7. Surgical treatment and outcome in nontuberculousmycobacterial keratitis in patients of Asociación Para Evitar La Ceguera en México "Dr. Luis Sánchez Bulnes" I.A.P.

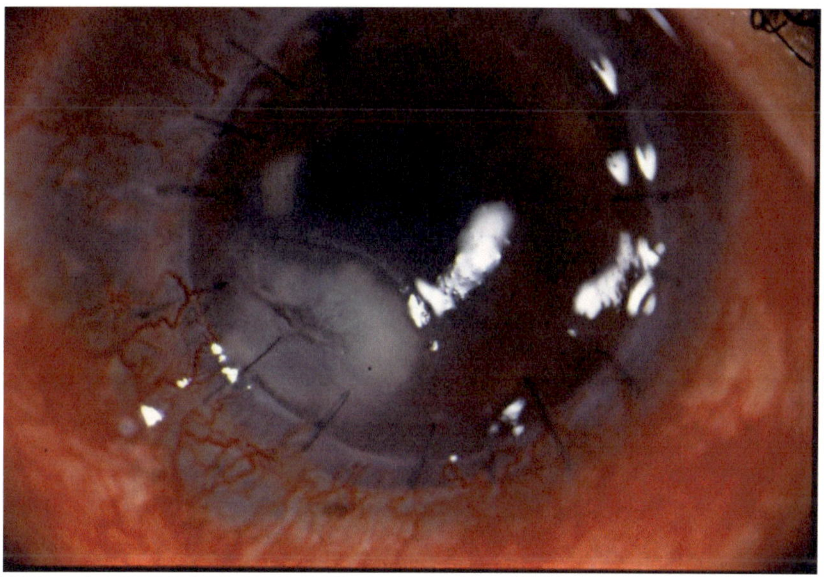

Figure 8. Patient 2, clinical examination 4 weeks after penetrating keratoplasty with conjunctival hyperemia and corneal infiltrate (3.0 x 2.0 mm) in graft-host junction caused by *Mycobacterium chelonae*.

8. Treatment

Management of this type of infectious keratitis often traduces in a medical challenge. In cases of identified NTM corneal infection, there is considerable benefit from the use of combined antibiotics, since atypical mycobacteria have a slower growth rate compared to other bacteria and may become resistant to a single antibiotic class during the course of extended treatment.

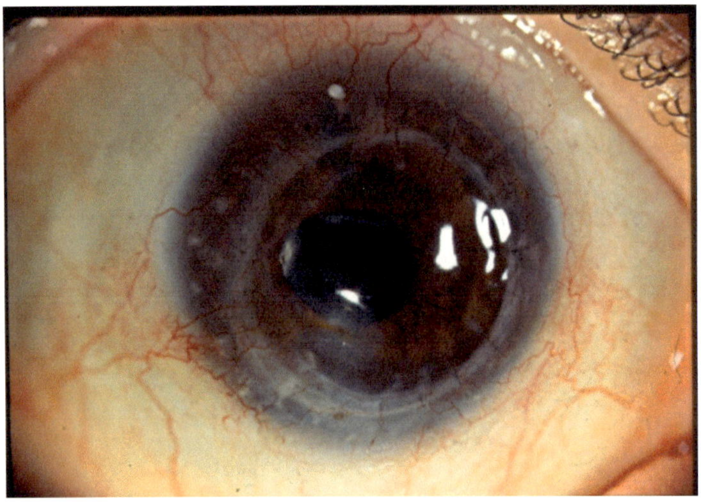

Figure 9. Patient 2, eighteen months after therapy discontinuation. Corneal graft is infection-free and clear in the visual axis; best-corrected vision of 20/30 was attained with a +3.50-D contact lens.

The base of treatment consists of a double approach; appropriate antibiotic and judicious surgical intervention. Such antimicrobial choice becomes complicated since a poor correlation exists between *in vitro* susceptibility profiles and the final clinical response. We recommend surgical debridement, depending on the case, to facilitate drug penetration to the interlamellar space. In some cases, flap amputation may be necessary, the rationale for this procedure is to lower the bacterial load, remove necrotic as well as infected tissue, and permit better antibiotic penetration. We recommend this surgical procedures in recalcitrant post-LASIK NTM keratitis to maintain the infection under control.

De La Cruz et al. suggest initial combined antibiotic therapy that includes at least 2 of the 3 most susceptible agents (clarithromycin, amikacin, and fourth-generation fluoroquinolones) for rapidly growing mycobacteria specially if known resistance has been documented. The initial therapy recommended for many years has been the use of topical Amikacin sulfate 20-40mg/mL.This antibiotic is the most frequently used agent in the treatment of NTM keratitis. In our institution we use amikacin sulfate (Amikin® 500mg injectable solution. Bristol-Myers Squibb de México S. de R.L. de C.V.)diluted to a concentration of 20mg/mL, one drop every hour and dose-response. Even though this antibiotic constitutes the first line of treatment against atypical mycobacterial keratitis, only a success rate of 30-40% has been reported. This therapeutic agent has also been associated with high epithelium toxicity when it is applied for a prolonged course.

We recommend the addition of two additional antibiotics to the drug scheme, such as a macrolide like clarithromycin and a fourth-generation fluoroquinolone like gatifloxacin.[Table 6] In our hospital we employ oral clarithromycin Klaricid H.P.® 500mg (Abbott Laboratories de México S.A. de C.V. México, D.F.) twice daily, and Zymar® (gatifloxacin 0.3% Allergan Labs, Irvine, CA).

Fluoroquinolone antibiotics are concentration-dependent killers. Therefore, they require a minimum inhibitory concentration (MIC) to be reached in order to be effective. In vitro studies have shown that fourth-generation fluoroquinolones are effective against atypical mycobacteria, inhibiting 90% of isolates after reaching its proper concentration.[23,43]

The fourth-generation fluoroquinolones have significant advantages over earlier generation fluoroquinolones in treating mycobacterial infections, including superior bactericidal activity, higher corneal concentrations, and decreased risk for bacterial resistance.

The reason for adding a fourth-generation fluoroquinolone to the therapeutic scheme is that 8-metoxy-fluoroquinolones such as gatifloxacin and moxifloxacin has shown better in vitro activity against these organisms, in comparison to second-generation fluoroquinolones like ciprofloxacin.

Furthermore, the molecular structures of moxifloxacin and gatifloxacin have a greater binding affinity for 2 of the enzymes necessary for bacterial DNA synthesis (deoxyribonucleic acid gyrase [also called topoisomerase II] and tipoisomerase IV) in both gram-negative and gram-positive microorganisms. By inhibiting such enzymes, these bacteria require to undergo two genetic mutations in order to create resistance. Older fluoroquinolones adequately inhibit tipoisomerase II in gram-negative microorganisms but are not as effective in inhibiting topoisomerase IV in gram-positive organisms.

The great effectiveness of fourth-generation fluoroquinolones rely due to their superior bactericidal activity, the ability to reach higher corneal concentration, and better resistance pattern.In a rabbit model, fourth-generation fluoroquinolones were found to be synergistic to our first-line drug options, amikacin and clarithromycin against *M. chelonae.* Lastly, considering antibiotic resistance as an emerging problem; Ford et al. reported in their study that more than 60% of atypical mycobacteria are unresponsive to second-generation fluoroquinolones. [5,34]

Lazar et al reported a torpid answer to the use of Rifampin in nontuberculous mycobacteria ocular infections. In our experience, we required to add a new antibiotic drug in patient 1 (Table 6), when we reached the three antibiotics suggested by diverse authors in literature (Amikacin, Clarythromicin and Gatifloxacin). We added topical rifampin to the scheme obtaining positive outcomes. We prepared a topical solution of Rifampin at our hospital by dissolving 300mg of Rifampin (Rifadin®) (SANOFI-AVENTIS de México, S.A. de C.V.) with 10mL of Sodium Hyaluronate (Lagricel® SOPHIA, S.A. de C.V., Laboratorios. Guadalajara, México) indicating a drop every hour and dose-response.

Management of mycobacterial keratitis usually requires a prolonged and intensive therapy consisting of topical and systemic medication. In our experience, medical treatment of NTM keratitis can prolong as long as 30 months. Shih et al have reported full months of therapy even when the appropriate antibiotic, chosen by drug sensitivity test results, is used. In [Table 8]we summarize our suggested treatment for the proper management of nontuberculous Mycobacterial keratitis.

		Suggested treatment
Triple Antibotic Therapy	*Topical*	1. Amikacin 20 mg/mL 2. Fourth-generation fluoroquinolone (gatifloxacin)
	Systemic	3. Clarithromycin 500mg PO BID
		* *In case of resistance addition of Rifampin 30mg/mL.*
SurgicalTherapy		1. Flap lift and irrigation 2. Flap amputation in post-LASIK 3. Biopsy and culture 4. Penetrating keratoplasty

Table 8. We suggest a triple antibiotic treatment combined if needed with surgical therapy.

9. Modification to initial therapy

The medical response of mycobacterial keratitis to antibiotic therapy can be achieved by constant clinical observance. This can be difficult to appreciate in the first days of treatment due to increase in inflammation and local reaction to topical agents. The clinical response varies depending on the microorganism and pathogenicity of the mycobacteria, duration of the infection, risk factors involved and the patient's individual response (immunosuppresion).

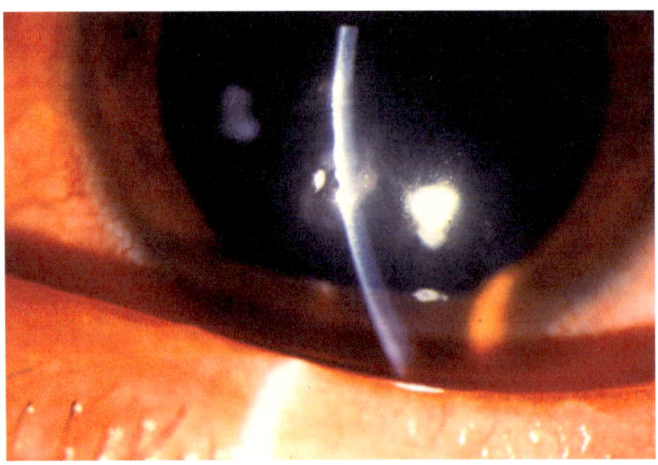

Figure 10. Patient 4 presented in the first clinical examination a paracentral infiltrate caused by *Mycobacteria chelonae*. Previous to initiation of proper antibiotic treatment. At this moment visual acuity was count fingers 2 meters.

http://dx.doi.org/10.5772/45964

If the chosen therapy is effective, some response should manifest within the first of 24 to 72 hours of appropriate treatment. [Figure 10,11]. Said response manifests with the decrease of stromal infiltrates and less anterior chamber inflammation in case it exists. [Figure 12, 13]

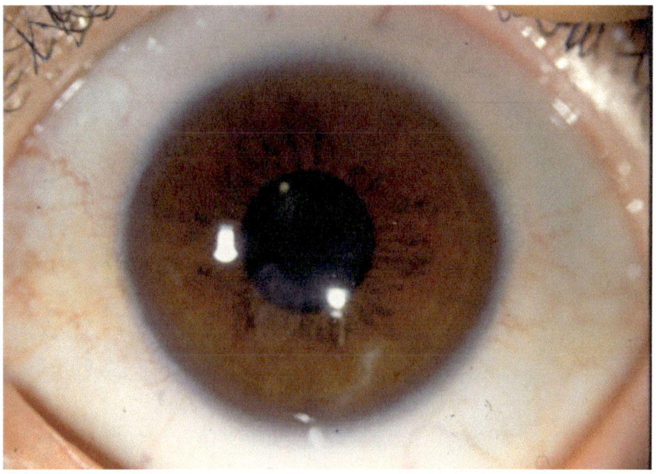

Figure 11. Patient 4 at 3 months follow-up after proper antibiotic treatment was applied. Final visual acuity was 20/30.

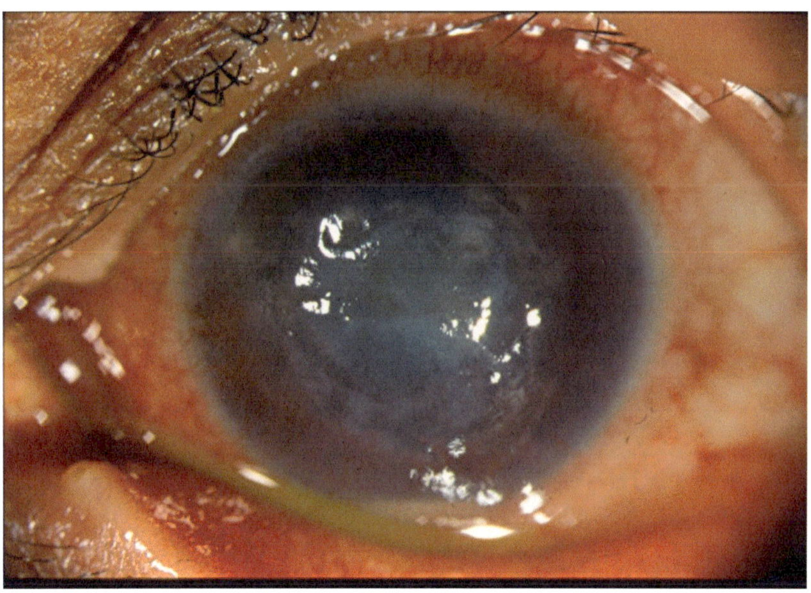

Figure 12. Patient 1 with preceding hypopyon (black arrow) and anterior chamber reaction who underwent a therapeutic flap amputation procedure.

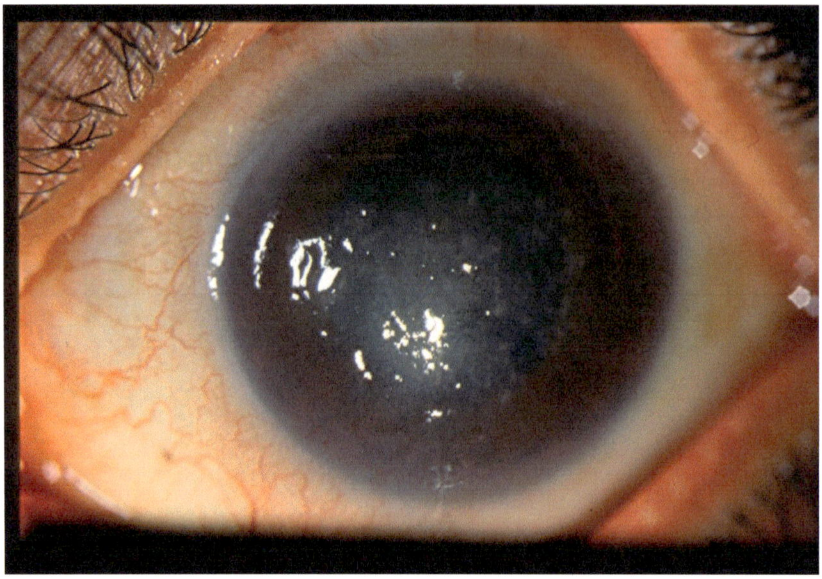

Figure 13. Absence of ahypopyon seen in Patient 1 as a manifestation of positive response to antibiotic treatment.

If clinical improvement exists at 48 hours of initiation of treatment, we encourage to continue the same pharmacological agents, reducing the administration time to 1 drop every 2 hours until completion of 5 days with night rest. After the 5 days, if further improvement exists, antibiotic doses should be decreased progressively in function of clinical response, drug tolerance and sensitivity tests results. Antibiotic with the best sensitivity should be the one chosen to continue the treatment for 2-3 more weeks.

Special caution should be kept when therapy is suspended, as some microorganisms may remain in corneal tissue. In this case, a prolonged treatment may be required.

If lesion progression occurs after 48 hours of initiation of treatment, manifested by evident increase in size, stromal thinning or incomplete resolution of symptoms, the ophthalmologist should consider a lack of sensitivity to the chosen treatment or a failure in the patient's attachment to the therapy. Culture results should be rechecked as well as sensitivity test results, as an addition of a different antimicrobial agent might be needed.[Table 9]

Positive clinical response parameters	Negative clinical response parameters
Peripheral corneal clearance of infiltrates and density reduction.	Increase in size or depth.
Decrease in stromal edema.	Stromal thinning.
Less anterior chamber inflammation.	Partial resolution of symptoms.
Corneal epithelial regeneration.	

Table 9. Response parameters associated with antibiotic therapy

http://dx.doi.org/10.5772/45964

10. Complementary therapy

Pain management: The cornea is a highly innervated tissue. Despite most of the times, these lesions tend to have an indolent course, on occasions, patients can refer any degree of pain, ranging from mild to severe. The clinician should administer a cyclopegic agent to ease the symptoms caused by ciliary spasms and to prevent the formation of sinequiae. We recommend the employment of cyclopentolate 1% eye drops or Atropine 1% collyrium every 12 hours.

Topical corticosteroids: Its role and appropriate moment of use is a controversial topic. Corticosteroids are applied to diminish the host's inflammatory response, capable of producing tissue destruction. Its use is also aimed to decrease the subsequent corneal cicatrization. Nevertheless, some potential adverse effects of these agents include bacterial growth stimulation by local immunosuppression, decrease in phagocytic activity, inhibition of collagen synthesis, drug-induced glaucoma and secondary cataract formation. Several experimental studies have shown a lack of harmful effects associated by addition of steroids to the preexistent bactericidal regime in keratitis. However, other studies documented an increase in bacterial growth with the addition of topical steroids to previous therapy. Due to the uncertain role of these agents in keratitis caused by nontuberculous mycobacteria, we recommend the use of low doses of steroids like fluorometholone (Flumetol® SOPHIA, S.A. de C.V., Laboratorios. Guadalajara, México) if it is considered appropriate, only when certainty exists of the infectious process being under control or in an inactive phase.

Alternate medical treatment: Authors have recommended the use of Azithromycin 2mg/mL or 1%, prepared Clarithromycin eye drops 10mg/mL, imipenem, tobramycin and systemic doxyciclin. We do not have experience with these drugs. [1,5]

Surgical treatment Conjunctival flap: Its purpose is aimed to provide blood vessels to the infected area, thus promoting curation. It is indicated in uncontrolled progression of the corneal lesion or infiltrates, limbal compromise with imminent scleritis or elevated risk of corneal perforation.

Therapeutic penetrating keratoplasty: It is difficult to perform in the initial stages of mycobacterium keratitis, furthermore it involves a higher incidence of complications and an inferior graft survival rate in comparison to optical PKP in an inactive process. We recommend to avoid this surgical option when possible. The indications for urgent therapeutic PKP are:

- Uncontrolled progression of the infection.
- Imminent risk of corneal perforation
- Confirmed cornealperforation.

We recommend maximal antibiotic therapy for 48 hours prior to surgery to decrease the number of bacterial colonies as much as possible and consequently the diminish the risk of endophthalmitis. Additional to topical antibiotics, we suggest the use of systemic antimicrobial and antiinflammatory agents in the preoperative period. The trepan employed on the recipient's cornea should be of enough size to extract the entire infected area, and the donor's corneal graft should be 0.5mm bigger than the measurement made on the recipient's cornea. It is advisable to obtain cultures from one half of the obtained cornea tissue (including stains and special culture media), and the other half should be sent for histopathological study. Sutures should be placed separately due to intense inflammatory reaction. In the postoperative period, corticosteroid therapy should be continued as well as specific antibiotics. Systemic therapy should continue. Posterior to the complete resolution of corneal infection, an optical PKP is an option of treatment to seek visual rehabilitation, as seen in out patient that appears on [Table 7]. As a consequence of the long term infectious process caused by mycobacterium keratitis, secondary cataract formation can be induced by the production of toxins, iridocyclitis, treatment toxicity and corticosteroid usage. For this complication, and optic PKP combined with a cataract extraction and Ahmed valve implantation can be considered as a treatment option, as seen in patient 1 who developed glaucoma.[Table 6,7]

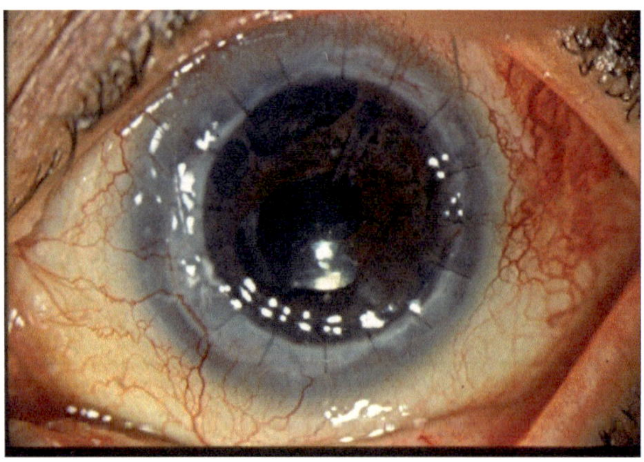

Figure 14. Patient 1 treated with optic PKP combined with Ahmed valve implantation and cataract extraction with colocation of intraocular lens posterior to the resolution of nontuberculous mycobacterial keratitis.

11. Conclusion

We describe our experience in patients who developed keratitis caused by nontuberculous mycobacteria. As the most common cause of post-LASIK keratitis is NTM, a greater degree of suspicion, recognition of typical clinical course and presentation, and knowledge of similar cluster of NTM keratitis prompts rapid institution of appropriate antibiotic therapy, granting this cases with a better prognosis in comparison with those of late diagnosis. Antibiotic resistance continues to be an emerging problem, thus a limitation in the coverage of this pharmacological agents exists. We emphasize the need for vigilance in the follow-up of patients. Appropriate adjustment of antimicrobial therapy may be required based on cultures and sensitivity tests when atypical mycobacteria are responsible for corneal infection.

We believe that fourth-fluoroquinolones adequately combined with first-line antibiotics constitute the best option so far to treat keratitis caused by atypical mycobacteria.

Acknowledgements

We express our gratitude to the cornea service and pathology service at Asociación Para Evitar La Ceguera en México "Hospital Dr. Luís Sánchez Bulnes" for their valuable contribution with images that helped making this chapter possible. Also to Miss. Elia Portugal for her assistance in the translation of this work.

Author details

Ana Lilia Pérez-Balbuena[1], David Arturo Ancona-Lezama[1], Lorena Gutiérrez-Sánchez[1] and Virginia Vanzzini-Zago[2]

1 Cornea Service. Asociación para Evitar la Ceguera en México I.A.P. "Hospital. Dr. Luis Sánchez Bulnes". Vicente García Torres,México D.F., México

2 Laboratory of Microbiology. Asociación para Evitar la Ceguera en México I.A.P. "Hospital. Dr. Luis Sánchez Bulnes". Vicente García Torres, México D.F., México

References

[1] Moorthy RS, Valluri S, Rao NA. Major Review; Nontuberculous Mycobacterial Ocular and Adnexal Infections.SurvOphthalmol 2012;57:202-235.

[2] Pallikaris IG, Papatzanaki ME, Stathi EZ, et al. Laser in situ keratomileusis. Lasers Surg Med 1990;10:463-468.

[3] Krachmer JH, Mannis MJ, Holland EJ. Cornea, Chapter 82. Nontuberculous Mycobacteria Keratitis. 3rd edition. ElSevier Mosby.

[4] Chandra NS, Torres MF, Winthrop KL, Bruckner DA, Heidemann DG, Calvet HM, Yakrus M, Mondino BJ, Holland GN. Cluster of Mycobacterium chelonae keratitis cases following laser in-situ keratomileusis. Am J Ophthalmol. 2001:132(6):819-830.

[5] Ford JG, Huang AJ, Pflugfelder SC, Alfonso EC, Forster RK, Miller D. Nontuberculous mycobacterial keratitis in south Florida. Ophthalmology. 1998:105(9):1652-1658.

[6] Freitas D, Alvarenga L, Sampaio J, Mannis M, Sato E, Sousa L, Vieira L, Yu MC, Martins MC, Hoffling-Lima A, Belfort R Jr. An outbreak of Mycobacterium chelonae infection after LASIK. Ophthalmology. 2003:110(2):276-285.

[7] Garg P, Bansal AK, Sharma S, Vemuganti GK. Bilateral infectious keratitis after laser in situ keratomileusis: a case report and review of the literature. Ophthalmology. 2001;108(1):121-125.

[8] Kouyoumdjian GA, Forstot SL, Durairaj VD, Damiano RE. Infectious keratitis after laser refractive surgery. Ophthalmology. 2001 Jul;108(7):1266-1268.

[9] Maloney RK. Cluster of Mycobacterium chelonae keratitis cases following laser in situ keratomileusis. Am J Ophthalmol. 2002:134(2):298-299.

[10] Solomon A, Karp CL, Miller D, Dubovy SR, Huang AJ, Culbertson WW. Mycobacterium interface keratitis after laser in situ keratomileusis. Ophthalmology. 2001:108(12):2201-2208.

[11] Sossi N, Feldman RM, Feldman ST, Frueh BE, McGuiere G, Davis C. Mycobacterium gordonae keratitis after penetrating keratoplasty Arch. Ophthalmol. 1991:109(8): 1064-1065.

[12] Winthrop KL, Steinberg EB, Holmes G, Kainer MA, Werner SB, Winquist A, Vugia DJ. Epidemic and sporadic cases of nontuberculous mycobacterial keratitis associated with laser in situ keratomileusis. Am J Ophthalmol. 2003;135(2):223-224.

[13] Pfyffer GE, Palicova F. Mycobacterium: General characteristics, laboratory detection, and staining procedures. In Versalovic J, Carrol KC, Funke G, Jorgensen JH, Landry ML, Warnock DW. Manual of Clinical Microbiology 10th ed. ASM press. Washington DC. 472-502.

[14] Runyon EH. Identification of mycobacterial pathogens using colony characteristics. Am J ClinPathol. 1970;54:578-586.

[15] Vincent V, Brown-Elliot BA, Jost KC Jr, et al. Mycobacterium: Phenotypic and Genotypic Identification, in Murray PR, Baron EJ, Jorgensen JH, Pfaller MA, Yolken RH (eds) Manual of Clinical Microbiology. Vol. 1. Washington, DC, ASM Press, 2003, 8th ed, pp 560-658.

[16] Broadway DC, Kerr-Muir MG, Eykyn SJ, Pambakian H. Mycobacterium chelonei keratitis: a case report and review of previously reported cases. Eye 1994; 8: 134-142.

[17] Fowler AM, Dutton JJ, Fowler WC, et al. Mycobacterium chelonaecanaliculitis associated with SmartPlug use. Ophthal Plast ReconstrSurg. 2008;24:241-243.

[18] Chang WJ, Tse DT, Rosa RH Jr, et al. Periocular atypical mycobacterial infections. [see comment]. Ophthalmology. 1999;106:86-90.

[19] Mauriello JA Jr. Atypical Mycobacterial Study G. Atypical mycobacterial infection of the periocular region after periocular and facial surgery. OphthalPlastReconstr Surg. 2003;19:182-188

[20] Margo CE, Pavan PR. Mycobacterium chelonae conjunctivitis and scleritis following vitrectomy. Arch Ophthalmol. 2000;118:1125—1128.

[21] Nash KA, Zhang Y, Brown-Elliott BA, et al. Molecular basis of intrinsic macrolide resistance in clinical isolates of Mycobacterium fortuitum. J AntimicrobChemother. 2005; 55:170-177.

[22] Benz MS, Murray TG, Dubovy SR, et al. Endophthalmitis caused by Mycobacterium chelonaeabscessus after intravitreal injection of triamcinolone. Arch Ophthalmol. 2003;121:271-273.

[23] Velotta JT. Nontuberculous (atypical) mycobacterial keratitis after LASIK: current status and clinical implications. Cornea. 2005;24:245-255

[24] Rola NH, Baha N, Hayham IS,Randa H, Johnny MK. Recalcitrant post-LASIK Mycobacterium chelonae Keratitis Eradicates after the Use of Fourtn–Generation Fluoroquinolone .Ophthalmology 2006;113:950-954.

[25] Lazar M, Nemet P, Bracha R, et al. Mycobacterium fortuitum keratitis. Am J Ophthalmol 1974;78:530-532.

[26] Reviglio V, Rodriguez ML, Picotti GS, et al. Mycobacterium Chelonae Keratitis Following Laser in situ Keratomileusis. J Refract Surg 1998;14:357-360.

[27] Mirate D, Hull D, Steel J, et al. Mycobacterium chelonei keratitis: a case report. Br J Ophthalmol 1983;67:324-327.

[28] Zabel R, Mintsioulis G, MacDonald I. Mycobacterium keratitis in a soft contact lens wearer. Can J Ophthalmol. 1988;23:315-317.

[29] Chang MA, Jain S, Azar DT. Infections following laser in situ keratomileusis: an integration of the published literature. SurvOphthalmol. 2004;49:269-280.

[30] Solomon R, Donnenfeld ED, Azar DT. Infectious keratitis after laser in situ keratomileusis: Results of an ASCRS survey. J Cataract Refract Surg 2003;29:2001-2006

[31] Lin RT, Maloney RK- Flap complications associated with lamellar refractive surgery. Am J Ophthalmol 1999;127(2):129-136.

[32] Machat J. LASIK complications and their management. In Machat J, editor: Excimer laser refractive surgery: practice and principles, Thorofare, NJ 1996, Slacc 359-400.

[33] Alvarenga L, Fretias D, Hofling-Lima AL, et al. Infectious post-LASIK crystalline keratopathy caused by nontuberculous mycobacteria. Cornea. 2002;21:426-429.

[34] De La Cruz J, Behlau I, Pineda R. Atypical mycobacteria keratitis after laser in situ keratomileusis unresponsive to fourth-generation fluoroquinolone therapy. J Cataract ReractSurg 2007;33:1318-1321.

[35] Shukla PK, Kumar M, Keshava GBS. Mycotic keratitis: an overview of diagnosis and therapy. Mycoses. 2008;51:183-199.

[36] Dart JKG, Saw VPJ, Kilvington S. Acanthamoeba keratitis: diagnosis and treatment update 2009. Am J Ophthalmol. 2009;148:487-499.

[37] Knickelbein JE, Hendricks RL, Charukamnoetkanok P. Management of herpes simplex virus stromal keratitis: An evidence-based review. SurvOphthalmol. 2009;54:226-234.

[38] Schonherr U, Naumann GO, Lang GK, et al. Sclerokeratitis caused by Mycobacterium marinum. Am J Ophthalmol. 1989;108:607-608

[39] Donnenfeld ED, Kim TK, Holland EJ Azar DT, Palmon FR, Rubenstein JB, Daya S, Yoo SH. American Society of Cataract and Refractive Sugery Cornea Clinical Committee. ASCRS White Paper. Management of infectious keratitis following laser in situ keratomileusis. J Cataract Refract Surg 2005;31:2008-2011.

[40] Llovet F, de Rojas V, Interlandi E, Martín C, Cobo-Soriano R, Ortega-Usobiaga J, Baviera J. Infectiouskeratitia in 204586 LASIK procedures. Ophthalmology 2010;117:232-238.

[41] Pérez-Balbuena AL, Vanzzini-Zago V, Garza M, Cuevas-Cancino D. Atypical Mycobacterium Keratitis Associated With Penetrating Keratoplasty: Case Report of Successful Therapy With Topical Gatifloxacin 0.3%. Cornea 2010;29:468-470.

[42] Bullington RH Jr, Lanier JD, Font RL. Nontuberculous mycobacteria keratitis; report of two cases and review of the literature. Arch Ophthalmol 1992;110:519-524.

[43] Hu F-R, Luh K-T. Topical ciprofloxacin for treating nontuberculous mycobacterial keratitis. Ophthalmology 1998;105:269-272.

[44] Schlech BA, Alfonso E. Overview of the potency of moxifloxacin ophthalmic solution 0.5% (VIGAMOX®). SurvOphthalmol 2005;50(suppl):S7-S15.

[45] Hamam RN, Noureddin B, Salti H, et al. Recalcitrant post-LASIK Mycobacterium chelonae keratitis eradicated after the use of fourth-generation fluoroquinolones. Ophthalmology 2006;113:950-954.

[46] Hyon JY, Joo MJ, Hose S, et al comparative efficacy of topical gatifloxacin with ciprofloxacin, amikacin, and clarithromycin in the treatment of experimental Mycobacterium chelonae keratitis. Arch Ophthalmol 2004,122:1166-1169.

[47] Shih et al have reported full months of therapy even when the appropriate antibiotic, chosen by drug sensitivity test results, is used. (Shih MH, Huang FC. Effects of Photodynamic Therapy on Rapidly Growing Nontuberculous Mycobacteria Keratitis. Invest Ophthalmol Vis Sci. 2011; 52:223-229.

[48] Banoch PR, Hay GJ, McDonellPJ, et al. A rat model of bacterial keratitis :effects of antibiotics and corticosteroids. Arch Ophthalmol 1980,98:718-20.

[49] Leibowitz HM, Kupferman A. Topically administered corticosteroids: effect with antibiotic treated bacterial keratitis. Arch opthalmol 1980, 98: 1287-1290.

http://dx.doi.org/10.5772/45964

[50] Pérez-Balbuena AL, Santander-García D, Vanzzini-Zago V. Therapeutic Keratoplasty for Microbial Keratitis. In: MoscaL. Keratoplasties. Surgical Techinques and Complications. Rijeka: InTech; 2011.

Chapter 9

Endophthalmitis: Experience from a Tertiary Eye Care Center

Imtiaz A. Chaudhry, Hassan Al-Dhibi,
Waleed Al-Rashed, Hani S. Al-Mezaine,
Yonca O. Arat and Wael Abdelghani

Additional information is available at the end of the chapter

http://dx.doi.org/10.5772/54431

1. Introduction

Endophthalmitis is a devastating ocular inflammatory process that can lead to blindness. In endophthalmitis, there is inflammation of the vitreous cavity along with the retinal and uveal components of the eye. [1] In the vast majority of cases of endophthalmitis, inflammation is triggered by an infectious agent. [1, 2] The source of such infectious agent could be an exogenous such as following trauma or after an eye surgery (Figures 1 & 2). Eye surgeries may be either intraocular (such as cataract, glaucoma, retina) or extra-ocular such as refractive or muscle surgery. Post-operative endophthalmitis could be either sterile or infectious. The infectious agent encountered following the eye surgery or trauma is usually the organisms harboring the outer surface of the eye. [2, 3] Bacterial infections are the most common cause of post-operative endophthalmitis, and Gram-positive isolates account for the majority of these cases. [2] Fungal infections may occur, particularly in association with the use of contaminated ocular irrigation fluids. [4, 5] Patients having previous history of glaucoma surgery with thin blebs and penetrating keratoplasty may also be vulnerable to risks of developing endophthalmitis. Endogenous endophthalmitis is less common and occur secondary to hematogenous dissemination and spread from a distant infective source in the body. [2, 3, 6, 7] In patients with endogenous endophthalmitis, some of the predisposing risk factors may include diabetes, cardiac disease, and malignancy. [2, 3] The common foci of infection may be urinary tract infection, septic arthritis, pneumonia, and endocarditis. Less common causes of endogenous endophthalmitis include orbital and periorbital cellulitis and in rare cases facial cellulitis. [8] Recently, endophthalmitis was a major reason for evisceration among the 187 cases reported from a tertiary eye care center. [9]

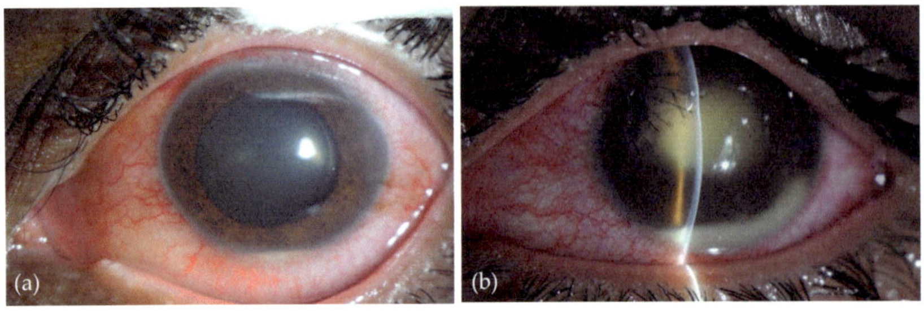

Figure 1. Signs of early post-operative endophthalmitis in patients after intraocular surgery (a) and after repair of traumatic eye injury (b) after injury.

2. The etiology of endophthalmitis

The spectrum of the microorganisms causing endophthalmitis may differ in different parts of the World. According to the Western literature, over 75% of culture positive cases of endophthalmitis are due to Gram-positive bacteria that includes, Staphylococcus species, Streptococcus species, Enterococcus species, and other Gram-positive species. [2, 3] Gram-negative species may account for up to 6% of endophthalmitis cases. Studies from other countries such as India reveal that Gram-positive bacteria may account for 53% of post-operative cases of endophthalmitis and up to 26% may be due to Gram-negative bacteria, while rest 17% may be due to fungal infection. [2, 3, 10, 11]

3. Presenting features of endophthalmitis and diagnosis

An eye with inflammation that is out of proportion to the predicted post-operative clinical course or previous trauma than expected should be suspected of having endophthalmitis. [1-3, 12] Majority of patients with post-operative endophthalmitis present with an acute onset usually within a week after surgery. [12] Most common presentations include decreased vision, ocular pain, photophobia, redness, corneal edema, hypoyon and vitritis (Figure 2). In addition, retinal vasculitis, retinal hemorrhages, and posterior pole hypoyon may also occur. Chronic post-operative endophthalmitis is characterized by insidious inflammation and appears less common than the acute type. Patients with chronic post-operative endophthalmitis usually present several weeks after surgery and often these patients have infection with less virulent bacterial and fungal pathogens. [13]

Progressive vitritis is one of the key findings in cases of infectious and non-infectious endophthalmitis, and in the vast majority of cases, a hypopyon can be seen at the time of initial presentation. [2, 3] Absence of a fundus red-reflex, presence of relative afferent pupillary defect (RAPD) and light perception vision at the time of initial presentation may be associated with worse final visual outcome (Figure 3). Infections with virulent organisms present with

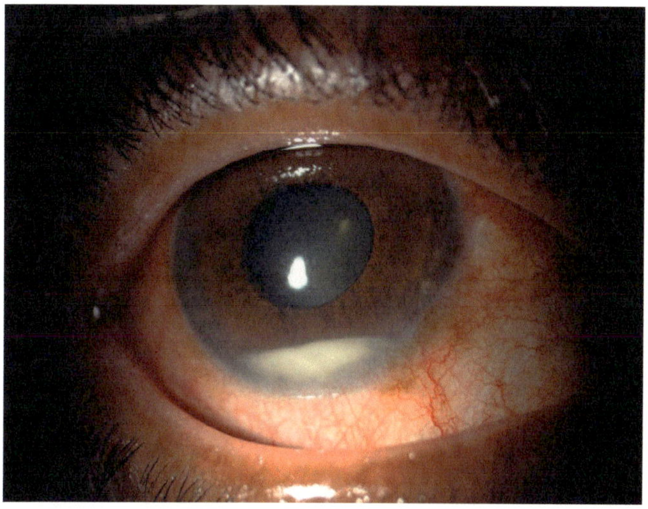

Figure 2. Anterior chamber reaction and hypopyon in a patient with endophthalmitis.

aggressive signs and symptoms of endophthalmitis. Other risk factors associated with worse visual outcome may include presence of corneal infiltrate, wound abnormalities after cataract surgery and virulent pathogens. According to the Endophthalmitis Vitrectomy Study (EVS), [10] a prospective, randomized clinical trial of post-operative acute endophthalmitis, hypopyon was documented in 75% of the enrolled patients and according to the European Society of Cataract and Refractive Surgeons Endophthalmitis Study (ESCRS), hypopyon was present in 72% of patients having endophthalmitis. [11, 14] Pain was absent in almost one-fourth of patients enrolled in the EVS at the time of their initial presentation. Untreated endophthalmitis may lead to panophthalmitis which may present with increased pain, proptosis, limitation of eye movements, eyelid edema, intense conjunctival chemosis, corneal edema, infiltrate, complete anterior chamber hypopyon and even eye perforation. [15]

Patients having full blown endophthalmitis within days after the surgery often have infection due to Staphylococcus or Streptococcus species or alpha-hemolytic Streptococci species of the 'viridans' group during which vision can be lost over 12 hours if no intervention is undertaken. [10, 16-18] A diagnosis of endophthalmitis should be entertained for any patient presenting within 6 weeks after surgery with pain and loss of vision. In most cases, the diagnosis of endophthalmitis is made on clinical grounds. Ultrasonography is necessary for the clinical evaluation of patients with suspected infectious endophthalmitis in the absence of a good fundus view. Rapid detection and identification of the causative pathogens is crucial for vision-saving treatment. [19] Conjunctival and corneal swabs are usually not helpful, as the correlation with the microorganisms isolated is very low. [2, 10, 11, 18] Similarly, microorganism identification from the anterior chamber is less successful as compared to vitreous tap in cases of suspected endophthalmitis. Depending on the visual acuity, an anterior chamber tap and a vitreous tap along with intra-vitreal antibiotics may be indicated to confirm the infection and treat the cause. Samples of aqueous and vitreous should be collected

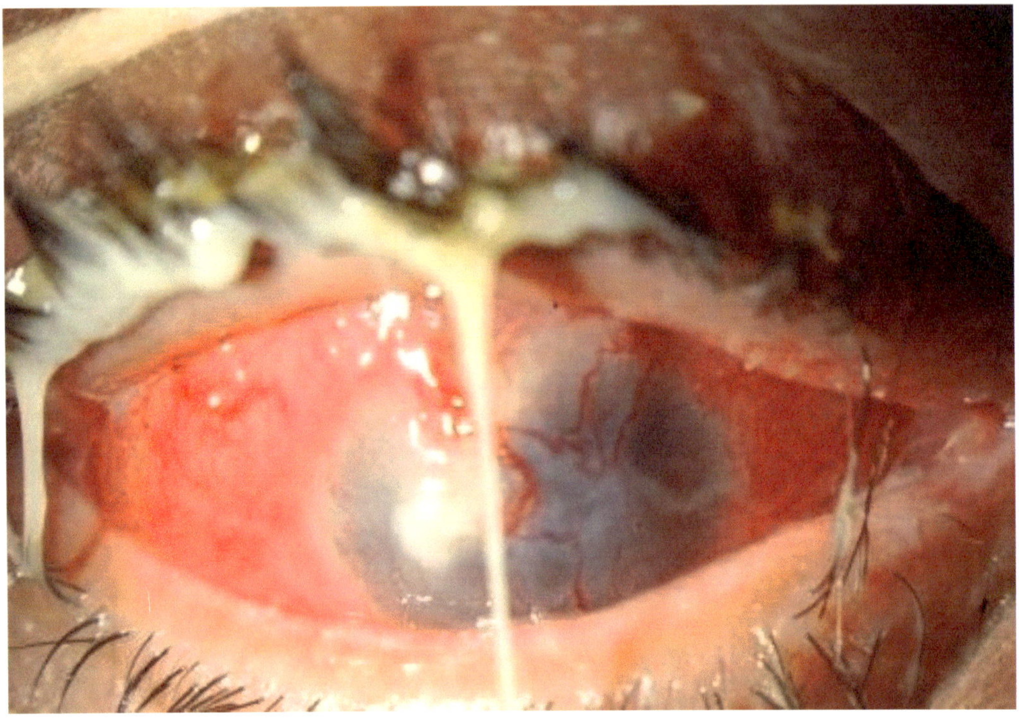

Figure 3. External photograph of a patient with history of cataract surgery who presented with severe conjunctivitis, corneal opacification and vascularization was found to have evidence of endophthalmitis.

from these patients for Gram staining, culture, and Polymerase Chain Reaction (PCR) assay. [20] Anterior chamber and vitreaous specimens obtained should be directly inoculated on to the culture media at the time of procedure. If any of these investigations yield a positive result, the case can be classified as a proven case of infective endophthalmitis; otherwise the case should be classified as presumed unproven endophthalmitis. Each unproven case should be carefully considered if there is evidence of the Toxic Anterior Segment Syndrome (TASS) or non-infective uveitis when the case is not considered infective otherwise. [21, 22]

Patients presenting late after surgery with uveitis that has not responded to a course of corticosteroids need to be investigated for chronic infectious endophthalmitis. One should always consider the possibility of having an infection within the capsular sac with Propionibacterium species, Corynebacterium species, or coagulase negative Staphylococci. [1, 3, 23, 24] Such infections may persist years after the ocular surgery and require an anterior chamber and vitreous tap. Some of the bacterial organisms may be sequestered within macrophages surrounded by lens capsule. In these circumstances, removal of the intraocular lens or exchange to prevent recurrent or persistent endophthalmitis may be necessary. These patients may present initially as having uveitis and hypopyon within 6-8 weeks of surgery, which fails to respond to corticosteroids and needs eventual vitrectomy with intra-vitreal antibiotics and often the removal of the intraocular lens (IOL). In chronic saccular endophthalmitis, there is granulomatous inflammation and characteristic white capsular plaque.

[13, 23] A"trial of therapy"with Clarithromycin or Azithromycin may be considered since these drugs penetrate well into the tissue, and Propionibacterium acnes is very sensitive to these drugs. [13, 24, 25] For unknown reasons, culture-negative endophthalmitis may respond well when the patient is treated with clarithromycin. [25] One needs to be aware, that Propionibacterium acnes may appear as a Gram-variable coccobacillus when the specimen is obtained from the anterior chamber or vitreous. The PCR technique has been found to be more sensitive to identify bacteria in these situations. [20] Molecular techniques using multiplex or broad-range PCR may enable rapid detection and identification of causative pathogens in ocular infectious diseases. In certain circumstances, PCR technique may provide the results of the causative micro-organism within 6 hours of biopsy. The PCR method offers much improved pathogen detection especially in the case of chronic endophthalmitis with low pathogen counts. PCR was extensively evaluated in the multi-center European prophylaxis study of postoperative endophthalmitis following cataract surgery and was found to be useful in identifying 6 out of 20 pathogens causing endophthalmitis where standard Gram-stain and cultures results were found to be negative. [11] Multiplex PCR has the drawback of allowing only a limited number of genes to be analyzed in one reaction, and pre-identification of the species level is required. Analysis of amplicons by DNA sequencing after broad-range PCR, are the most used techniques for identifying DNA, but the time and effort associated with data analysis lead to some limitations. Therefore, improved high-throughput genotyping methods that are sensitive and discriminative may be desired. DNA microarray technology has been found to be a promising genotyping method that allows simultaneous identification of a wide variety of genes and rapid determination of the genetic profile of a microorganism in a single experiment. DNA microarray technique may be useful for genetic screening and identification of microorganisms in cases of suspected infectious endophthalmitis. [26]

4. Exogenous bacterial endophthalmitis

Patients may present days or several weeks following cataract or other ocular surgery with reduced visual acuity (VA) and signs of inflammation in the anterior chamber along with other evidence suggestive of endophthalmitis. [27, 28] Intraocular surgery remains the most common cause of endophthalmitis considering the number of cataract surgeries being performed around the World. [12] The infection may also occur following glaucoma surgery, retina surgery and even following strabismus surgery. [29, 30] Ocular trauma remains another major source of endophthalmitis especially in cases of Retained Intraocular Foreign Body (IOFB). Symptoms of acute endophthalmitis in these patients may include decreased vision, pain, swollen eye lids, conjunctival chemosis with discharge and photophobia. [31] There may be signs of conjunctival and corneal edema, anterior chamber inflammation with inflammatory cells, hypopyon or fibrin clot (Figure 4). Presence of vitreous haze may prevent clear view of the fundus. Loss of the red reflex may be a poor guide to the general state of the vitreous, which may be most opaque anteriorly where the inflammatory process has begun. In some instances, signs of endophthalmits following ocular surgery or trauma may appear soon. For example, acute suppurative endophthalmitis due to Streptococcus pyogenes may occur days after cataract surgery in which case the patient may present with swollen eyelid, opaque cornea, conjunctival chemosis and significant pain. [2, 3] Endophthalmitis elicits an aggressive inflammatory reaction that can result in the breakdown of the blood-ocular barrier. Such acute inflammatory process may need to be controlled in order to preserve vision by protecting the uveal tissue. Intra-vitreal Dexamethasone at the time of vitreal biopsy and intra-vitreal antibiotics has been found to be very helpful in minimizing uveal tissue damage.

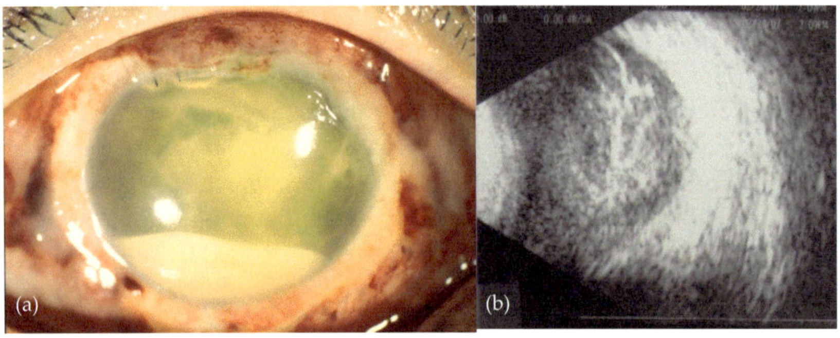

Figure 4. External photograph of a patient's right eye who presented with decreased vision, pain, tearing, redness and photophobia several days after having penetrating trauma to his right eye. He was found to have conjunctival chemosis along with anterior chamber hypopyon (a). Ultrasonography revealed evidence of vitreous opacification suggestive of endophthalmitis (b).

5. Risk factors for the development of the post-operative endophthalmitis

The relative risks of developing post operative endophthalmitis depend on a number of factors, including the presence of eyelid or conjunctival diseases, the patient's general health, the use of immunosuppressant medications, the type of intraocular surgery, the type of intra-ocular lens (IOL) used and intra-operative complications. [31] Diabetes has been associated with endophthalmitis; one study revealed that among the 162 patients who were treated for endophthalmitis, 21% of them had evidence of diabetes. In that study, patients with diabetes had poor visual outcome and the possibility was related to these patient's having poor wound healing ability. This association was also observed in the EVS trial, patients with diabetes had a trend toward worse vision at baseline, higher incidence of positive cultures and need for additional surgeries during follow-up. [33] Specific eyelid or peri-orbital diseases such as blepharitis, ectropion, entropion and paralytic disorders may enhance the chance of post-operative endophthalmitis. It is recommended that minimizing the contact between IOL and the ocular surface may reduce the risk of endophthalmitis at the time of its implantation. Risk of developing endophthalmitis has been reported to be lower with the introduction of injectable IOLs as compared with foldable lenses since injectable lenses avoid the contact with ocular surface. There is also evidence that certain kinds of materials used for manufacturing intraocular lenses may have higher incidence of endophthalmitis. For example, PMMA lenses may be associated with a higher rate of endophthalmitis as compared with acrylic IOLs. [5,

34, 35] Intra-operative complications, specifically posterior capsular break or vitreous loss may also be a cause of increased risk of post-operative endophthalmitis.

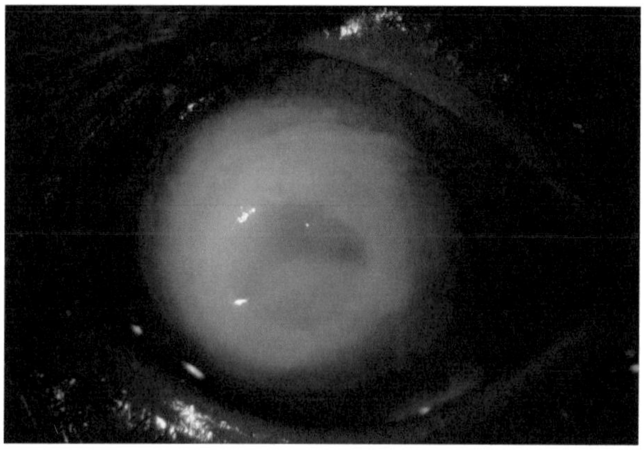

Figure 5. External photograph of a patient's left eye showing failed corneal graft due to infectious keratitis and endophthalmitis.

Procedures, such as penetrating keratoplasty, trabeculectomy, and glaucoma drainage device implantation have all been reported to cause endophthalmitis which are higher than simple cataract operation (Figure 5). [36] Endophthalmitis can occur in 0.2-9.6% of cases following glaucoma surgery depending on the procedure and the use of 5-fluorouracil or mitomycin-C as anti-fibrotic agents. [3, 29, 30] Rare causes of endophthalmitis have been reported following phakic IOL implantation for refractive errors and extra-ocular surgeries such as excision of pterygium, strabismus surgery and sclera buckling procedure. [4] Secondary IOL implantation has been found to be associated with the highest risk for developing endophthalmitis (0.2%–0.37%) and PPV with the lowest (0.03%–0.05%). Other sources of infection include, contaminated surgical equipment, irrigation fluids and poor patient hygiene. Other risk factors for the development of post-operative endophthalmitis include canaliculitis, acute and chronic dacryocystitis and anti-glaucoma aqueous drainage devices. [36-39] It is recommended that patient having any evidence of chronic canaliculitis, dacryocystitis should only undergo any intraocular surgery after resolution of their infection. Patients having chronic dacryocystitis may harbor multiple micro-organisms which may be resistant to the commonly prescribed post-cataract surgery prophylactic antibiotics. It has been reported that almost 10% of patients having chronic dacryocystitis in the setting of nasolacrimal duct obstruction may develop acute dacryocystitis requiring systemic antibiotics. [37-39]

6. Endophthalmitis following cataract surgery

Over 90% of post-operative endophthalmitis develop as a complication of cataract surgery since it is the most common intraocular surgery performed by ophthalmologists worldwide

(Figure 6). [3, 40] A century ago, the incidence of endophthalmitis after cataract operations was over 10% which has dramatically decreased since the advent of antibiotics and the utilization of aseptic techniques. During the era of extra capsular cataract extraction under improved hygiene conditions, the infection rate has fallen below 0.1% in the developed countries. [2] In the absence of prospective randomized case-controlled studies, the true incidence of endophthalmitis may be difficult to determine given its rare occurrence within a single center. [1-3] Recently, clinical features, microbiology and final visual outcome as well as the incidence of acute-onset post-operative endophthalmitis after cataract surgery have been reported from Saudi Arabia by Al-Mezaine et al, [12] from a single tertiary eye care center over a 10-year period. According to their retrospective series, the incidence of acute-onset endophthalmitis after cataract surgery was 0.068% and the most common presenting features were pain and poor red reflex. Staphylococcus species and Streptococcus species were the most common micro-organisms encountered. Visual outcomes were good in cases of endophthalmitis following phacoemulsification and in those caused by Staphylococcus epidermidis and worse in cases that were caused by Streptococcus species. Overall, clear corneal phacoemulsification had a 1.73-fold higher risk for acute endophthalmitis than extra-capsular cataract extraction but the visual outcome was worse in post-extra capsular cataract extraction cases. In this series, the poor visual outcome was associated with more virulent organisms and delayed presentation. [12]

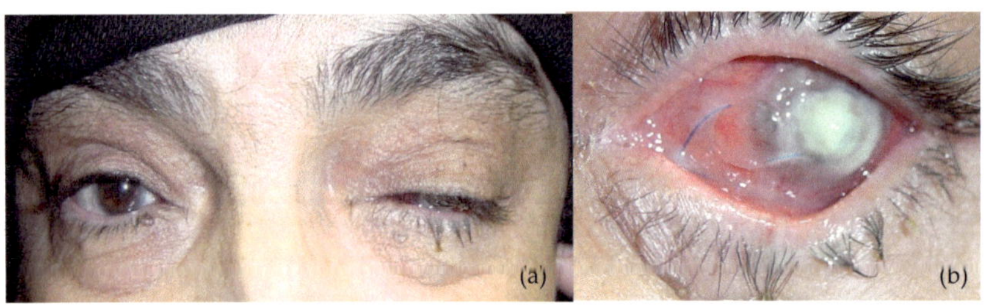

Figure 6. External photograph of a 65-years-old female who underwent uneventful cataract extraction along-with intraocular lens implantation in her left eye. Two weeks later, she presented with painful left eye and complete loss of vision (a). She was found to have necrosis of her left corneal wound and extrusion of the implanted intra-ocular lens (b).

A review of the literature has provided a greater number of patients with risk factors for the development of endophthlamitis. [2, 3, 40] In a systematic review of the literature by Taban et al, [41] of 215 studies of 3,140,650 cataract extractions published between 1963 and 2003, a higher overall post-cataract endophthalmitis rate occurred between 2000 and 2003 (0.265%) as compared with between 1963 and 2000 (0.128%). The rate of endophthalmitis was higher with clear cornea incision (0.189%) versus scleral incision (0.079%) between 1992 and 2003. In another large population-based review of United States Medicare beneficiary claims between 1994 and 2001 of 447,627 cataract operations, 1026 cases of presumed endophthalmitis were noted and an increased incidence was associated with the introduction of clear cornea incision. [42] The incidence of endophthalmitis was higher from 1998 to 2001 (2.5 per 1000) as compared with between 1994 and 1997 (1.8 per 1000), possibly reflecting the increasing

http://dx.doi.org/10.5772/54431

use of clear corneal incisions during this time period. Some limitations to these larger studies are their being retrospective in nature that may differ in methodology and definitions. In addition, decreased preoperative use of povidine-iodine and fewer administrations of sub-conjunctival injections at the end of surgery may have occurred as ophthalmologists converted from retro-bulbar or peri-bulbar anesthesia to topical anesthesia during this time period which may be confounding factors leading to an increased rate of endophthalmitis. [2, 3, 42]

Following intraocular surgery, leak-proof closure of the corneal incision is recommended to limit access of microorganisms to the anterior chamber. [43] Evidence indicates that with the clear corneal incision, in the absence of sutures, the wound appears to be loose allowing microorganisms to enter into the eye and subsequent development of endophthalmitis. Type of wound closure may also be an important determinant of the endophthalmitis following PPV. [3, 44] As compared to the cataract surgery, the incidence of endophthalmitis following PPV is low and ranges between 0.03-0.05%. [3] However, even after PPV, the use of sutureless and minimal incision techniques have been found to be associated with higher incidence of post-operative endophthalmitis than standard closure technique.

7. Intra-operative antibiotic prophylaxis

Antibiotics are used in the irrigating solution as a prophylaxis by many ophthalmologists around the world during the routine cataract surgery operations. While it is suggested that the addition of antibiotics to the irrigating solution may have a protective effect, it has not been possible to reduce the incidence of endophthalmitis in any prospective clinical study. [45] Most of the studies on the incidence of endophthalmitis following intraocular surgery have been obtained either from the retrospective studies or from studies of antibiotic use where there was no control group. Prophylactic intra-cameral irrigation of antibiotics such as Cefuroxime and Vancomycin has been found to be beneficial against post-operative endophthalmitis. [46] The ESCRS demonstrated that the prophylactic use of intra-cameral antibiotics may help to reduce the incidence of post-operative endophthalmitis after cataract surgery by 75%. [47]

8. Post-operative antibiotic prophylaxis

Over the past several decades, sub-conjunctival antibiotics injection has been advocated as a prophylaxis against infection after most of the intraocular surgeries. [1-3] At the time of sub-conjunctival antibiotic injection, corticosteroids are frequently used as adjunctive treatment to reduce the inflammatory response due to infection that might help to reduce secondary damage. No study, however has proven that this method has any prophylactic effect on the prevention of endophthalmitis. [1] A retrospective report found one case of endophthalmitis after 8856 surgeries using sub-conjunctival antibiotics and 9 cases of endophthalmitis following 5030 surgeries without having sub-conjunctival injections. [48] Sub-conjunctival antibiotics may temporarily provide therapeutic levels in the anterior segment but do not penetrate sufficiently into the vitreous cavity, and hence larger retrospective studies did not reveal any additional benefit compared with intra-vitreal antibiotic application.

A careful wound construction with a minimum wound leakage and the placement of sutures when necessary is recommended to prevent incident of any post-operative infection. [19, 43] Optical coherence tomography may show variations in gaping of un-healed wounds and Indian ink may migrate through un-healed wound into the anterior chamber. Experience has shown that it may take upto a week before the epithelial surface heals completely to have the wound become water-tight. Therefore, it may be necessary that post-operatively one may consider addition of topical antibiotics drops. Some studies have suggested that silicone IOLs may have a three times higher risk of developing post-operative endophthalmitis than acrylic IOLs. On the other hand, hydrophilic heparin-coated IOLs have demonstrated their lower adherence for Staphylococcal organisms to the lens surface. [1-3] In order to reduce the risk of infection following clear corneal incisions, the use of topical antibiotic drops for 1-2 weeks after the surgery has been recommended. [49] Usually broad spectrum antibiotics are used to cover the most commonly encountered microorganism. These antibiotics are administered topically 4-6 times daily.

9. Toxic anterior segment syndrome (TASS)

One may need to differentiate between the postoperative endophthalmitis from the less common cases of TASS. The TASS presents acutely within the first 48-hours after surgery with pain and blurred vision. In these cases, there may be diffuse corneal edema of the whole cornea along with endothelial cell damage. One may see evidence of a small hypopyon along with signs of iritis that may result in iris atrophy. TASS is usually a toxic reaction in the absence of any infectious process and occurs in groups following intraocular surgery. [21] Acute endopthalmitis due to Bacillus cereus after cataract surgery have a fulminant onset with extremely high intraocular pressure, corneal edema and intense pain which may look like TASS. [22] However these eyes rapidly progress to develop corneal infiltrates, scleral and uveal tissue necrosis with hyphema, brownish exudates in anterior chamber and necrotizing retinitis within hours despite immediate intra-vitreal antibiotics and vitrectomy. One may see gram-positive bacilli from the aqueous. The organism is sensitive to conventional antibiotics except penicillin. Because acute onset endophthalmitis due to Bacillus cereus has an onset within 12 to 24 hours of intraocular surgery, it simulates TASS in the first few hours but then the clinical course of endophthalmitis due to Bacillus cereus is marked by rapidly worsening necrotizing infection, leading to very poor outcomes despite early institution of appropriate therapy. [22] One must closely observe every case of TASS that presents with intense pain and extremely high IOP and rule out acute post-operative endophthalmitis due to Bacillus cereus with microbiologic testing.

Different causes of TASS have been reported and timely action is required for proper diagnosis and treatment. Variety of stimuli including bacterial endotoxin (lipopolysaccharide cell wall of Gram-negative bacteria) from water within the ultrasound machine used for instruments cleaning or even from contaminated but sterile water used to make steam in an autoclave and viscoelastic materials used can cause TASS. TASS may also be due to agents stuck to devices that have become denatured, the wrong concentration of antibiotics used in the Basic Saline Solution (BSS) irrigating solution during intraocular surgery, use of drugs containing preservatives, BSS made up at the wrong pH, or ethylene oxide residue left on plastics. It is recommended that if an outbreak of several cases of TASS occurs, one should investigate the cause and consider stopping similar operative techniques and use of materials. [3, 21] Techniques of instrument cleaning, sterilization, type of water used for cleaning, autoclaving, and the use of reusable instruments and cannulae may need to be investigated. In these circumstances, representative samples should be collected for endotoxin assay from the various potential sources of TASS. Treatment is given with corticosteroids, which can be used aggressively once infection is excluded by making an anterior chamber tap for microscopy and culture and PCR testing if available. [21] Early diagnosis and treatment with a course of topical corticosteroids may yield a good visual prognosis.

10. Management of acute post-operative bacterial endophthalmitis

Evaluation and treatment of acute post-operative bacterial endophthalmitis is initiated when such infection is suspected, generally within few hours of patient's presentation. [1-3] In severe cases, 3-port PPV is recommended depending on the level of visualization. Posterior capsulotomy should be performed and pus and the fibrin material need to be aspirated. Aggressive surgery is not recommended in these circumstances since these eyes may have concomitant retinal vasculitis and edema which may result in retinal breaks and retinal detachment. Following PPV, intra-vitreal antibiotics are injected. [2, 3] Doses of antibiotics are reduced in cases of complete vitrectomy. In addition, intra-vitreal dexamethasone is also injected to reduce inflammation. [3] The procedure can be performed under general, peribulbar, or retro-bulbar anesthesia. General anesthesia may be indicated in cases of severely inflamed eyes. The use of vitrector may be required in cases of infected vitreous. Following the sampling, antibiotics and corticosteroids are injected through the sclerotomy and the sclerotomy incision may not require any suturing.

11. Late-onset post-operative endophthalmitis

Late cases of endophthalmitis after cataract operation are the 2nd most common form of endophthalmitis accounting for up to one-third cases of endophthalmitis. [1, 13] In the late-onset cases of endophthalmitis, the symptoms are milder and Propionibacterium acnes has been reported to be the cause in majority of cases (Figure 7). Because of the difficulty in culturing Propionibacterium acnes and the high rate of recurrence, anterior vitrectomy may be necessary. In these cases, one has to perform capsulectomy to remove the nidus of infection and make the area more accessible for the antibiotic penetration. A further advantage of vitrectomy is that adequate material for culturing the causative organism can be obtained besides obtaining of the capsular bag material as well. [3]

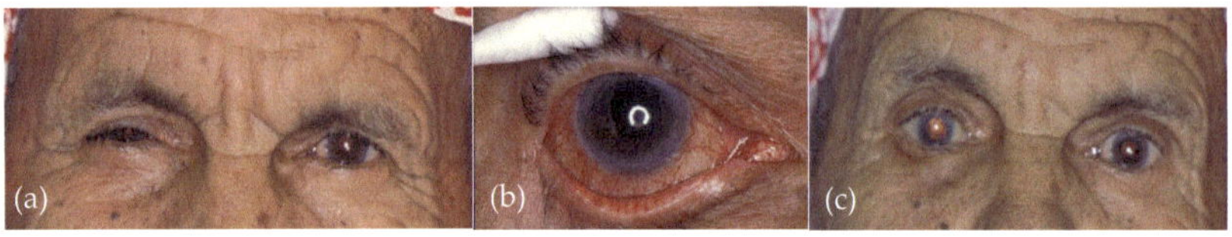

Figure 7. An elderly male patient presented with right eye pain, redness and photophobia (a), which was attributed to delayed onset post-operative endophthalmitis requiring intervention (b). After treatment of intraocular infection, patient's symptoms improved (c).

12. Bleb-related endophthalmitis

Bleb-related endophthalmitis usually follows a chronic course of infection (Figure 8). In these infections, commonest causative organisms are Streptococcus species and Gram-negative bacteria, especially Haemophilus influenzae. [29] Because of the existing history of glaucoma, visual prognosis in these cases is expected to be poor requiring early aggressive intervention. [3] These patients require immediate vitrectomy along with intra-vitreal antibiotic injection. These patients may also require systemic antibiotics. Most frequent causative organisms isolated in cases of delayed-onset bleb-related endophthalmitis include, Streptococcus species, Enterococcus and Gram-negative bacteria. [29] A retrospective consecutive case series of delayed-onset bleb-associated endophthalmitis seen at Bascom Palmer Eye Institute over a 14 year period identified 86 eyes of 85 patients from which 63% eyes were culture-positive. [50] The most common organisms recovered from cultures among these patients were: Streptococcus, 25%; Gram-negative, 18%; coagulase-negative Staphylococcus, 11%; Enterococcus, 7%; Moraxella, 10%; Pseudomonas, 4%; and Serratia, 4%. This large study revealed that culture-positive cases were associated with worse presenting visual acuity, higher presenting intraocular pressure, and worse visual outcomes than culture-negative cases. Streptococcus, Pseudomonas, and Serratia cases were associated with poor presenting view of the fundus and worse visual outcomes than coagulase-negative Staphylococcus and Moraxella cases. [50] Worse view of the fundus in the Streptococcus cases likely compelled the treating clinician to more frequently favor PPV.

13. Endophthalmitis vitrectomy study (EVS)

Endophthalmitis Vitrectomy Study, a multicenter randomized prospective clinical trial of 420 patients with acute post-operative endophthalmitis, showed that immediate PPV provided a clear benefit in a well defined subgroup; patients with light perception vision only at the time of presentation had a significant, 3-fold improved chance of obtaining 20/40 vi-

http://dx.doi.org/10.5772/54431

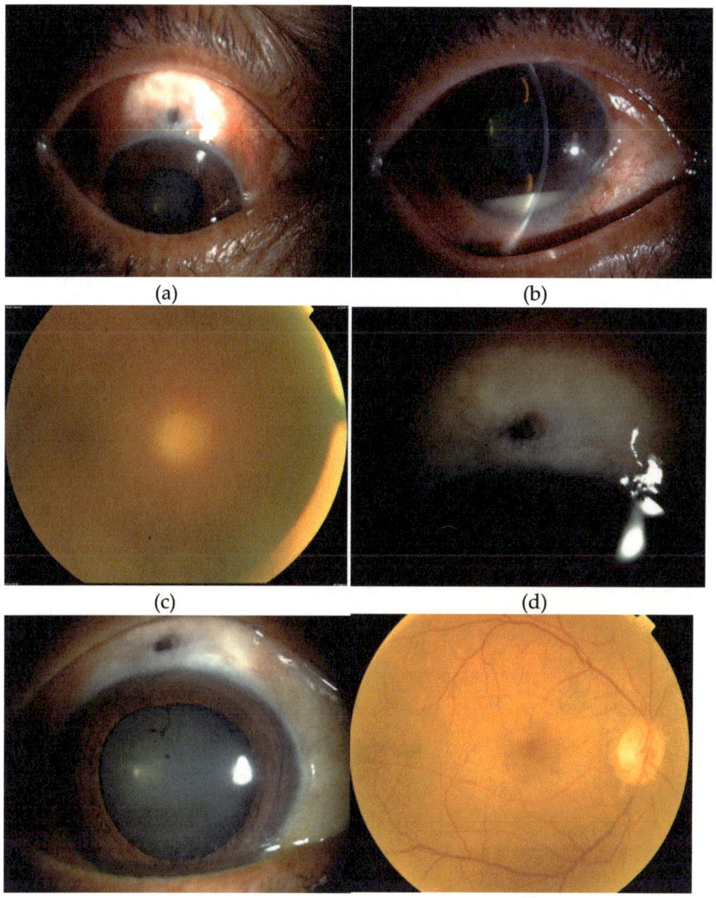

(a) (b) (c) (d) (e) (f)

Figure 8. External (a), slit-lamp (b) and fundus (c) photographs of a patient who developed bleb-related endophthalmitis which was treated with topical and intra-vitreal antibiotics resulting in resolution of infection as evident by external (d,e) and fundus photograph (f).

sion or better after PPV. [10] For diabetic patients with hand movement or better vision, at least a trend toward better final VA after PPV was documented compared with vitreous tap and biopsy only. Patients with diabetes had a trend toward worse vision at baseline, higher incidence of positive cultures and need for additional surgeries and worse final visual outcome. [33, 51, 52] According to the EVS recommendations, patients with acute post-operative endophthalmitis after a cataract operation with an initial vision of hand movements or better can be treated by vitreous biopsy and intra-vitreal antibiotics. [10] On the other hand patients having vision at presentation worse than hand movement should undergo immediate PPV. Further, patients with suspected aggressive pathogens such as acute Streptococcal endophthalmitis, immediate PPV may be necessary even though vision is better than light perception at their initial presentation. Immediate PPV can remove the highly inflammatory bacterial pathogens from the vitreous cavity. Retrospective studies have confirmed this notion that affected eyes can benefit from early PPV. Data has shown that there may be difference in how diabetic and non-diabetic patients behave with similar endophthalmitis. [53] Generally, diabetic patients having hand movement or better visual acuity obtain vision of 20/40 more often by PPV than after by only vitreous biopsy and the intra-vitreal injection of antibiotics. Type of infecting organism may have prognostic effect on the final visual outcome. Due to their ability to induce significant inflammation, Staphylococcus aureus, Streptococci, and Gram-negative isolates seem to result in a worse visual outcome. [2, 10] Infections with coagulase-negative Staphylococci had final visual acuity of 20/100 or better in the EVS population (84%). Additionally, 80% cases of culture-negative endophthalmitis resulted in a final visual acuity of 20/100 or better. Other strong predictors for poor visual outcome were initial visual acuity of light perception only, older age, corneal ring ulcers, compromised posterior capsule, abnormal intraocular pressure, presence of RAPD, rubeosis iridis, and absence of the red fundus reflex. [51] Benefits of vitrectomy include a better sample for cultures, reduction of pathogen load, toxins and inflammatory material.

14. Limitations of EVS

The EVS study recommendations do not apply to late-onset post-operative endophthalmitis, bleb-related endophthalmitis, post-traumatic endophthalmitis and endogenous endophthalmitis. [7, 52] In these circumstances and in the absence of any prospective studies, careful evaluation of each case may be recommended by the treating ophthalmologist. Generally, endophthalmitis in these cases may have more aggressive set of bacterial pathogens and therefore require vitrectomy along with intra-vitreal as well as systemic antibiotics. Although, the principles of management in cases of post-traumatic and endogenous endophthalmitis may be the same as for acute post-operative endophthalmitis, the visual outcome is usually dismal.

15. Endophthalmitis associated with microbial keratitis

Many cases of infectious keratitis may progress to endophthalmitis if not treated early in the course of the diseases. [4, 9] Patient with underlying conditions may have propensity to poor response to non-aggressive treatment of infectious keratitis. Infections due to some pathogens may be very difficult to treat in patients with diabetes and other systemic conditions (Figure 9). Patients with chronic diseases, past history of corneal trauma, cataract surgery with lack of posterior capsule, having used topical corticosteroids, compromised immune system and trachoma have a poor visual prognosis. The bacterial species include Mycobacterium chelonae, Nocardia species, Staphylococcus aureus, streptococci and Coliforms as well as Capnocytophaga. [3] In these patients, fungi are the most frequently reported organisms, of which Fusarium species are the commonest. Management in these patients may require early intervention that includes intra-vitreal antibiotics guided by the organisms seen on Gram and Ziehl-Neelsen stains of anterior chamber and vitreal taps.

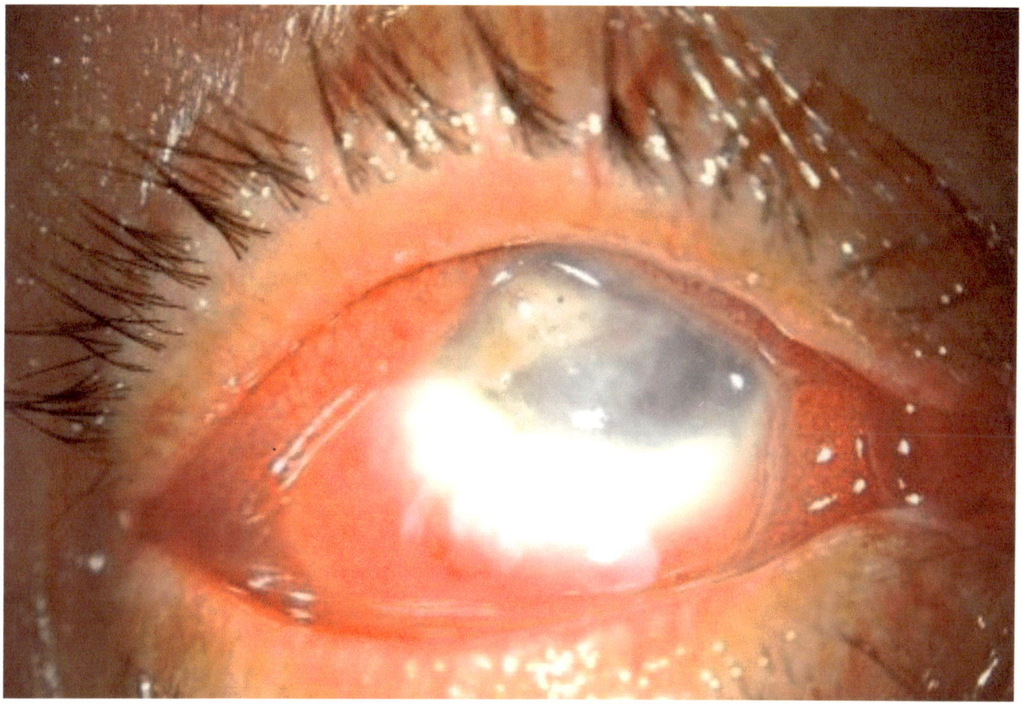

Figure 9. External photograph of a 55-years-old male patient who presented with corneal ulcer which progressed to endophthalmitis despite aggressive medical management.

16. Post-operative endophthalmitis: treatment

According to the EVS, 38% of eyes with post-operative endophthalmitis demonstrated Gram-positive cocci. [10] Since systemically administered antibiotics do not reach sufficient concentrations in vitreous, intravitreal injections have become the accepted primary route of delivery biotic delivery. Desired therapy includes antibiotics which cover most common Gram-positive organisms as well as Gram-negative bacteria. Current protocol includes Gram positive coverage by Vancomycin (1.0 mg/0.1 mL) along with Gram-negative coverage by Ceftazidime (2.25 mg/0.1 mL). If indicated, alternative drugs such as Amikacin (400 ug/0.1 mL), might be considered instead of Ceftazidime. In recent years sensitivity of Gram-negative bacterial species has decreased to the administered Amikacin or Ceftazidime. Potential alternate of Amikacin and Ceftazidime may include 3rd and 4th generation fluoroquinolones, such as Levofloxacin and Moxifloxacin, with their enhanced activity against Gram-positive pathogens having broad-spectrum activity that covers most organisms encountered in bacterial endophthalmitis. [54] Anterior chamber levels achieved using

Moxifloxacin may be higher than those obtained with any other topically administered fluoroquinolone antibiotics, however, these levels are too low for effective treatment of intraocular infections. [55]

Depending on the pharmacokinetics of the drugs selected, intra-vitreal antibiotics may be repeated as needed according to the clinical response at intervals of 48 to 72 hours. The doses selected needs to be appropriate to prevent retinal toxicity. In cases of total vitrectomy, the doses of the intra-vitreal antibiotics are reduced. According to the EVS, systemic antibiotics do not appear to have any effect on the course and outcome of endophthalmitis after cataract surgery. [10] Vancomycin provides a good coverage for Gram-positive bacteria including Methicillin-resistant Staphylococcus aureus. While, Ceftazidime provides a good coverage for Gram-negative bacteria, Clindamycin, Vancomycin, or Cefuroxime are effective for Propionibacterium acnes endophthalmitis. [3] Anti-inflammatory therapy in the form of corticosteroids at the time of intra-vitreal antibiotics can limit the tissue destruction by infiltrating leukocytes due to their cytokines. Intra-vitreal Dexamethasone injection (400 mg/0.1 mL) after vitrectomy may lead to a rapid subsidence of the intraocular inflammation. [3]

17. Post traumatic endophthalmitis

The incidence of endophthalmitis after open globe injuries ranges between 2-17% of cases depending on the design of the study and geographical location. [31] For example, a major collective review of 4795 post-traumatic eyes evaluated in 15 tertiary care centers in China over a 5 years period revealed an incidence of 8.4%. [56] In cases of initial evaluation of post-traumatic endophthalmitis, one must exclude presence of an IOFB, as in cases of IOFB, there is much greater risk of developing endophthalmitis than in cases where no IOFB is involved. The incidence of endophthalmitis associated with IOFB may be even higher in the setting of having a ruptured globe in the rural areas as compared with trauma in the urban setting (Figure 10). In the rural areas, the occurrence of post-traumatic endophthalmitis may be as high as 80% after an injury. In contrast, post-traumatic endophthalmitis occurred in 11% of 204 patients in non-rural districts. Depending on the virulent nature of the infecting organism, post-traumatic endophthalmitis may occur within hours or several weeks after trauma. [57] In these eyes, the signs of infection usually occur early but may be masked by the post-traumatic reactions of the injured tissue. [58] The initial symptoms are usually pain, intraocular inflammation, hypopyon, and vitreous clouding. Risk factors for endophthalmitis after ocular trauma include, delayed presentation, older age, unclean wound, lens capsule rupture and the presence of IOFB. [31, 57, 59] Appropriate history should be obtained regarding the setting of the trauma and likely nature of the IOFB present. When the fundus view is not possible, imaging studies in the form of ultrasonography and computed tomography should be requested. Magnetic resonance imaging is avoided in cases of suspected metallic IOFBs. Without an imaging study, the IOFB can be missed. To save vision, the IOFB needs prompt removal along-with intra-vitreal antibiotics injections.

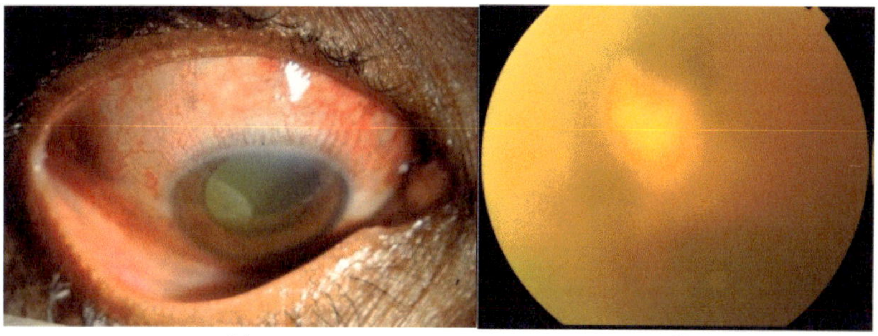

(a) (b)

Figure 10. External photograph of a 63-years-old patient who presented with decreased vision, redness, tearing and pain in his right eye after having trauma several days earlier (a). He was found to have cloudy vitreous and no clear view of the fundus (b). A diagnosis of endophthalmitis was made and patient was treated with intra-vitreal antibiotics after obtaining vitreous biopsy.

Similar to post-operative endophthalmitis, two thirds of the bacteria in post-traumatic endophthalmitis are Gram-positive and 10% to 15% are Gram-negative. [31] In contrast to post-operative endophthalmitis, virulent Bacillus species are the commonest pathogens in post-traumatic endophthalmitis and can be present in 20% of all cases. In the rural population, they are also found in 42% of cases of post-traumatic endophthalmitis. They are thus the second commonest cause of all cases of endophthalmitis. Most Bacillus infections are associated with IOFB. Infections that are caused by Bacillus species usually commence with rapid loss of vision together with severe pain (Figure 11). Bacillus species are resistant to Penicillin and Cephalosporins, but are sensitive to Gentamicin and Vancomycin. Other bacteria include Staphylococcus species, Streptococci, Coliforms, and Clostridium species. [1, 6] Fungi are the causative organisms in 10% to 15% of cases of endophthalmitis after trauma and may occur weeks to months after the trauma. [13]Although mixed microbial infections tend to be less common in post-operative cases of endophthalmitis, they have been isolated in up-to 42% of the trauma-associated endophthalmitis. [1-3]

As compared to post-operative endophthalmitis, the prognosis of post-traumatic endophthalmitis is usually poor. [28, 31] Poor prognosis stems from the presence of more virulent pathogens, presence of mixed infections, traumatic tissue injury and the failure to start prophylactic antibiotics. Microbiologic spectrum and visual outcome of culture-positive cases of infectious endophthalmitis after open globe injuries have been presented from two tertiary eye care centers in the Middle East by Al-Omran et al. [59] The most common isolates were coagulase-negative staphylococci and Streptococcus species (26.9% of isolates each). Gram-negative organisms and fungi comprised 12.8% and 3.8% of isolates, respectively. The most common organisms identified were coagulase-negative staphylococci and Streptococcus species. Clinical features associated with better visual acuity outcomes included better presenting visual acuity, early presentation to the eye clinics, and isolation of a nonvirulent organism. Post-traumatic endophthalmitis is associated with a poor visual prognosis.

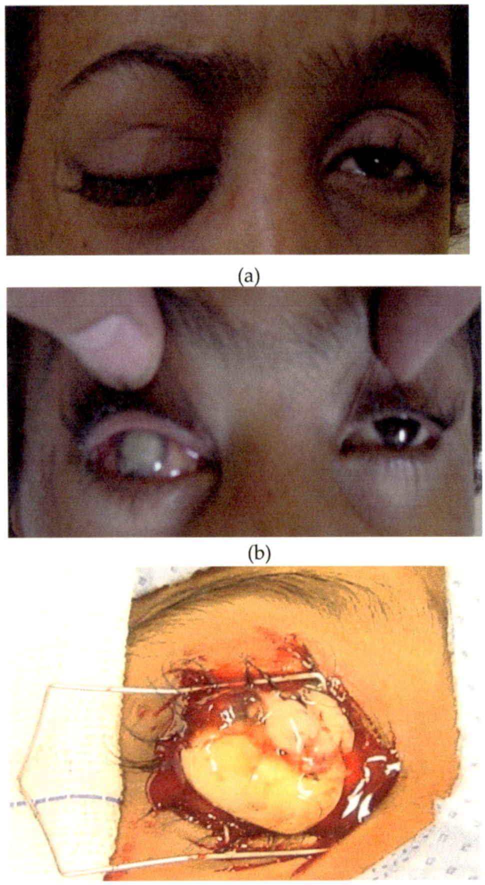

(a) (b) (c)

Figure 11. External photographs of a 13-years-old male who presented one week after trauma to his right eye (a and b). He was found to have no light perception vision and evidence of pus filled right eye which required evisceration (c).

18. Risks of endophthalmitis with retained IOFB and prevention

Intraocular penetration of a dirty or soil-contaminated foreign body requires an emergent intervention. Delayed removal of IOFB following trauma may result in a significant increase in the development of clinical endophthalmitis. Risk factors for poor visual outcome may include poor initial presenting VA, posterior location of IOFB and the lack of vitrectomy at the time of initial IOFB removal. [27, 28, 59] A retrospective study of a 20-year review found that 8% of patients with an IOFB developed endophthalmitis, of whom half lost all light perception. [1, 6] One of the largest study of penetrating eye trauma and retained IOFB in eyes of 565 patients managed at a large tertiary eye care center over a 22 year period revealed that 7.5% of them developed clinical evidence of endophthalmitis at some point after trauma. [31] In these patients, the initial presenting VA of 20/200 or better was recorded in only 18.1% of eyes and the remaining 81.9% had VA ranging from 20/400 to light perception. On-

http://dx.doi.org/10.5772/54431

ly 25% of these eyes underwent IOFB removal and repair within 24 hours after trauma while 75% had IOFB removal 24 hours or more after trauma. From this group, 70% underwent primary PPV at the time of removal of posteriorly located IOFB and only 38.6% had positive cultures. Improvement in vision was only possible in 47.7% of eyes and 38.7% had deterioration of their vision, including 22.7% that had complete loss of vision. Predictive factors for the good visual outcome in these patients included good initial presenting VA, early surgical intervention to remove IOFB (within 24 hours), and PPV. Predictors of poor visual outcome included IOFB removal 48 hours or later, posterior location and no PPV at the time of initial surgery (Figure 12). [31]

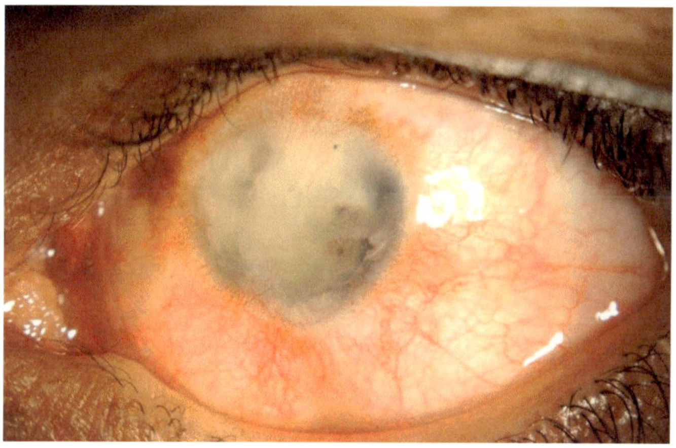

Figure 12. External photograph of a 43-years-old male who developed post-traumatic endopthalmitis resulting in phthisis of his left eye despite aggressive medical and surgical intervention.

Antibiotic prophylaxis has been advocated for IOFB removal. All patients suspecting of an IOFB should require antibiotic prophylaxis. Beside virulent infections caused by Bacillus species in the setting of IOFB which can cause severe visual loss, Staphylococcus aureus, Coliforms, Streptococci, and, sometimes Clostridium perfringens can also cause sight-threatening endophthalmitis. [60] If trauma takes place in a rural area, there is more likelihood of infection to be a polymicrobial infection. [27, 28, 31, 59] If the patient presents early with good vision and the IOFB is recognized and treated as soon as possible, then the chances of endophthalmitis are reduced.

19. Exogenous fungal endophthalmitis

Exogenous fungal endophthalmitis has been reported more often from countries in the tropical region. Most common causes of exogenous fungal endophthalmitis include Aspergillus and Fusarium species. [3] These infections are usually associated with trauma, but can follow intraocular surgery especially in the rural settings. [61] The filamentous fungus especially Aspergillus as well as Fusarium cause infection following trauma with soil contaminated objects. [61]According to some studies, up to 50% of central corneal ulcers may be caused by fungi and almost 50% of these cases may be associated with fungal endophthalmitis. [62] The fungal endophthalmits can also occur due to the failed treatment of contact lens-associated keratitis. Exogenous fungal endophthalmitis is mostly sight threatening unless aggressive intervention by antifungal therapy and surgery initiated. Effective therapy requires proper identification of the causative organisms and their sensitivity to the desired antifungal agents (Figure 13). Currently, some of the effective antifungal drugs include Amphotericin B, Natamycin, Flucytosine, Thiabendazole, Miconazole, Ketoconazole, Clotrimazole, Econazole, Fluconazole, Itraconazole, Voriconazole, and Posaconazole. Amphotericin B is the only fungicidal depending on concentration achieved, and is active against a wide range of fungi including Aspergillus species, Fusarium species and Candida species. It may be given topically, sub-conjunctivaly, and intra-vitreally. [63] In addition to intra-vitreal therapy, Amphotericin B is given systemically by a slow intravenous infusion for the treatment of fungal endophthalmitis. For fungal endophthalmitis, Amphotericin or Miconazole is usually used following vitrectomy. Amphotericin B can be administered intravenously combined with oral Flucytosine for severe Candida endophthalmitis associated with retino-choroiditis. For Candida retinochoroiditis without endophthalmitis, treatment is effective with systemic Ketoconazole, Fluconazole, or Voriconazole. [64]

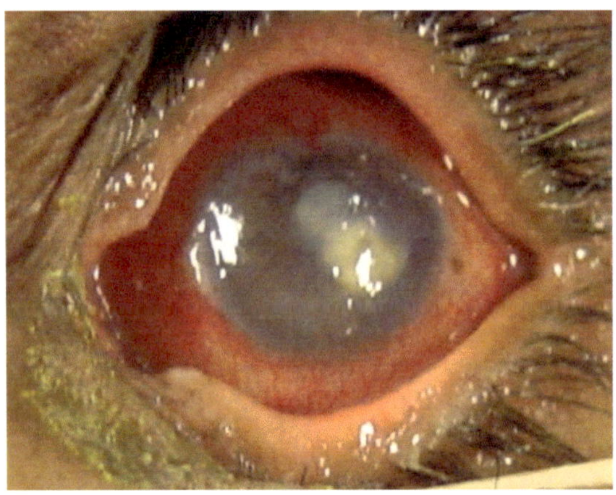

Figure 13. External photograph of left eye of an elderly female who developed fungal keratitis and endophthalmitis requiring surgical as well as systemic antifungal treatment.

Treatment for minimal fungal chorioretinitis and vitritis include systemic antifungal therapy along with serial ophthalmic evaluations. [3, 61, 64] In cases of moderate to severe vitritis due to fungal endophthalmitis, intra-ocular antifungal therapy along-with systemic as well as surgical intervention may be necessary to treat fungal endophthalmitis (Figure 14). Recommended treatment protocols include, Amphotericin B and Voriconazole as primary therapeutic options. [61, 64] Both can be given systemically and intra-vitreally. Since the intraocular penetration of Amphotericin B after topical or systemic treatment is limited, and many fungal pathogens are not susceptible to these agents, Voriconazole seem to be promising alternative. Systemically administrated Voriconazole has a good intraocular penetration

http://dx.doi.org/10.5772/54431

with minimal systemic side effect profile as compared with amphotericin B. In general in vitro susceptibility of Candida, Aspergillus, and Fusarium species appears to be almost 100% to the administered Voriconazole. [63] Candida endophthalmitis seems to result in better outcome than Aspergillus endoophthalmitis. Caspofungin appears to have a very good activity against Candida and Aspergillus species and when administered systemically along with Voriconazole, it has been found to be very effective in treating endophthalmitis caused by these organisms. Due to its unique mechanism of action and high activity against yeast and molds, Caspofungin may show more promise in future treatment strategies for fungal endophthalmitis. Fusarium endophthalmitis is particularly difficult to treat, requiring both surgical removal of the inoculums along with Amphotericin and Imidazoles therapy. Generally, Voriconazole or Fluconazole (to cover Candida albicans) or Itraconazole (to cover other Candida species, Aspergillus or Cryptococcus) can be considered. [65, 66]

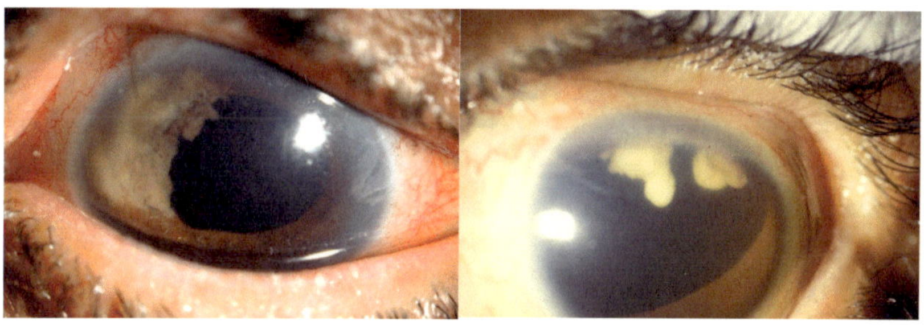

(a) (b)

Figure 14. Post-operative delayed fungal endophthalmitis; photograph (a) showing sectoral iris infiltration with Aspergillus niger requiring pars-plana vitrectomy, total capsulectomy, total iridectomy and removal of intraocular lens, photograph (b) showing white plaque extending from the upper capsule equator caused by Aspergillus terreus requiring 3 PPVs and intra-viteal Amphotericin B injections and eventual enucleation because of recurrent fungal infection. (Figures reproduced with permission: Al-Mezaine HS, Al-Assiri A, Al-Rajhi AA. Incidence, clinical features, causative organisms, and visual outcomes of delayed-onset pseudophakic endophthalmitis. Eur J Ophthalmol 2009;19:804-811).

20. Endogenous endophthalmitis

Endogenous endophthalmitis is a severe vision-threatening intraocular infection that spreads through bloodstream from a concurrent infection somewhere else in the body. Endogenous endophthalmitis is relatively uncommon, accounting for 2% to 8% of all reported cases of endophthalmitis. [67] The outcome of endogenous bacterial endophthalmitis has not improved over the last several decades and clinicians need to have a high level of suspicion of this commonly misdiagnosed condition. [67, 68] The majority of patients with endogenous endophthalmitis are initially misdiagnosed and many have an underlying disease known to predispose to infection. Blood cultures may be the most frequent means for establishing the infective cause. Endogenous bacterial endophthalmitis usually leads to total loss of vision. Although most cases of endogenous endophthalmitis present as unilateral, bilateral cases have also been reported. [69, 70] In a large study of endophthalmitis from a major center over a 10-

year period, 86 cases were reported; 10 of these were due to endogenous causes. [71] The poor visual outcome in these patients has been related to the delay in the early diagnosis and appropriate timely treatment. [72] Systemic symptoms rather than acute ocular symptoms may be the most common reasons for a patient to present to a physician and many of these cases may be initially misdiagnosed. Jackson et al. reviewed 267 reported cases of endogenous bacterial endophthalmitis and also presented a 17-year prospective series. [67]

21. Risk factors for endogenous endophthalmitis

The most frequent risk factors for developing endogenous endophthalmitis include a prior history of diabetes mellitus, gastrointestinal disorders, hypertension, heart valve diseases, endocarditis, chronic obstructive lung disease, previous wound infection, meningitis, urinary tract infection, cystic fibrosis, immune-compromised status, splenectomy, organ transplantation and indwelling intravenous catheters, hepatic abscess, hemodialysis fistula, peritonitis and intravenous drug abuse (Figure 15). [71-78] Less frequent risk factors include, otitis media, dental infection, septic arthritis, abortion, pharyngitis and Hemoglobin SC disease. [79-83] Other chronic diseases such as immunosuppressive status, HIV infection, cancer, renal failure requiring dialysis, long-term use of broad-spectrum antibiotics, use of steroids and other immunosuppressive drugs, intravenous hyper-alimentation and indwelling intravenous catheters can lead potential pathogens access to the circulatory system and septicemia. History of chronic intravenous drug abuse, dental work, otitis media, soft-tissue infection including orbital cellulitis, and septic arthritis may lead to septicemia and endogenous endophthalmitis. [3, 79, 80]

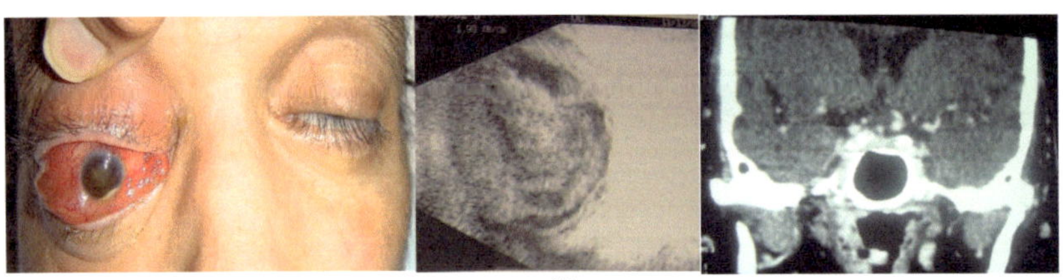

(a) (b) (c)

Figure 15. External photograph of a diabetic patient who presented with loss of vision and painful ophthalmoplegia of his right eye along with fever and mental status changes (a). He was found to have severe panophthlamia of his right eye and ultrasonography revealed endophthalmitis (b). Computed tomography (coronal view) of his brain revealed evidence of septic emboli (c). Patient was treated with systemic antibiotics and right eye evisceration.

22. Endogenous endophthalmitis: presenting features and diagnosis

New onset of floaters, blurred vision, photophobia and ocular discomfort in a patient with underlying systemic risk factors may be the presenting features of endogenous endophthalmitis. Clinical findings in endogenous endophthalmitis may include decreased VA, ocular pain, conjunctival injection, hypopyon, corneal edema, vitritis and reduced fundus view (Figure 16). Endogenous bacterial endophthalmitis is bilateral in approximately 14- 25% of cases. In bilateral infection, simultaneous ocular involvement is the rule; however, one eye is characteristically more severely affected than the other eye. Delayed involvement of the second eye can occur even in patients already being treated with systemic antibiotics. The right eye is involved twice as often as the left, probably because of this eye's proximity and more direct blood flow from the right carotid artery. There is no gender predisposition in cases of endogenous endophthalmitis. For prognostic purposes, endogenous endophthalmitis has been classified based on location (anterior or posterior) and extent (focal or diffuse). [72] According to this classification, focal and anterior cases appear to have a good prognosis, while posterior and diffuse endophthalmitis nearly always leads to blindness. In panophthalmitis, severe involvement of both the anterior and posterior segment is associated with inflammation of orbital structures, indicated by marked eyelid edema, chemosis, proptosis and limitation of eye movements. Ultrasonography may be helpful in the diagnosis; the combination of thickening of the retinochoroid layer and echoes in the vitreous supports the diagnosis of endophthalmitis. [72, 84] On MRI of the orbits, intra-ocular hyperintensity on fluid-attenuated inversion recovery and diffusion-weighted images have been found to be very useful for diagnosing endophthalmitis. [85] No eyes that have suffered posterior, diffuse or panophthalmitis has received any useful vision regardless of management. [7] Pathological examination of the enucleated globes in panophthalmitis has revealed that most of the retina is necrotic resulting in devastating visual outcome. [72]

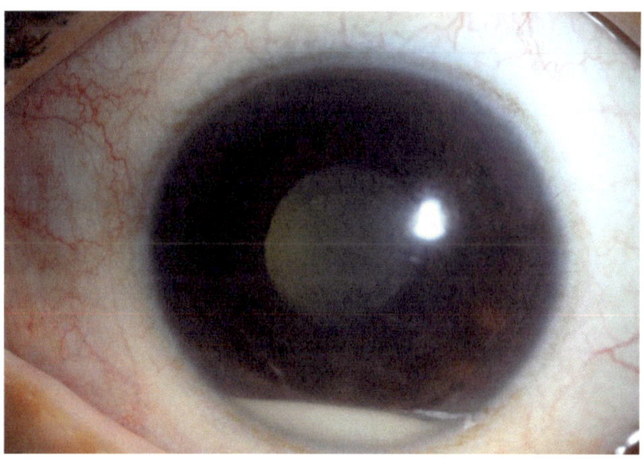

Figure 16. External photograph of a patient's eye who presented with pain, conjunctival chemosis and decreased vision. His examination was significant for having an evidence of anterior chamber reaction in the form of hypopyon and vitritis. A diagnosis of endogenous endophthalmitis was made in the absence of patient's having no prior history of ocular trauma or surgery.

The majority of patients with endogenous endophthalmitis are initially misdiagnosed and many have an underlying systemic diseases frequently overlooked by ophthalmologists (Figure 17). Blood cultures may be the most frequent means for establishing the infective cause. If not diagnosed early on and therapy initiated, endogenous bacterial endophthalmitis usually leads to total loss of vision. [7] In Candida infections, localized fluffy creamy white retinal or sub-retinal nodules may be associated with vitreous haze. [82, 83] In advanced cases of fungal endogenous endophthalmitis, one may encounter areas of peri-vascular infiltrates, retinal infarction, hemorrhages and retinal necrosis. Patients having evidence of systemic fungal infection need to be screened for any peripherally located fungal lesions as these patients may be asymptomatic initially.

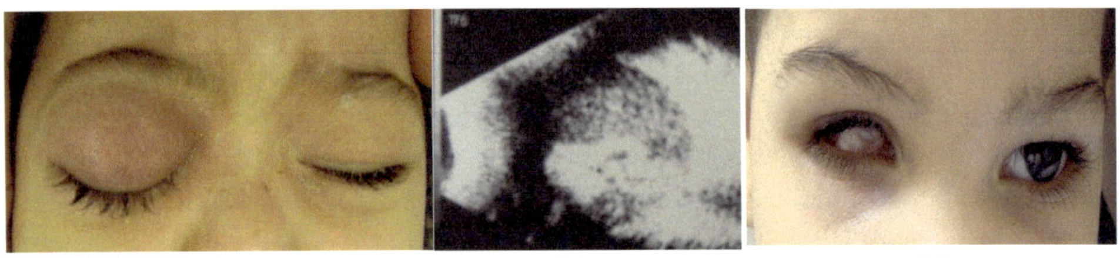

(a) (b) (c)

Figure 17. External photograph of a child who presented with gradual swelling of his right eyelids, pain and loss of vision over one month period after a bout of gastrointestinal illness. There was no prior history of eye trauma or surgery (a). Based on ultrasonography (b), a diagnosis of panophthalmitis was made and the child was treated with intravitreal antibiotic injection after obtaining vitreous biopsy to which patient responded well. Culture results revealed evidence of Enterococcus faecalis and the eye became rapidly phthisical (c).

Early diagnosis of endogenous endophthalmitis can be suspected only if there are ocular symptoms associated with concomitant systemic infection. [86] While in adults, early ocular symptoms may prompt patients to see an ophthalmologist and perhaps endogenous endophthalmitis diagnosed and treated early in the course, in cases of pediatric endogenous endophthalmitis delay in early diagnosis and treatment may result in no light perception vision or loss of an eye. [7, 87] The earliest symptoms of adult endogenous endophthalmitis include pain and decreased vision. However, because of poor communication in pediatric patients diagnosing endogenous endophthalmitis at an early stage is very difficult. Unfortunately, in pediatric patients endogenous endophthalmitis is often not suspected and may be even misdiagnosed as uveitis, persistent hyperplastic primary vitreous, cataract, retinopathy of prematurity, Toxocariasis, Coat's disease, retinal detachment and retinoblastoma. [7, 72]

Patients suspected of having endogenous endophthalmitis require immediate investigation with blood cultures along with anterior chamber and vitreous taps and possibly vitrectomy along with intravitreal antibiotic injections. [88] Gram stain of the specimens along with cultures and sensitivity as well as PCR if possible should be performed. Isolation of any bacterial colonies on direct inoculation of agar plates cultured aerobically or anaerobically may be indicative of culture-positive endophthalmitis. Blood cultures may be the most frequent means for establishing the infective cause. Identification of the causative pathogen by blood, urine, or cerebrospinal fluid culture may be successful in over 75% of endogenous endophthalmitis cases. Positive cultures from vitreous samples can be achieved much less frequently in endogenous endophthalmitis than in exogenous endophthalmitis. [3, 67, 71, 72] Vitrectomy has the advantage of obtaining material for cytologic and microbiologic studies to make the correct diagnosis and allowing removal of the offending organisms. Vitreous specimens for culture obtained by vitrectomy have been found to be more sensitive in detecting the causative organism than the vitreous needle biopsy. [88, 89] In some cases, the culture of the vitreous samples may not grow any bacteria probably due to effect of antibiotics. Vitreous biopsy should be considered because a culture of the vitreous sample is useful for identifying the responsible bacteria. The positive rate for identification of any causative organism may be 87% for vitreous, 32% for aqueous humor, and 33% for blood. In addition to cultures, in certain cases and for fastidious organisms, bacterial and fungal DNA can be detected by PCR assay in specimens obtained from the ocular tissues. [90 -92] DNA extracted using a single-extraction protocol from 50 microL of vitreous and amplified with broad-range bacterial and fungal primers (targeting the conserved 16S and 18S ribosomal RNA gene sequences of bacteria and fungi, respectively) may enable the rapid differentiation between bacterial and fungal endophthalmitis and allow tailoring of therapy to individual patients. [91, 93] RNA-based Reverse Transcriptase PCR (RT-PCR) can be utilized to confirm presence of viable bacteria in intraocular specimens obtained from patients with infectious endophthalmitis. RT-PCR can serve as a rapid and reliable tool to detect viable bacteria causing endophthalmitis. [20]

23. Bacteriology of endogenous endophthalmitis

Depending on location, a wide range of organisms have been shown to cause endogenous endophthalmitis. Causative organisms of endogenous endophthalmitis may be bacteria, as well as fungi, which vary depending on the geographical location. For example in Europe and the United States, Streptococcus species, Staphylococcus aureus, and other Gram-positive bacteria account for two-thirds of bacterial endogenous endophthalmitis cases and Gram negative isolates are found in only 32% of cases. [71, 82] These numbers differ significantly from East Asia, where most cases of endogenous endophthalmitis are caused by Gram-negative organisms especially Klebsiella species accounting for 80% to 90% of positive cultures. [67, 94] The difference might be associated with higher incidence of cholangio-hepatitis and liver abscess in these patients. Some of the other reported organisms include, Candida albicans, Neisseria meningitis, Enterococcus, Haemophilus influenzae, Klebsiella, Salmonella, Streptococcus, Staphylococcus aureus, Escherichia coli, Kingella Kingae, Pseudomonas aeroginosa, Propionibacterium acnes, Serratia, Bacillus cereus, Brucella melitensis and Actinobacillus. [67, 71-73, 77, 78, 81, 84, 95-98] Studies from East Asian countries have reported liver abscess as the major source of infection and Klebsiella pneumoniae as the causative organism. [81, 94] Incidence of fungal endogenous endophthalmitis has increased in recent years, Candida albicans and Aspergillus species being the prominent causative agents. Candida species are the most common cause of nosocomial fungal infections in compromised hosts. Candida chorioretinitis occur predominantly as a result of candidemia seeding the eye. Cryptococcus and Fusarium species have also been reported to the cause of endogenous fungal endophthalmitis. Compared with published series of post-operative or post-traumatic endophthalmitis, patients with endogenous endophthalmitis are more likely to have fungal isolates with a predominance of Candida albicans. The most common Gram positive organisms are Staphylococcus aureus, group B streptococci, Streptococcus pneumoniae,and Listeria monocytogenes; the most common Gram negative organisms are Klebsiella spp., Escherichia coli, Salmonella, Pseudomonas aeruginosa, and Neisseria meningitidis. [2, 3, 69, 91]

24. Management of endogenous endophthalmitis

The optimal treatment for endogenous endophthalmitis is controversial. When indicated, these patients may require systemic antibiotics in addition to the PPV. While EVS has provided guidelines for the role of early vitrectomy and intra-vitreal antibiotics in post-operative endophthalmitis, no such study has addressed endogenous endophthalmitis. Data from the EVS may not be applicable to cases of endogenous endophthalmitis because the spectrum of causative organisms differs significantly in endogenous endophthalmitis as compared to post-operative endophthalmitis. Although systemic and intra-vitreal antibiotics may be sufficient in milder forms of infection, PPV has been shown to be helpful in severe cases of endogenous endophthalmitis. More virulent organisms such as endotoxin-producing Streptococcus and Bacillus species are commonly involved in endogenous endopthalmitis. [67, 71] In addition, material from vitrectomy may provide a better source for culture. This is particularly true in children because of the variety of pediatric cases and lack of sufficient experience in diagnosing in this age group. [7] In the adults, early intervention with PPV has been found to be highly effective, no such data has been proven for cases of pediatric endogenous endophthalmitis. Suggested medical treatment in these patients include topical, sub-conjunctival and intra-vitreal injection of antibiotics having broad coverage with consideration for corticosteroids in cases of severe inflammation. Patients with endogenous endophthalmitis should be evaluated for underlying systemic conditions. Systemic anti-microbial therapy is the mainstay of endogenous endophthalmitis. Intravitreal antibiotic selection is similar to exogenous endophthalmitis including Vancomycin (1.0 mg/0.1 mL) for Gram-positive coverage or in combination with Ceftazidime (2.25 mg/0.1 mL) or Amikacin (400 ug/0.1 mL) for Gram-negative coverage.. In general, systemic therapy must be continued for several weeks to ensure eradication of the infection. Generally, a combination of intra-vitreal antibiotics is injected that may include Vancomycin, Cephazolin or Ceftazidime and Amikacin after the tap has been performed. Systemic antibiotics are administered according to the focus of the infection. Infectious diseases consultation may be sought in cases of endocarditis and early vitrectomy should be planned if indicated. [88] Immediate vitrectomy is performed in eyes with light-perception-only vision at the initial visit. Routine immediate vitrectomy is not necessary in eyes presenting with better than light-perception vision. Aggressive therapy and early vitrectomy may be considered in endogenous endophthalmitis caused by virulent pathogens such Pseudomonas aeruginosa and in cases of Klebsiella endophthalmitis. [81, 97, 99] Patients with endogenous endophthalmitis who undergo PPV early in the course of endogenous endophthalmitis may end up with some useful vision.

25. Visual outcome in endogenous endophthalmitis

Endogenous endophthalmitis is generally associated with high mortality and poor visual outcomes, particularly when caused by more virulent species such as Aspergillus. [98] Fungal endopthalmitis has a poor visual outcome as compared to bacterial endophthalmitis. [100] The visual outcome in cases of treated Streptococcal endophthalmitis is generally poor than some of the Staphylococcal species. Patients with good initial VA typically have good final VA. It is believed that an active therapeutic approach including intra-vitreal antibiotics and vitreo-retinal surgery may save eyes from blindness. In the past, the visual outcome has been poor with most cases leading to blindness in the affected eye. [70, 81] In an experimentally model of endogenous endophthalmitis, infant rats inoculated by either intra-nasal or intra-peritoneal injection of Haemophilus influenzae type b, suppurative endophthalmitis occurred in 50% of bacteremic animals who survived. [101] This experimental induced endogenous endophthalmitis ultimately progressed to panophthalmitis followed by organization of the exudate and phthisis bulbi. Recent data for the effectiveness of vitrectomy and intra-vitreal antibiotics to save some vision has been encouraging. [88] Endophthalmitis due to Streptococcal species may result in earlier onset and perhaps worse visual outcome. On the other hand, endophthalmitis which yields no positive results from culture usually have delayed onset of infection and better visual results.

26. Endogenous fungal endophthalmitis

In fungal endophthalmitis, some of the most important metastatic sources of infections include endocarditis, gastrointestinal tract, genitourinary tract, skin wound infections, pulmonary infections, meningitis, and septic arthritis. [102] Other predisposing factors include chronic invasive procedures, such as hemodialysis, bladder catheterization, total parenteral nutrition, chemotherapy, dental procedures, and intravenous drug abuse (Figure 18). In the past, the incidence of endogenous fungal endophthalmitis has been estimated to range between 9- 45% of patients with disseminated fungus infection which has decreased in recent years to less than 3%. [1, 102] Candida albicans is by far the most frequent cause (75-80% of fungal cases), followed by Aspergillus species. Because of advanced medical care and a longer life-span of patients with chronic diseases in the Western countries along with frequent use of long-term intravenous access, Candida albicans retino-choroiditis has become more common in clinical practice and less common in those with organ transplants and immunosuppression as the result of early ophthalmological screening of all susceptible patients. [81, 99] Endophthalmitis may occur in patients with candidemia depending on the population studied, especially those with an organ transplant and having a highly immunocompromised status. [1, 3] Aspergillosis is the second most common cause of fungal endophthalmitis, particularly in intravenous drug abusers. Less frequent causes are other Candida species, Torulopsis glabrata, Cryptococcus neoformans, Sporothrix schenckii, Scedosporium apiospermum (Pseudallescheria boydii), Blastomyces dermatitidis, Coccidioides immitis, and Mucor.

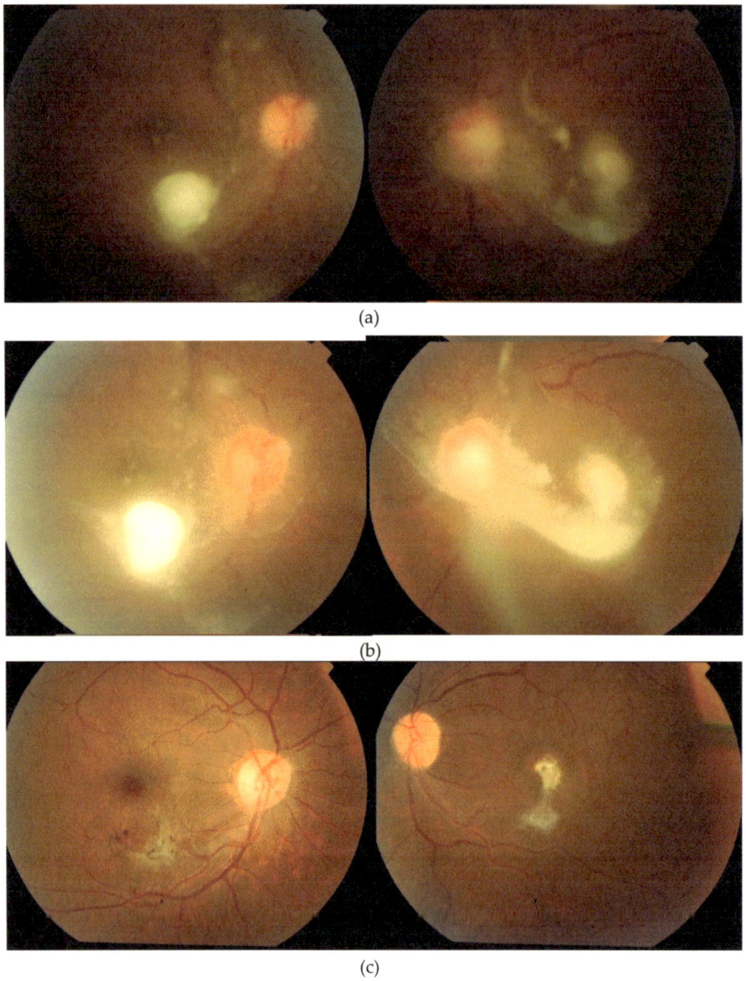

Figure 18. Fundus photographs of a 35-years-old immuno-compromised male patient who presented with bilateral decreased vision. He was found to have evidence of bilateral fungal endophthalmitis (a). Initially the patient was treated by intra-vitreal antifungal agents (b). Because of worsening of infection, bilateral pars-plana vitrectomy along-with systemic antifungal therapy resulted in clearance o f his eye infection (c). (Photographs: Curtsy of Essam Al-Harthi, MD).

27. Orbital and peri-orbital cellulitis as a cause of endogenous endophthalmitis

Orbital and peri-orbital cellulitis have been reported as causes of endogenous endophthalmitis. [8, 37] Facial cellulitis is rarely reported as a focus of infection leading to endogenous endophthalmitis. Facial cellulitis usually appears more rapidly than other deep infections, so treatment is required early on. However, facial cellulitis can be a direct or indirect causative infection. The indirect pathway involves distant spread through the blood stream via the internal jugular vein. Microorganisms are then able to spread through the heart to the internal carotid artery and ophthalmic artery. Furthermore, they can follow a retrograde pathway toward the cavernous sinus of the skull, establishing thrombophlebitis in the facial vessels. These anatomical characteristics explain how facial cellulitis can be a primary infection site of endogenous endophthalmitis. Kang et al, [8] reported a case of 51-year-old unconscious woman presenting with fever, facial swelling, and decreased VA secondary to facial cellulitis, endogenous endophthalmitis and end-stage renal disease. These authors reported successful treatment with intra-vitreal (Vancomycin, Ceftazidime) and intravenous antibiotics (Vancomycin, Meropenem). The authors reported a successful outcome in their patient's bilateral endogenous endophthalmitis following timely treatment with the intra-vitreal as well as systemic antibiotic administration.

28. Endophthalmitis after intra-vitreal injections

In recent years, increasing number of iatrogenic cases of endophthalmitis have been reported as a result of increased used of intra-vitreal injections for various retinal conditions. [103-108] Studies have suggested that coagulase-negative Staphylococci, like postoperative endophthalmitis, appear to be the predominant organism in the pathogenesis in the development of endophthalmitis after intra-vitreal injection. Variety of other organisms have been implicated in the development of endophthalmitis following intra-vitreal injections of anti-VEGF agents as well as intra-vitreal Triamcinolone injections (Figure 19). Alkuraya et al, [106] reported a case of culture-positive endophthalmitis after intra-vitreal injection of bevacizumab (Avastin) in a 51-year-old diabetic women. In their case, the patient presented with decreased vision, redness, and mild pain in her eye 3 days after intra-vitreal injection of Avastin for macular edema due to a branch retinal vein occlusion. A clinical diagnosis of endophthalmitis was made, a vitreous tap was performed and intra-vitreal antibiotics were administered. Because of worsening of the endophthalmitis, PPV was undertaken followed by repeat intra-vitreal antibiotic injection. The patient's ocular condition improved dramatically; however, her VA did not improve. The cultures from vitreous taps revealed Staphylococcus lugdunesis. An up-to-date overview of all patients reported in the literature with

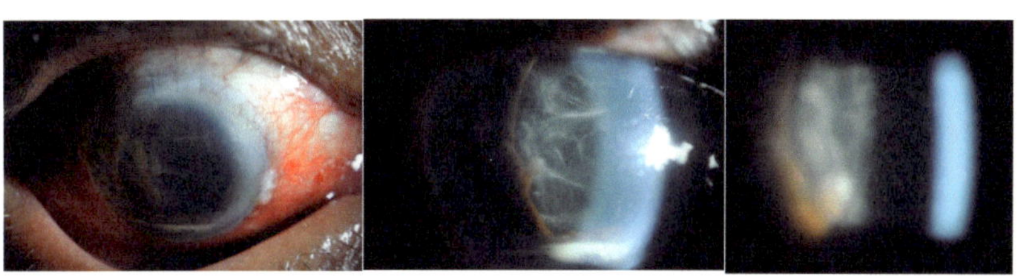

(a) (b) (c)

Figure 19. External (a) and slit-lamp (b,c) photographs of a patient's eye who developed endopthalmitis after intraviteal Triamcinolone injection to treat post-operative macular edema.

suspected bacterial endophthalmitis along-with specific symptoms and signs which could differentiate between infectious and non-infectious causes following anti-VEGF injection has been reported by Hoevenaars et al. [108] These authors reviewed case series of 118 patients from the PubMed data along with records of their own 15 patients from the Rotterdam Eye Hospital with suspected bacterial endophthalmitis after anti-VEGF injection. Their study revealed that patients presenting with a VA of 20/200 (logMAR 1.0) or less and later than 24 hours after injection were more likely to have bacterial endophthalmitis and suggested that in order to prevent under-treatment in these patients, the threshold to proceed to vitreous biopsy and empirical intra-vitreous antibiotics should be low.

29. Conclusion

Patients suspected of having endophthalmitis following ocular surgery or trauma require prompt evaluation and treatment. Patients having ocular symptoms and signs in the absence of trauma or ocular surgery and presence of risk factors such as diabetes, cardiac disease, renal disease, organ transplantation, immunodeficiency status and malignancy should be evaluated for endogenous endophthalmitis. Since endophthalmitis can be caused by a large number of bacterial as well as fungal species, it requires rapid identification of the causative organism. Visual prognosis depends mainly on the underlying microorganisms, and it is particularly poor in cases of infection with Gram-positive bacteria or Aspergillus species. Experience has shown that early Vitrous biopsy along with intra-vitreal antibiotics may save vision in some patients while in other patients pars-plana vitrectomy may be necessary to prevent total loss of vision and perhaps an eye.

Author details

Imtiaz A. Chaudhry[1], Hassan Al-Dhibi[2], Waleed Al-Rashed[3], Hani S. Al-Mezaine[4], Yonca O. Arat[5] and Wael Abdelghani[6]

1 Houston Oculoplastics Associates, Memorial Herman Medical Plaza, Texas Medical Center, Houston, Texas, USA

2 Vitreo-Retina Division, King Khaled Eye Specialist Hospital, Riyadh, Saudi Arabia

3 AL-Imam Muhammad ibn Saud Islamic University Faculty of Medicine, Riyadh, Saudi Arabia

4 Department of Ophthalmology, King Saud University, Riyadh, Saudi Arabia

5 Department of Ophthalmology, Univ. of Wisconsin, Madison, Wisconsin, USA

6 The Woodlands Retina Center, Woodlands, Texas, USA

http://dx.doi.org/10.5772/54431

References

[1] Peyman G, Lee P, Seal DV. Endophthalmitis: Diagnosis and Management. Taylor & Francis, London & New York: 2004:1–278.

[2] Kresloff MS, Castellarin AA, Zarbin MA. Endophthalmitis. Surv Ophthalmol. 1998;43:193–224.

[3] Kernt M, Kampik A. Endophthalmitis: Pathogenesis, clinical presentation, management, and perspective. Clin Ophthalmol. 2010;4:121-135.

[4] Peponis V, Rosenberg P, Chalkiadakis SE, Insler M, Amariotakis A. Fungal scleral keratitis and endophthalmitis following pterygium excision. Eur J Ophthalmol. 2009;19:478–480.

[5] Abu el-Asrar AM, Kadry AA, Shibl AM, al-Kharashi SA, al-Mosallam AA. Antibiotics in the irrigating solutions reduce Staphylococcus epidermidis adherence to intraocular lenses. Eye (Lond). 2000;14 (Pt 2):225-30.

[6] Peyman GA, Meffert SA, Conway MD, Chou F. Vitreoretinal Surgical Techniques. Martin Dunitz, London 2001, 1–605.

[7] Chaudhry IA, Shamsi FA, Al-Dhibi H, Khan AO. Pediatric endogenous bacterial endophthalmitis: case report and review of the literature J AAPOS. 2006;10:491-3.

[8] Kang MH, Seong M, Lee JH, Cho HY. Endogenous Endophthalmitis Associated with Facial Cellulitis after a Tongue Bite. Open Journal of Ophthalmology, 2012;2, 85-88.

[9] Chaudhry IA, Shamsi FA, Kurraya HA, Elzaridi E, Riley FC. Current Indications for Evisceration in a Tertiary Eye Care Center. Ophthalmic Epidemiology 2007;14:93-97.

[10] Endophthalmitis Vitrectomy Study Group. Results of the EVS study: a randomised trial of immediate vitrectomy and of intravenous antibiotics for the treatment of postoperative bacterial endophthalmitis. Arch Ophthalmol 1995;113:1479–96.

[11] Seal D, Reischl U, Behr A, Ferrer C, Alió J, Koerner RJ, Barry P; ESCRS Endophthalmitis Study Group. Laboratory diagnosis of endophthalmitis: comparison of microbiology and molecular methods in the European Society of Cataract & Refractive Surgeons multicenter study and susceptibility testing. J Cataract Refract Surg. 2008;34:1439-50.

[12] Al-Mezaine HS, Kangave D, Al-Assiri A, Al-Rajhi AA. Acute-onset nosocomial endophthalmitis after cataract surgery: incidence, clinical features, causative organisms, and visual outcomes. Cataract Refract Surg. 2009;35:643-9.

[13] Al-Mezaine HS, Al-Assiri A, Al-Rajhi AA. Incidence, clinical features, causative organisms, and visual outcomes of delayed-onset pseudophakic endophthalmitis. Eur J Ophthalmol 2009;19:804-811.

[14] Seal DV, Barry P, Gettinby G et al. ESCRS study of prophylaxis of postoperative endophthalmitis after cataract surgery. Case for a European multicenter study. J Cataract Refract Surg. 2006; 32:396–406.

[15] Chaudhry IA, Shamsi FA, Elzaridi E, Al-Rashed W. Al-Amri AM, Al-Anezi F, Arat YO, Holck DEE. Outcome of treated orbital cellulitis from a tertiary eye care center in the Middle East. Ophthalmology. 2007;114:345-354.

[16] Miller JJ, Scott IU, Flynn HW et al. Endophthalmitis caused by Streptococcus pneumoniae. Am J Ophthalmol. 2004; 138:231–36.

[17] Verbraeken H. Treatment of post-operative endophthalmitis. Ophthalmologica. 1995;209:165–71.

[18] ESCRS Endophthalmitis Study Group. Prophylaxis of postoperative endophthalmitis following cataract surgery: results of the ESCRS multicentre study and identification of risk factors. J Cataract Refract Surg. 2007; 33:978–88.

[19] Packer M, Chang DF, Dewey SH, Little BC, Mamalis N, Oetting TA, Talley-Rostov A, Yoo SH; ASCRS Cataract Clinical Committee. Prevention, diagnosis, and management of acute postoperative bacterial endophthalmitis. J Cataract Refract Surg. 2011;37:1699-714.

[20] Aarthi P, Bagyalakshmi R, Therese KL, Malathi J, Mahalakshmi B, Madhavan HN. Optimization and Application of a Reverse Transcriptase Polymerase Chain Reaction to Determine the Bacterial Viability in Infectious Endophthalmitis. Curr Eye Res. 2012 Jul 3. [Epub ahead of print]

[21] Mamalis N, Edelhauser H, Dawson DG et al. Toxic Anterior Segment Syndrome. J Cataract Refract Surg. 2006; 32:324–32.

[22] Rishi E, Rishi P, Sengupta S, Jambulingam M, Madhavan HN, Gopal L, Therese KL. Acute Postoperative Bacillus cereus Endophthalmitis Mimicking Toxic Anterior Segment Syndrome. Ophthalmology. 2012 Sep 15. pii: S0161-6420(12)00633-1. [Epub ahead of print]

[23] Warheker PT, Gupta SR, Mansfield DC, Seal DV, Lee WR. Post-operative saccular endophthalmitis caused by macrophage-associated staphylococci. Eye. 1998;12:1019–1021.

[24] Warheker PT, Gupta SR, Mansfield DC, Seal DV. Successful treatment of saccular endophthalmitis with clarithromycin. Eye. 1998; 12:1017–1019.

[25] Okhravi N, Guests S, Matheson MM et al. Assessment of the effect of oral clarithromycin on visual outcome following presumed bacterial endophthalmitis. Curr Eye Res. 2000; 21:691–702.

[26] Cleven BEE, Palka-santini M, Gielen J, et al. Identification and characterization of bacterial pathogens causing bloodstream infections by DNA microarray. J Clin Microbiol. 2006;44:2389–2397.

[27] Al-Mezaine HS, Osman EA, Kangave D, Abu El-Asrar AM. Risk factors for culture-positive endophthalmitis after repair of open globe injuries. Eur J Ophthalmol. 2010;20:201-8.

[28] Abu el-Asrar AM, al-Amro SA, al-Mosallam AA, al-Obeidan S. Post-traumatic endophthalmitis: causative organisms and visual outcome. Eur J Ophthalmol. 1999;9:21-31.

[29] Al-Turki TA, Al-Shahwan S, Al-Mezaine HS, Kangave D, Abu El-Asrar AM. Microbiology and visual outcome of bleb-associated endophthalmitis. Ocul Immunol Inflamm. 2010;18:121-6.

[30] Al-Torbak AA, Al-Shahwan S, Al-Jadaan I, Al-Hommadi A, Edward DP. Endophthalmitis associated with the Ahmed glaucoma valve implant. Br J Ophthalmol. 2005;89:454–458.

[31] Chaudhry IA, Shamsi FA, Al-Harthi E, Al-Theeb A, Elzaridi E, Riley FC. Incidence and visual outcome of endophthalmitis associated with intraocular foreign bodies. Graefes Arch Clin Exp Ophthalmol. 2008;246:181-6.

[32] Ou JI, Ta CN. Endophthalmitis prophylaxis. Ophthalmol Clin N Am. 2006;19:449-456.

[33] Doft BH, Wisniewski SR, Kelsey SF, et al. Diabetes and postoperative endophthalmitis in the endophthalmitis vitrectomy study. Arch Ophthalmol. 2001;119:650–6.

[34] Abu el-Asrar AM, Shibl AM, Tabbara KF, al-Kharashi SA. Heparin and heparin-surface-modification reduce Staphylococcus epidermidis adhesion to intraocular lenses. Int Ophthalmol. 1997;21:71-4.

[35] Pinna A, Zanetti S, Sechi LA, Usai D, Falchi MP, Carta F. In vitro adherence of Staphylococcus epidermidis to polymethyl methacrylate and ACRYSOF intraocular lenses. Ophthalmology. 2000;107:1042–1046.

[36] Chaudhry IA, Shamsi FA, Morales J. Orbital cellulitis following implantation of aqueous drainage devices for glaucoma. Eur J Ophthalmol. 2007;17:136-140.

[37] Lopez PF, Beldavs RA, al-Ghamdi S, Wilson LA, Wojno TH, Sternberg P Jr. Pneumococcal endophthalmitis associated with nasolacrimal obstruction. Am J Ophthalmol. 1993;116:56–62.

[38] Chaudhry IA, Shamsi FA, Al-Rashed W. Bacteriology of chronic dacryocystitis in a tertiary eye care center. Ophthal Plast Reconstr Surg. 2005;21:207-10.

[39] Chaudhry IA, Al-Rashed W, Shamsi FA, Elzaridi E, Riley FC. Microbial Profile and Prevalence of Acute Dacryocystitis in Adult Patients with Chronic Dacryocystitis. Saudi J Ophthalmol. 2005;19:93-8.

[40] Nichamin LD, Chang DF, Johnson SH et al. What is the association between clear corneal cataract incisions and postoperative endophthalmitis ? J Cataract Refract Surg. 2006; 32:1556–59.

[41] Taban M, Behrens A, Newcomb RL et al. Acute endophthalmitis following cataract surgery. A systematic review of the literature. Arch Ophthalmol. 2005; 123: 613–20.

[42] West ES, Behrens A, McDonnell PJ, et al. The incidence of endophthalmitis after cataract surgery among the US Medicare population increased between 1994 and 2001. Ophthalmology. 2005;112:1388–94.

[43] Ku JJ, Wei MC, Amjadi S, Montfort JM, Singh R, Francis IC. Role of adequate wound closure in preventing acute postoperative bacterial endophthalmitis. J Cataract Refract Surg. 2012;38:1301-2.

[44] Lundstrom M, Wejde G, Stenevi U et al. Endophthalmitis after cataract surgery. A nationwide prospective study evaluating incidence in relation to incision type and location. Ophthalmology. 2007; 114:866–70.

[45] Ciulla TA, Starr MB, Masket S. Bacterial endophthalmitis prophylaxis for cataract surgery: an evidence based update. Ophthalmology. 2002;109:13–24.

[46] Masket S. Preventing, diagnosing, and treating endophthalmitis. J Cataract Refract Surg. 1998;24(6):725–726.

[47] Prophylaxis of postoperative endophthalmitis following cataract surgery: Results of the ESCRS multicenter study and identification of risk factors. J Cataract Refract Surg. 2007;33:978–988.

[48] Colleaux KM, Hamilton WK. Effect of prophylactic antibiotics and incision type on the incidence of endophthalmitis after cataract surgery. Can J Ophthalmol. 2000; 35:373–78.

[49] Nagaki Y, Hayasaka S, Kadoi C et al. Bacterial endophthalmitis after small-incision cataract surgery. Effect of incision placement and intraocular lens type. J Cataract Refract Surg. 2003; 29:20–26.

[50] Jacobs DJ, Leng T, Flynn HW, Shi W, Miller D, Gedde SJ. Delayed-onset bleb-associated endophthalmitis: presentation and outcome by culture result. Clin Ophthalmol. 2011;5:739–744.

[51] Doft BH, Kelsey SF, Wisniewski SR. Additional procedures after the initial vitrectomy or tap-biopsy in the Endophthalmitis Vitrectomy Study. Ophthalmology. 1998;105:707–716.

[52] Kuhn F, Gini G. Ten years after... are findings of the Endophthalmitis Vitrectomy Study still relevant today? Graefes Arch Clin Exp Ophthalmol. 2005;243:1197–1199.

[53] Phillips WB II, Tasman WS. Postoperative endophthalmitis in association with diabetes mellitus. Ophthalmology. 1994;101:508–18.

[54] Callegan MC, Ramirez R, Kane ST, Cochran DC, Jensen H. Antibacterial activity of the fourth-generation fluoroquinolones gatifloxacin and moxifloxacin against ocular pathogens. Adv Ther. 2003;20:246–252.

[55] Hariprasad SM, Blinder KJ, Shah GK, et al. Penetration pharmacokinetics of topically administered 0.5% moxifloxacin ophthalmic solution in human aqueous and vitreous. Arch Ophthalmol. 2005;123:39–44.

[56] Zhang Y, Zhang M, Jiang C, Yao Y, Zhang K. Endophthalmitis following open globe Injury. Br J Ophthalmol. 2010;94:111-4.

[57] Thompson JT, Parver LM, Enger CL, Mieler WF, Liggett PE. Infectious endophthalmitis after penetrating injuries with retained intraocular foreign bodies. National Eye Trauma System. Ophthalmology. 1993;100:1468–1474.

[58] Spoor TC. An Atlas of Ophthalmic Trauma. Martin Dunitz, London 1997, 1–207.

[59] Al-Omran AM, Abboud EB, Abu El-Asrar AM. Microbiologic spectrum and visual outcome of posttraumatic endophthalmitis. Retina. 2007;27:236-42.

[60] Abu el-Asrar AM, Tabbara KF. Clostridium perfringens endophthalmitis. Doc Ophthalmol. 1994;87:177-82.

[61] Narang S, Gupta A, Gupta V, et al. Fungal endophthalmitis following cataract surgery: Clinical presentation, microbiological spectrum, and outcome. Am J Ophthalmol. 2001;132:609–617.

[62] Wykoff CC, Flynn HW Jr, Miller D, Scott IU, Alfonso EC. Exogenous fungal endophthalmitis: Microbiology and clinical outcomes. Ophthalmology 2008;115:1501-1507.

[63] Bunya VY, Hammersmith KM, Rapuano CJ, Ayres BD, Cohen EJ. Topical and oral voriconazole in the treatment of fungal keratitis. Am J Ophthalmol. 2007;143:151–153.

[64] Pappas PG, Kauffman CA, Andes D, et al. Clinical practice guidelines for the management of candidiasis: 2009 update by the Infectious Diseases Society of America. Clin Infect Dis. 2009;4:503–535.

[65] Agarwal MB, Rathi SA, Ratho N, Subramanian R. Caspofungin: Major breakthrough in treatment of systemic fungal infections. J Assoc Physicians India. 2006;54:943–948.

[66] Durand ML, Kim IK, D'Amico DJ, et al. Successful treatment of Fusarium endophthalmitis with voriconazole and Aspergillus endophthalmitis with voriconazole plus caspofungin. Am J Ophthalmol. 2005;140:552–554.

[67] Jackson TL, Eykyn S, Graham EM et al. Endogenous bacterial endophthalmitis: a 17-year prospective series and review of 267 reported cases. Surv Ophthalmol 2003; 48:403–23.

[68] Chaudhry IA, Al-Harthi EA, Shamsi FA, Alkuraya H, Al-Mezaine H, Al-Dhibi H, El-zaridi E, Buhaimad M, Arat Y, Al-Rashed W. Visual outcome of patients with endogenous endophthalmitis presenting to a tertiary eye care center. Association of Research in Visual Sciences and Ophthalomology (ARVO), Ft. Lauderdale, Florida, USA, May, 2009.(Paper Presentation).

[69] Park P, Khawly JA, Kearney DL, Altman CA, Yen KG. Bilateral endogenous endophthalmitis secondary to endocarditis with negative transesophageal echocardiogram. Am J Ophthalmol. 2004;138:151-3.

[70] Christensen SR, Hansen AB, La Cour M, Fledelius HC. Bilateral endogenous bacterial endophthalmitis: a report of four cases. Acta Ophthalmol Scand. 2004;82:306-10.

[71] Okada AA, Johnson RP, Liles WC, D'Amico DJ, Baker AS. Endogenous bacterial endophthalmitis: Report of a ten-year Retrospective study. Ophthalmology. 1994;101:832-838.

[72] Greenwald MJ, Wohl LG, Sell CH. Metastatic bacterial endophthalmitis: A contemporary reappraisal. Surv Ophthalmol. 1986;31:81–101.

[73] Leibovitch I, Lai T, Raymond G, Zadeh R, Nathan F, Selva D. Endogenous endophthalmitis: a 13-year review at a tertiary hospital in South Australia Scand J Infect Dis. 2005;37:184-9.

[74] Motley WW 3rd, Augsburger JJ, Hutchins RK, Schneider S, Boat TF. Pseudomonas aeruginosa endogenous endophthalmitis with choroidal abscess in a patient with cystic fibrosis. Retina. 2005;25:202-7.

[75] Nahata SK, Saffra NA, Genovesi MH, Connolly MW, Cunningham JN Jr. Endogenous endophthalmitis resulting from sternal wound infection after coronary artery bypass grafting. : J Thorac Cardiovasc Surg. 1998;116:176-7.

[76] Tufail A, Weisz JM, Holland GN. Endogenous bacterial endophthalmitis as a complication of intravenous therapy for cytomegalovirus retinopathy. Arch Ophthalmol. 1996;114:879-80.

[77] Chou FF, Kou HK. Endogenous endophthalmitis associated with pyogenic hepatic abscess. J Am Coll Surg. 1996;182:33-6.

[78] Al-Mahmood AM, Al-Binali GY, Alkatan H, Abboud EB, Abu El-Asrar AM. Endogenous endophthalmitis associated with liver abscess caused by Klebsiella pneumoniae. Int Ophthalmol. 2011;31:145-8.

[79] Ziakas NG, Tzetzi D, Boboridis K, Georgiadis NS. Endogenous group G Streptococcus endophthalmitis following a dental procedure. Eur J Ophthalmol. 2004;14:59-60.

[80] Siegersma JE, Klont RR, Tilanus MA, Verbeek AM, Schulin T, Cruysberg JR, Deutman AF. Endogenous endophthalmitis after otitis media. Am J Ophthalmol. 2004;137:202-4.

[81] Chen YJ, Kuo HK, Wu PC, Kuo ML, Tsai HH, Liu CC, Chen CH. A 10-year comparison of endogenous endophthalmitis outcomes: an east Asian experience with Klebsiella pneumoniae infection. Retina. 2004;24:383-90.

[82] Chee SP, Jap A. Endogenous endophthalmitis. Curr Opin Ophthalmol. 2001;12:464-70.

[83] Werner MS, Feist RM, Green JL. Hemoglobin SC disease with endogenous endophthalmitis. Am J Ophthalmol. 1992;113:208-9.

[84] Margo CE, Mames RN, Guy JR. Endogenous Klebsiella endophthalmitis: a report of two cases and review of the literature. Ophthalmology.1994;101:1298-1301.

[85] Rumboldt Z, Moses C, Wieczerzynski U, Saini R. Diffusion-weighted imaging, apparent diffusion coefficients, and fluid-attenuated inversion recovery MR imaging in endophthalmitis. AJNR Am J Neuroradiol. 2005;26:1869-72.

[86] Romero CF, Rai MK, Lowder CY, Adal KA. Endogenous endophthalmitis: case report and brief review. Am Fam Physician. 1999;60:510-4.

[87] Al-Rashaed SA, Abu El-Asrar AM. Exogenous endophthalmitis in pediatric age group. Ocul Immunol Inflamm. 2006;14:285-92.

[88] Zhang YQ, Wang WJ. Treatment outcomes after pars plana vitrectomy for endogenous endophthalmitis. Retina 2005; 25:746-50.

[89] Binder MI, Chua J, Kaiser PK, Procop GW, Isada CM. Endogenous endophthalmitis: an 18-year review of culture-positive cases at a tertiary care center. Medicine (Baltimore). 2003;82:97-105.

[90] Jaeger EE, Carroll NM, Choudhury S, et al. Rapid detection and identification of Candida, Aspergillus, and Fusarium species in ocular samples using nested PCR. J Clin Microbiol. 2000;38:2902–2908.

[91] Lohmann CP, Linde HJ, Reischl U. Improved detection of microorganisms by polymerase chain reaction in delayed endophthalmitis after cataract surgery. Ophthalmology. 2000;107(6):1047–1051; discussion 1051–1052.

[92] Okhravi N, Adamson P, Carroll N, et al. PCR-based evidence of bacterial involvement in eyes with suspected intraocular infection. Invest Ophthalmol Vis Sci. 2000;41:3474–3479.

[93] Varghese B, Rodrigues C, Deshmukh M, Natarajan S, Kamdar P, Mehta A. Broad-range bacterial and fungal DNA amplification on vitreous humor from suspected endophthalmitis patients. Mol Diagn Ther. 2006;10:319-26.

[94] Wong JS, Chan TK, Lee HM, Chee SP. Endogenous bacterial endophthalmitis: An east Asian experience and a reappraisal of a severe ocular affliction. Ophthalmology. 2000;107:1483–1491.

[95] al-Hazzaa SA, Tabbara KF, Gammon JA. Pink hypopyon: a sign of Serratia marcescens endophthalmitis. Br J Ophthalmol. 1992;76:764-5.

[96] de la Fuente J, Fernandez-Catalina P, Sopena B, Cadarso L. Endogenous endophthalmitis caused by Propionibacterium acnes. Arch Ophthalmol. 1993;111:1468.

[97] Reedy JS, Wood KE. Endogenous Pseudomonas aeruginosa endophthalmitis: a case report and literature review. Intensive Care Med. 2000;26:1386-9.

[98] Schiedler V, Scott IU, Flynn HW Jr, Davis JL, Benz MS, Miller D. Culture-proven endogenous endophthalmitis: clinical features and visual acuity outcomes. Am J Ophthalmol. 2004;137:725-31.

[99] Chen KJ, Wu WC, Sun MH, Lai CC, Chao AN. Endogenous fungal endophthalmitis: causative organisms, management strategies, and visual acuity outcomes. Am J Ophthalmol. 2012;154:213-4.

[100] Keswani T, Ahuja V, Changulani M. Evaluation of outcome of various treatment methods for endogenous endophthalmitis. Indian J Med Sci. 2006;60:454-460.

[101] Myerowitz RL, Klaw R, Johnson BL. Experimental endogenous endophthalmitis caused by Haemophilus influenzae type b. Infect Immun. 1976;14:1043-51.

[102] Tanaka M, Kobayashi Y, Takebayashi H, Kiyokawa M, Qiu H. Analysis of predisposing clinical and laboratory findings for the development of endogenous fungal endophthalmitis. A retrospective 12-year study of 79 eyes of 46 patients. Retina. 2001;21:203–9.

[103] Bhavsar AR, Stockdale CR, Ferris FL 3rd, Brucker AJ, Bressler NM, Glassman AR; Diabetic Retinopathy Clinical Research Network. Update on risk of endophthalmitis after intravitreal drug injections and potential impact of elimination of topical antibiotics. Arch Ophthalmol. 2012;130:809-10.

[104] Moshfeghi DM, Kaiser PK, Scott IU, et al. Acute endophthalmitis following intravitreal triamcinolone acetonide injection. Am J Ophthalmol. 2003;136:791–796.

[105] Erbahçeci IE, Ornek K. Endophthalmitis after intravitreal anti-vascular endothelial growth factor antagonists: a six-year experience at a university referral center". Retina. 2012;32:1228.

[106] Alkuraya HS, Al-Kharashi AS, Alharthi E, Chaudhry IA. Acute endophthalmitis caused by Staphylococcus lugdunesis after intravitreal bevacizumab (Avastin) injection. Int Ophthalmol. 2009;29:411-3.

[107] Jager RD, Aiello LP, Patel SC et al. Risks of intravitreous injection: a comprehensive review. Retina. 2004; 24:676–98.

[108] Hoevenaars NE, Gans D, Missotten T, van Rooij J, Lesaffre E, van Meurs JC. Suspected Bacterial Endophthalmitis following Intravitreal Anti-VEGF Injection: Case Series and Literature Review. Ophthalmologica. 2012;228:143-7.

Chapter 10

Eye Infection Complications in Rheumatic Diseases

Brygida Kwiatkowska and Maria Maślińska

Additional information is available at the end of the chapter

http://dx.doi.org/10.5772/52968

1. Introduction

Rheumatic diseases are a group of illnesses characterized by the inflammation of the connective tissue, usually of autoimmunological origin. Although most of the symptoms of the rheumatic diseases concern primarily musculoskeletal system, in many of these disorders pathological changes take also place in various other organs. Changes in the organ of sight in the rheumatic diseases may result from the inflammatory process taking place in the course of immunological dysfunctions and their manifestations may precede typical in these illnesses musculoskeletal symptoms. Damage to the organ of sight may also be secondary to vascular lesions occurring in the course of its inflammation or may be the result of complications arising from the therapy of the rheumatic disease. (Table 1).

Rheumatic diseases with arthritis	Rheumatoid arthritis Spondyloarthropathies: Ankylosing spondylitis Psoriatic arthritis Reactive arthritis Arthritis associated with inflammatory bowel disease (Colitis ulcerosa, Leśniowski - Crohn's disease) undifferentiated spondyloarthropathy Juvenile idiopathic arthritis
Connective tissue diseases	Systemic lupus erythematosus Sjogren's syndrome Systemic scleroderma relapsing polychondritis

Systemic vasculitis	Polyarteritis nodosa Churg-Strauss syndrome Wegener's granulomatosis Behçet's disease Takayasu's disease Giant cell arteritis Cogan syndrome

Table 1. Rheumatic diseases with changes occurring in the organ of sight.

2. Characteristics of rheumatic diseases, in which the most frequent changes in the organ of sight occur

The rheumatoid arthritis (RA) and spondyloarthropathies (SpA) are the most common inflammatory rheumatic diseases. Significantly less frequently uvenile idiopathic arthritis (JIA), Sjögren's syndrome (SS), systemic lupus erythematosus (SLE) and other less frequent connective tissue diseases as scleroderma, dermato-and polymiositis, recurrent inflammation of the cartilage and systemic vasculitis are observed.

2.1. Rheumatoid arthritis

Rheumatoid arthritis is an autoimmune connective tissue disease that manifests itself mostly with symmetrical swelling of the joints (particularly of the hands) - and with morning stiffness. The incidence of RA in the world is estimated at about 0.33 -1.5% of the total population [1,2,3,4,5,6]. The diagnosis of RA is based on the current 2010 ACR / EULAR criteria. The diagnosis of RA is definite when the summary point record for all criteria (A + B + C + D) reaches ≥ 6 out of 10. (Table 2) [7].

A. Joint involvement	1 large joint	0
	2-10 large joints	1
	1-3 small joints (with or without involvement of large	2
	joints)	3
	4 - 10 small joints (with or without involvement of	5
	joints)	
	"/ 10 joints (at least 1 small joint affected)	
B. serological tests (at least one required)	Negative results for the presence of RF and ACPA	0
	Positive results in the presence of low-titer RF and	2
	ACPA	3
	Positive results in the presence of high titers of RF	
	and ACPA	

http://dx.doi.org/10.5772/52968

C. indicators of acute fase (at least one required)	Valid values for CRP and ESR	0
	Incorrect values of CRP and ESR	1
D. duration of symptoms	<6 weeks	0
	≥ 6 weeks	1

RF – Rheumatoid Factor, ACPA – Anti-Citrullinated Protein Antibodies, CRP – C-Reactive Protein, ESR – Erythrocyte Sedimentation Rate

Table 2. ACR/EULAR 2010 classification criteria for rheumatoid arthritis

Approximately 40% of patients with RA present not only joint inflammation but also clinical symptoms resulting from other organ involvement [8].

Frequently, in as many as about 30% of patients with rheumatoid, rheumatoid nodules occur [9]. The changes in the lungs, such as pleural involvement, take place in approximately 50% of patients, but only in 10% of cases are identified [10]. Similarly frequently autopsy reveals changes in the heart.

In echocardiography pericardial effusion is revealed in 31% of patients [11]. 1 - 5% of patients with RA are diagnosed with vasculitis, while autopsy studies detect these changes in 15-31% of patients [12,13]. Changes in the eyes in the course of RA are observed in approximately 25% of patients [14, 15]. The treatment of RA is based on disease-modifying drugs (DMARDs) such as methotrexate, sulfasalazine. leflunomide, cyclosporine, cyclophospamide, hydroxychloroquine or chloroquine and gold salts. Furthermore, patients often have glucocorticoids and non-steroidal anti-inflammatory drugs (NSAIDs) administered orally or locally (intra-articularly). In the contemporary rheumatology in case of ineffectivness of the traditional DMARDs therapy second line treatment is implemented - based on biological agents. These include TNF-alpha (tumor necrosis factor) inhibitors such as adalimumab, certolizumab pegol, etanercept, golimumab, infliximab as well as drugs with other mechanism of action such as abatacept (anti-CTL-4), rituximab (anti-CD 20) and tocilizumab (anti-IL-6) [16].

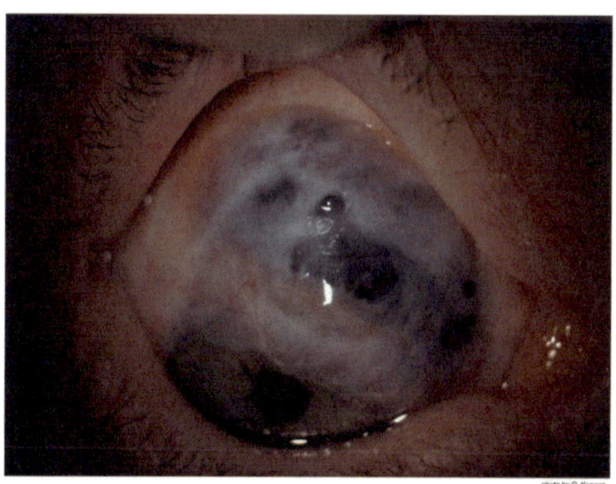

Figure 1. Scleromalacia perforans in patient with long-term RA (photo by D. Kopacz).

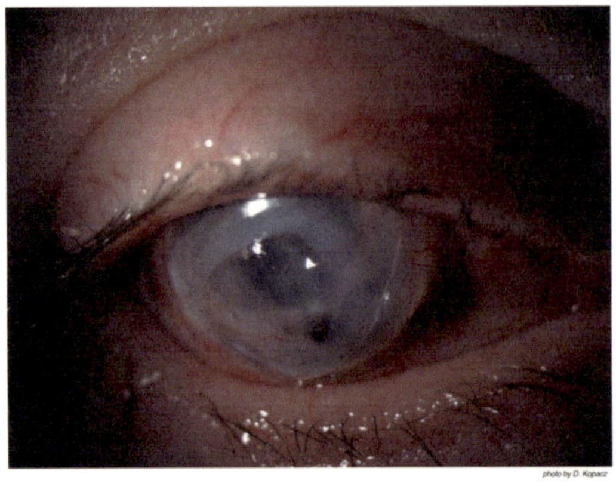

Figure 2. Scleromalacia perforans in patient with long-term RA (photo by D. Kopacz).

2.2. Spondyloarthropathies

Spondyloarthropathies (SpA) are a group of diseases are characterized by similar clinical symptoms and genetic predispositions.

Back pain lasting ≥ 3 months with the start in <45 years of age (with or without periferal symptoms of the disease

Sacroiliitis in imaging tests results + ≥ 1 symptom of spondyloarthropathy	or	Presence of HLA B27 antigen + ≥ 2 symptoms of spondyloarthropathy

Symptoms of SpA:

- The pain of an inflamed sites
- Arthritis
- Enthesitis
- Iritis
- Dactylitis
- Psoriasis skin
- Leśniowski-Crohn's disease / colitis ulcerosa
- Good response to non-steroidal anti-inflammatory drugs
- A history of SpA in the family
- The presence of HLA-B27 antigen
- Increased levels of CRP

Table 3. ASAS classification criteria for axial spondyloarthropathy

http://dx.doi.org/10.5772/52968

Spondyloarthropathies can be divided into 2 groups according to the predominant symptoms. The domination of symptoms suggestive of spinal involvement, such as inflammatory back pain (IBP) - i.e. pain escalating at night, decreasing after exercise, not alleviated by the period of rest - defines axial spondyloarthropathy. In patients with prevalence to enthesitis and peripheral arthritis, the peripheral sopndyloarthropathy is diagnosed. ASAS Group (Ankylosing spondylitis In Assessment) has developed diagnostic criteria common to these diseases (Table 3.4) [17, 18].

Peripheral arthritis (most commonly of the lower extremities and/or asymmetrical) or enthesitis (enthesitis), or sausage fingers (dactylitis)
AND ≥ 1 symptom of SpA ≥ 2 other symptoms SpA - Psoriasis - arthritis - Crohn's disease-Lesniewski / colitis ulcerosa **or** - inflammation of the tendon - Prior to infection - dactilitis , sausage fingers - presence of HLA-B27 antigen - inflammatory back pain (ever) - Uveitis - a history of SpA in the family - Inflammation of the sacroiliac joints in imaging tests (X-ray or MRI)

Table 4. ASAS classification criteria for peripheral spondyloarthropathy

There separate classification criteria for particular spondyloarthropathies such as ankylosing spondylitis (AS), psoriatic arthritis (PsA), reactinve arthritis (ReA), arthritis in course of ulcerative colitis and Leśniowski- Crohn's disease are also established.

Spondyloarthropathies incidence is similar to that of RA and ranges from 0.15 to 1.8% of the general population [19,20,21].

The uveitis affects approximately 0.5% of patients with spondyloarthropathies, and frequency of its occurence varies depending on the type of spondyloarthropathies. In AS uveitis occurs in 0.8% of patients, while in about 2.3% of patients with the PsA [22]. Ocular changes in SpA related to non-specific inflammatory bowel disease (ulcerative colitis, Leśniowski Crohn's disease) occur in up to 4-12% of patients [23,24].

Conjunctivitis occurs in 33-100% of patients with reactive arthritis [25] and 20 to 33% of patients with PsA [26].

The treatment of spondyloarthropathies is based on non-steroidal anti-inflammatory drugs, disease-modifying drugs such as methotrexate, leflunomide, sulfasalazine, cyclosporyna and biological agents from the group of anti-TNF-alpha. The glucocorticoids are also used in intraarticular injections [27,28].

2.3. Juvenile idiopathic arthritis

Juvenile idiopathic arthritis is the most common form of chronic inflammation of the connective tissue in children. Prevalence in the population is 43-148 cases per 100 000 persons [29,30,31]. The diagnosis of JIA is based on the 1997 ILAR criteria. For the arthritis do be diagnosed as JIA the onset of the disease must take place until 16 years of age, arthritis symptoms must last more than 6 weeks and other diseases in which arthritis occurs have to be excluded (e.g.infectious, reactive, toxic and allergic and neoplastamatic diseases and other conditions with joint involvment). Ocular complications - mainly uveitis - occur in approximately 12-17% of juvenile patients [32]. Treatment, as in RA, is based on DMARDs and biological agents.

2.4. Systemic lupus erythematosus (SLE)

Systemic lupus erythematosus (SLE) is a chronic inflammatory autoimmune disease with diverse symptomatology resulting from involvement of many organs and systems. The prevalence of SLE in the general population ranges from 0.016 to 0.092% [33,34,35]. The typical clinical features of SLE include facial erythema, discoid rash, photosensitivity, oral ulcers, arthritis, pleurisy or pericarditis, kidney changes, changes in the central nervous system, haematological disorders (such as hemolytic anemia, leukopenia, lymphopenia, thrombocytopenia), immune changes with presence of antinuclear, anti-DNA and anti-Sm autoantibodies, as well as false positive syphilis tests. SLE may be associated with antyphospolipid syndrome (APS) with thrombotic episodes in the arteries and veins and obstetrics failure in women. Diagnosis is based on the revised 1997 ACR classification criteria [36]. Changes in the organ of sight occur in approximately 25% of patients, mainly in the course of secondary Sjögren's syndrome but also as result of vasculitis and thrombosis [37]. Conjunctivitis, episcleritis and interstitial keratitis are rare [38].

2.5. Primary Sjögren's syndrome

Primary Sjögren's syndrome (pSS) is an inflammatory autoimmune disease that occurs most often in women between 40 and 50 years of age. The clinical symptoms of the disease result from B cell autoreactivity, polyclonal immunoglobulin overproduction and infiltration of exocrine glands by lymphocytes (CD4 cells predominate). The dominant symptom is dryness of the mouth and eyes. The nonerosive arthritis, vasculitis, peripheral neuropathy and different symptoms from central nervous system are also observed in pSS. According to different data Sjögren's syndrome prevalence rate ranges from 0.2 to 13.3% of the population [39,40,41]. Sjögren's syndrome is diagnosed on the basis of the revised 2002 American-European criteria[42]. Ocular symptoms associated with impaired secretion of tears occur in all patients with Sjögren's syndrome – either in the initial or more advanced stages of the dis-

http://dx.doi.org/10.5772/52968

ease – and constitute one of to the diagnostic criteria. Treatment is based on the use of both symptomatic drugs - moistening eyes and mouth – and of immunosuppressants.

2.6. Scleroderma

Scleroderma is an inflammatory connective tissue disease of unknown etiology characterized by the damage to blood vessels, the presence of autoantibodies (SCL 70 or anticentromeric autoantibodies for diffuse systemic sclerosis and localised systemic sclerosis respectively) and progressive fibrosis of the skin and internal organs. Systemic sclerosis prevalence rate in the world is ranging from 0.0007% to 0.265% [43,44,45]. Disease diagnosis based on the classification and diagnostic criteria of the 1980 ACR [46]. 71% of patients present changes in blood and conjunctival subepithelial fibrosis. In course of SS all structures of the eye may be affected [47,48]. Patient with SS may develop secondary Sjogren's syndrome and symptoms of dry eye, as well as complications due to the dryness of the conjunctiva [49].

2.7. Recurrent inflammation of the cartilage

Recurrent inflammation of the cartilage is a rare inflammatory autoimmune disease in which the inflammatory process involving mostly cartilage, causing changes and dysfunction of many tissues and organs. Onset of the disease usually affects people of 40-60 years of age and the prevalence of this disease in the world is estimated at about 3 cases per 1 million people in the population [50]. Currently, the diagnosis of this disease can be based on the diagnostic criteria of McAdam, 1976 [51]. Changes in the organ of vision occur in approximately 60% of patients and may include almost all structures of the eye [52, 53].

2.8. Systemic vasculitis

In the course of systemic vasculitis such as polyarteritis nodosa, Churga-Strauss syndrome, Wegener's granulomatosis, Behçet's disease, Takayasu disease, giant cell arteritis and Cogan syndrome there are changes in the organ of sight secondary to vascular changes. In polyarteritis nodosa ocular changes are observed in approximately 10-20% of patients [54,55], in Wegener's granuloma in 28-58% of patients [56,57] Behçet's disease in 68-85% of patients [58, 59, 60]. The ocular changes in course of inflammation of the large vessels, such as giant cell arteritis, are mainly associated with ischemia of optic nerve or retina. Ischemia causes impairment of vision and blindness, which may occur in 13 to 70% of patients [61,62]. The treatment of all systemic vasculitis requires agressive immunosuppressive therapy and high doses of glucocorticoids. In some cases of very active disease and no reaction to other treatment, especially in case of Wegener's granuloma, biological therapy (rituximab) is used [63,64]

3. Characteristic changes in the organ of sight in rheumatic diseases

The pathological changes can occur in all elements of the organ of sight in the course of rheumatic diseases. These can cause temporary or permanent damage (Table 5). Changes in the eyes are the first symptom of rheumatic fever observed in approximately 4% of patients [65].

type of symptoms and changes in the eye	rheumatic disease
conjunctivitis	Reactive arthritis
	Psoriatic arthritis
dryness	Sjögren's syndrome
	Rheumatoid vasculitis
	Rheumatoid arthritis
	Systemic vasculitis
Uveitis:	Spondyloarthropathies
Acute anterior uveitis	Behçet disease
Chronic anterior uveitis	colitis ulcerosa/ Leśniowski - Crohn's disease
Panuveitis	colitis ulcerosa/ Leśniowski-Crohn;s disease
	relapsing polychondritis
	Behçet disease
Scleritis	Rheumatoid arthritis
	systemic vasculitis
	Colitis ulcerosa/ Leśniewski- Crohn;s disease
	Relapsing polychondritis
Keratitis:	Sjögren's syndrome
Non-necrotizing corneal melt	Rheumatoid vasculitis
Necrotizing keratitis	Rheumatoid arthritis
	systemic vasculitis
Retinal vasculopathy	Systemic Lupus erythematosus
Microvasculopathy	Systemic lupus erythematosus
Diffuse vaso-occlusive disease	Antiphospholipid syndrome
	Behçet disease
Optic nerve disaease	Systemic vasculitis (particulary giant cell vasculitis)
Ischemic optic neuropathy	

Table 5. The most common ocular changes in the course of the rheumatic diseases.

Changes in the eyes in course of the rheumatic diseases may also be caused by the implemented treatment. Nonsteroidal anti-inflammatory drugs are medications most commonly used in alleviating the symptoms of rheumatic diseases. Cases of keratopathy (keratopathy) after indomethacin use have been reported [66], and diplopia (double vision) and amblyopia (amblyopia) after ibuprofen and naproxen treatment [67]. Antimalaric drugs such as hydroxychloroquine and more often chloroquine may aggregate in the cornea [68], in 13 - 40% of patients causing retinopathy [69,70]. Gold salts - administered parenterally over the total dose of 1000mg/kg of body weight – accumulate in various tissues of the body and have been observed in the eyes (conjunctiva, cornea, anterior lens and retina) in 97% of patients [71]. Gold salt deposits in the eyes may cause hypersensitivity reactions, induce inflammation and cause marginal ulceration [72]. After methotrexate therapy diffuse irritation of the cornea is observed [73]. Chronic glucocortycoid therapy often leads to cataracts, subcapsular cataracts and glaucoma [74, 75].

4. Infectious complications of the eyes in rheumatic diseases

Viral, bacterial and fungal infectious complications occur in the organ of sight in patients with rheumatic diseases more frequently than in healthy individuals due to the immunological system dysfunctions, immunosuppressive therapy and chronic use of corticosteroids.

4.1. Infective conjunctivitis

4.1.1. Bacterial conjunctivitis

Chlamydial conjunctivitis

Reactive arthritis, which belongs to spondyloarthropaties, may be caused by infection with Chlamydia trachomatis and Chlamydia pneumoniae [76]. In the course of the infection with Chlamydia trachomatis (serotypes DK) chronic conjunctivitis occurs in 6-19% of patients [77, 78]. Chlamydial conjunctivitis most commonly affects sexually active adults, especially men. Chlamydia DNA is detected by PCR (polymerase chain reaction) in 96% of patients with reactive arthritis concomitant conjunctivitis, leakage from the urethra and inflammation of asymmetric arthritis (former name of these symptoms is Reiter's syndrome) [79]. Eye involvement probably occurs by the way of self infection from the genitourinary system, or from one eye to another. In chlamydial conjunctivitis in adults symptoms initially occur in one of the eyes. It was also found that conjunctivitis may also occur (less frequently than in Chlamydia trachomatis) in the course of Chlamydia pneumoniae infection – as was demonstrated by confirming the presence of bacterial DNA from conjunctival scraping [80].

Clinical symptoms of chlamydial conjunctivitis in reactive arthritis are characterized by moderate redness of a single eye or less commonly of both eyes, tearing, photophobia and decreased vision. Ocular examination shows conjunctival hyperemia, chemosis and follicular reaction in conjunctiva and semilunar folds. Epithelial and subeopithelial infiltrates in cornea may develop.

The histopathology assessment reveals the presence of the chronic inflammation cells localized in submucosal layer, with the predominance of lymphocytes. In addition, fibrinogen deposits in the basal membrane of conjunctiva, infiltration of lymphocytes and macrophages around small blood vessels and lymphocytic infiltration of the walls of larger vessels of conjunctiva have been observed [81].

Diagnosis is based on the detection of IgM, IgG and IgA antibodies to these bacteria in the blood serum by ELISA method and confirmation with W-blot test. Classical method is a detection of Chlamydia basophilic intracytoplasmic inclusions in primary cells from the conjunctival swab or conjunctival scraping using DFA (direct immunofluorescence staining) method, DNA hybridization tests or PCR (polymerase chain reaction and LCR (Ligas chain reaction).

Treatment of chlamydial conjunctivitis infection in the course of reactive arthritis consists of systemic antibiotic therapy and topical use of tetracycline, erythromycin or fluorochinolones. In systemic treatment effectiveness of macrolides (azithromycin), tetracyclines and quinolones has been shown [82,83, 84]. Single dose of azithromycin (1000mg) showed efficacy in eradication of C. trachomatis infection [85] It's vital to stress that chlamydia infection is still the main cause of blindness on the African Continent. In the case of trachoma present drug of choice is azithromycin [86].

Because C.trachomatis infection is sexually transsmitted, other similarly transmitted co- infections should be considered, most commonly gonococcal.

4.1.2. Fungal conjunctivitis

Significantly higher incidence of fungal conjunctivitis is observed in patients with rheumatic diseases treated with systemic glucocorticoids (eg, RA) and in patients with primary Sjögren's syndrome. The most common pathogens are Candida albicans and Candida parapsilosis [87].

5. Infectious scleritis in rheumatic diseases

It has been shown that in patients with scleral inflammation lasting over 12 years, 7.5% of them had infectious complications, usually caused by herpes zoster virus [88]. Infectious complications can be even more frequent in patients with rheumatic diseases who are chronically treated with immunosuppressive drugs. The use of immunosuppressive drugs can cause reactivation of latent Mycobacterium tuberculosis infection which, in the form of nodular scleritis may occur in the eye [89]. There are reports of the occurrence of tuberculosis uveitis during treatment with etanercept (soluble anti TNF inhibitor) [90].

6. Infectious keratitis in rheumatic diseases

6.1. Viral keratitis

In RA patients inflammatory corneal ulceration may occur as a symptom of this disease. However, any such changes require the differentiation from herpes simplex infection, which presents the same clinical picture. The differentiation is important from the point of implemented treatment, because corneal ulceration in course of RA requires a very intensive immunosuppressive therapy, which exacerbates an inflammation caused by herpes simplex infection [91].

6.2. Bacterial keratitis

Bacterial keratitis in rheumatic diseases often is a complicated by erosive lesions of the cornea. Such changes are most commonly associated with primary and secondary Sjögren's syndrome. Most frequently - up to 73.9% - patients suffer from Gram-positive bacterial infections of as coagulase-negative Staphylococci, Staph. aureus and Spreptococcus pneumoniae. 0.3% of patients suffer from infections of Gram-negative Moraxella spp. Infections with Gram-positive bacteria are present in 17.4% of patients; most common are : Propionibacterium acnes, Corynebacterium spp. 6.5% patients reveal infections caused by Pseudomonas aeruginosa and Proteus spp [92,93].

6.3. Fungal keratitis

The fungal infections of the cornea may also develop in the primary and secondary Sjogren's syndrome due to improper hydration of the eye – both because of the composition of tears and rupture in the tear film. In 45.8% of patients with fungal infection of the cornea Candida albicans is the major pathogen, while Fusarium spp accouns for approximately 25% of the infections.

7. Comment

In the light of the wide use of immunosuppressive therapy, in particular in the era of biological therapies in rheumatic diseases, close attention should be paid to the possible reactivation of latent infections. Most commonly tuberculous infection should be considered, but viruses like Cytomegalovirus (CMV) may also be present in patients in their persistent form. In similar circumstances - in AIDS patients and patients after organ transplantations (e.g. bone marrow transpaltation) - CMV retinitis has been reported. Currently there are reports of CMV retinitis in the course of treatment RA with infliximab (anti TNF) [94].

Finally, it should be noted that biological drugs have proved effective in the treatment of ocular manifestations of many rheumatic diseases and the exclusion of potential infection is particularly important for the choice of treatment and safety of therapy.

Author details

Brygida Kwiatkowska and Maria Maślińska*

*Address all correspondence to: maslinskam@gmail.com

Institute of Rheumatology, Poland

References

[1] Helmic, C. G., Felson, D. T., Lawrence, R. C., et al. (2008). Estimates of prevalence of arthritis and other rheumatic conditions in the United States. *Part 1. Arthritis & Rheumatism*, 58(1), 15-25.

[2] Knox, S. A., Harrison, C. M., Britt, H. C., et al. (2008). Estimating prevalence of common chronic morbidities in Australia. *Medical Journal of Australia*, 189(2), 66-70.

[3] Symmons, D., Turner, G., Webb, R., et al. (2002). The prevalence of rheumatoid arthritis in the United Kingdom: New estimates for a new century. *Rheumatology*, 41(7), 793-800.

[4] Simonnson, M., Bergman, S., Jacobsson, L. T. H., et al. (1999). The prevalence of rheumatoid arthritis in Sweden. *Scandinavian Journal of Rheumatology*, 28(6), 340-343.

[5] Senna, E. R., De Barros, A. L. P., Silva, E. O., et al. (2004). Prevalence of rheumatoid diseases in Brazil: a study using the COPCORD approach. *Journal of Rheumatology*, 31(3), 594-597.

[6] Darmawan, J., Muirden, K. D., Valkenburg, H. A., et al. (1993). The epidemiology of rheumatoid arthritis in Indonesia. *British Journal of Rheumatology*, 32(7), 537-540.

[7] Aletaha, D., Neogi, T., Silman, A. J., et al. (2010). Rheumatoid arthritis classification criteria: an American College of Rheumatology/European League Against Rheumatism collaborative initiative. *Arthritis Rheum*, 62, 2569-2581.

[8] Cimmino, M. A., Salvarani, C., & Macchioni, P. (2000). Extra-articular manifestations of rheumatoid arthritis. *Rheumatol Int*, 19(6), 213-217.

[9] Young, A., & Koduri, G. (2007). Extra-articular manifestations and complications of rheumatoid arthritis. *Best Pract Clin Rheumatol*, 21(5), 907-927.

[10] Balbir-Gurman, A., Yigla, M., Nahir, A. M., et al. (2006). Rheumatoid pleural effusion. *Semin Arthritis Rheum*, 35, 368-378.

[11] Mac, Donald. W. J. Jr, Crawford, M. H., Klippel, J. H., et al. (1977). Echocardiographic assessment of cardiac structure and function in patients with rheumatoid arthritis. *Am J Med*, 63, 890-896.

[12] Genta, M. S., Genta, R. M., & Gabay, C. (2006). Systemic rheumatoid vasculitis: a review. *Semin Arthritis Rheum*, 36, 88-98.

[13] Bartels, C. M., & Bridges, A. J. (2010). Rheumatoid Vasculitis: Vanishing Menance or Target for New Treatments? *Curr Rheumatol Rep*, 12(6), 414-419.

[14] Harper, S. L., & Foster, C. S. (1998). The ocular manifestation of rheumatoid disease. *Int Ophtalmol Clin*, 38, 1-19.

[15] Zlatanovic, G., Veselinovic, D., Cekic, S., et al. (2010). Ocular manifestation of rheumatoid arthritis-different forms and frequency. *Bosn J Basic Med Sci*, 10, 323-327.

[16] Saag, K. G., Teng, G. G., Patkar, N. M., & Et, al. (2008). American College of Rheumatology recommendations for the use of nonbiologic and biologic disease-modifying antirheumatic drugs in rheumatoid arthritis. Arthritis Rheum.; , 59, 762-784.

[17] Rudwaleit, M., van der Heijde, D., & Landewé, R. et al. (2009). The development of Assessment of SpondyloArthritis International Society classification criteria for axial spondyloarthritis (partII)): validation and final selection. Ann Rheum Dis , 68, 777-783.

[18] Rudwaleit, M., van der Heijde, D., & Landewé, R. et al. (2011). The development of Assessment of SpondyloArthritis International Society classification criteria for peripheral spondyloarthritis and for spondyloarthritis in general. Ann Rheum Dis , 70, 25-31.

[19] Braun, J., Bollow, M., Remlinger, G., et al. (1998). Prevalence of the spondyloarthropaties in HLA-B27 positive and negative blood donors. *Arthritis & Rheumatism*, 41, 1483-1491.

[20] Saraux, A., Guillemin, F., Guggenbuhl, P., et al. (2001). Prevalence of the spondyloarthropathies in France. *Ann Rheum Dis*, 64, 1431-1435.

[21] Reveille, J. D. (2011). Epidemiology of Spondyloarthritis in North America. *Am J Med Sci*, 341(4), 284-286.

[22] Zeboulon, N., Dougados, M., & Gossec, M. (2008). Prevalence and characteristics of uveitis in the spondyloarthropathies: a systemic literature review. *Ann Rheum Dis*, 67, 955-959.

[23] Lampert, J. R., & Wright, V. (1976). Eye inflammation in psoriatic arthritis. *Ann Rheum Dis*, 35(4), 354-356.

[24] Bernstein, C. N., Blanchard, J. F., & Rawsthorne, P. (2001). The prevalence of extraintenstinal diseases in inflammatory bowel disease: a population based study. *Am J Gastroenterol*, 96, 1116-1122.

[25] Ardizzone, S., Puttini, P. S., Cassinotti, A., & at, . al. (2008). Extraintenstinal manifestations of inflammatory bowel disease. Givestive and Liver Disease , 40, 253-250.

[26] Lee, D. A., Barker, S. M., Su, W. P., et al. (1986). The clinical diagnosis of Reiter's syndrome. Ophthalmic and nonophthalmic aspects. *Ophtalmology*, 93(3), 350-356.

[27] Braun, J., van der Berg, R., & Baraliakos, X. et al. (2010). update of the ASAS/EULAR recommendations for the management of ankylosing spondylitis. Ann Rheum Dis. 2011; , 70, 896-904.

[28] Gossec, L., Smolen, J., Gaujoux-Viala, C., et al. (2012). European Legue Against Rheumatism recommendations for the management of psoriatic arthritis with pharmacological therapies. *Ann Rheum Dis*, 71, 4-12.

[29] Towner, S. R., Michet, C. J., O'Fallon, W. M., et al. (1983). The epidemiology of juvenile arthritis in Rochester, Minnesota, 1960-1979. *Arthritis Rheum*, 26(10), 1208-1213.

[30] von, Koskull. S., Truckenbrodt, H., Holle, R., et al. (2001). Incidence and prevalence of juvenile arthritis in an urban population of southern Germany: a prospective study. *Ann Rheum Dis*, 60(10), 940-945.

[31] Riise, Ø. R., Handeland, K. S., Cvancarova, M., et al. (2008). Incidence and characteristics of arthritis in Norwegian children: a population-based study. *Pediatrics*, 121(2), 299-306.

[32] Berk, A. T., Kocak, N., & Ünsal, E. (2001). Uveitie in Juvenile arthritis. *Ocular Immunol*, 9(4), 243-251.

[33] Dadoniene, J., Adamoviciute, D., Rugiene, R., et al. (2006). The prevalence of systemic lupus erythematosus in Lithuania: the lowest rate in Northern Europe. *Lupus*, 15(8), 544-546.

[34] Govoni, M., Castellino, G., Bosi, S., et al. (2006). Incidence and prevalence of systemic lupus erythematosus in a district of north Italy. *Lupus*, 15(2), 110-113.

[35] Boyer, G. S., Templin, D. W., & Lanier, A. P. (1991). Rheumatic diseases in Alaskan Indians of the southeast coast: high prevalence of rheumatoid arthritis and systemic lupus erythematosus. *Journal of Rheumatology*, 18(10), 477-484.

[36] Hochberg, M. C. (1997). Updating te American College of Rheumatology revised criteria for the classification of systemic lupus erythematosus. *Arthritis Rheum*, 40, 725-734.

[37] Jensen, J. L., Bergem, H. O., & Gilboe, I. M. (1999). Oral and ocular sicca symptoms and findings are prevalent in systemic lupus erythematosus. *J Oral Patho Med*, 28(7), 317-322.

[38] Nguyen, Q.d., & Foster, C. S. (1998). Systemic lupus erythematosus and the eye. *Int Ophtalmol Clin*, 38(1), 33-60.

[39] Bowman, S. J., Ibrahim, G. H., Holmes, G., et al. (2004). Estimating the prevalence among Caucasian women of primary Sjögrem syndrome in two general practices in Birmingham, UK. *Scandinavian Journal of Rheumatology*, 33(1), 39-43.

[40] Kabsakal, Y., Kitapcioglu, G., Turk, T., et al. (2006). The prevalence of Sjögren syndrome In adult women. *Scandinavian Journal of Rheumatology*, 35(5), 379-383.

[41] Sanchez-Guerrero, J., Perez-Dosal, M. R., et al. (2005). Prevalence of Sjögren syndrome In ambulatory patients according to the American-European Consensus Group criteria. *Rheumatology*, 44(2), 235-240.

[42] Vitali, C., Bombardieri, S., Jonsson, R., et al. (2002). Classification criteria for Sjögren's syndrome: a revised version of the European criteria proposed by the American-European Consensus Group. *Ann Rheum Dis*, 61, 554-558.

[43] Allcock, R. J., Forrest, I., Corris, P. A., et al. (2004). A study of prevalence of systemic sclerosis in northeast England. *Rheumatology*, 43(5), 596-602.

[44] Le Guern, V., Mahr, A., Mouyhon, L., et al. (2004). Prevalence of systemic sclerosis in French multi-ethnic county. *Rheumatology*, 43(9), 1129-1137.

[45] Robinson Jr, D., Eisenberg, D., Nietert, P. J., et al. (2008). Systemic sclerosis prevalence and comorbidities in US, 2001-2002. *Current Medical Research and Opinion*, 24(4), 1157-1166.

[46] Subcommittee for scleroderma criteria of the American Rheumatism Association Diagnostic and Therapeutic Criteria Committee. (1980). Preliminary criteria for the classification of systemic sclerosis (scleroderma). *Arthritis Rheum*, 23, 581-590.

[47] West, R. H., & Barnett, A. J. (1979). Ocular involvement in scleroderma. *Br J Ophtalmol*, 63(12), 845-847.

[48] Tailor, R., Herrick, A., & Kwartz, J. (2009). Ocular manifestations of scleroderma. *Survey of Ophtalmology*, 54(2), 292-304.

[49] Alarcon-Segovia, D., Ibanez, G., & Hernandez-Ortiz, J. (1974). Sjögren's syndrome in progressive systemic sclerosis (scleroderma). *Am J Med*, 57(1), 78-85.

[50] Kent, P. D., Michet, C. J., & Luthra, H. S. (2004). Relapsing polychondritis. *Curr Opin Rheumatol*, 16(1), 56-61.

[51] Mc Adam, L. P., O'Hanlan, MA, Bluestone, R., et al. (1976). Relapsing polychondritis: prospective study of 23 patients and a review of the literature. *Medicine (Baltimore)*, 55, 193-215.

[52] Isaak, B. L., Liesegang, T. J., & Michet, C. J. (1986). Ocular and systemic findings in relapsing polychondritis. *Ophtalmology*, 93(5), 681-189.

[53] Lahmer, T., Treiber, M., von Werder, A., et al. (2010). Relapsing polychondritis:. *An autoimmune disease with many faces*, 9, 540-546.

[54] Cohen, R. D., Conn, D. I., & Ilstrup, D. M. (1980). Clinical features, prognosis, and response to treatment in polyarteritis. *Mayo Clini Proc*, 55(3), 145-155.

[55] Hamideh, F., & Prete, P. E. (2001). Ophtalmologic Manifestations of Rheumatic Diseases. *Seminars in Arthritis and Rheumatism*, 30(4), 217-241.

[56] Bullen, C. L., Liesegang, T. J., Mc Donald, T. J., et al. (1983). Ocular complications of Wegener's granulomatosis. *Ophtalmology*, 90(3), 272-290.

[57] Montagnac, R., Nyandwi, J., Loiselet, G., et al. (2009). Ophtalmic manifestations in Wegener's granulomatosis. *Review of literature about an observation. Nephrol Ther*, 5(7), 603-613.

[58] Colvard, D. M., Robertson, D. M., & O'Duffy, J. D. (1997). The ocular manifestations of Behçet's disease. *Arch Ophtalmol*, 95(10), 1813-1817.

[59] Nussenblatt, R. B. (1977). Uveitis in Behçet's disease. *Int Rev Immunol*, 14(1), 67-79.

[60] O'Duffy, J. D. (1990). Vasculitis in Behçet's disease. *Rheum Dis Clin North Am*, 16(2), 423-431.

[61] Hayreh, S. S., Podhajsky, P. A., & Zimmerman, B. (1998). Ocular manifestations of giant cell arteritis. *Am J Ophtalmol*, 125(4), 506-520.

[62] Gordon, L.k., & Levin, L. A. (1998). Visual loss in giant cel arteritis. *JAMA*, 280(4), 385-386.

[63] Omdal, R., Wildhagen, K., Hansen, T., et al. (2005). Anti-CD20 therapy of treatment-resistant Wegener's granulomatosis: favourable but temporary response. *Scandinavian Journal of Rheumatology*, 34(3), 229-232.

[64] Cheung, C. M. G., Murray, P. I., & Savage, C. O. S. (2005). Successful treatment of Wegener's granulomatosis associated scleritis with rituximab. *Br J Ophtalmol*, 89(11), 1542.

[65] Hamideh, F., & Prete, P. E. (2001). Ophtalmologic Manifestations of Rheumatic Diseases. *Seminars in Arthritis and Rheumatism*, 30(4), 217-241.

[66] Blaho, K. (1992). Non-steroidal anti-inflammatory drugs: current trends in pharmacology and therapeutics. *J Am Optom Assoc*, 63(12), 875-878.

[67] Lyle, W. M., & Hayhoe, D. A. (1976). A literature survey of the potentially adverse effects of the drugs commonly prescribed for the elderly. *J Am Optom Assoc*, 47(6), 768-778.

[68] Mahoney, B. P. (1976). Rheumatologic disease and associated ocular manifestations. *J Am Optom Assoc*, 47(6), 403-415.

[69] Crues, A. F., Schachet, A. P., & Nicholl, J. (1985). Chloroquine retinopathy. *Ophtalmology* [928], 1127-1129.

[70] Grant, S., Greenseid, D. Z., & Leopold, I. H. (1989). Toxic retinopathies. *In: Duane TD, Jaeger EA editors. Clinical Ophtalmology.Philadelphia: Lippincott.*

[71] Mc Cormic, S. A., Dibartolomeo, A. G., & Raju, V. F. (1985). Ocular chrysiasis. *Ophtalmology*, 92(10), 432-435.

[72] Kincaid, M. C., Green, W. R., & Hoover, R. E. (1982). Ocular chrysiasis. *Arch Ophtalmol*, 100(11), 791-794.

[73] Loprinzi, C. L., Love, R. R., Garrity, J. A., et al. (1990). Cyclophosphamide, Methotrexate, and 5Fluorouracil (CMF)-Induced Ocular Toxicity. *Cancer Investigation*, 8(%), 459-465.

[74] Kersey, J. P., & Broadway, D. C. (2006). Corticosteroid-induced glaucoma: a review of the literature. *Eye*, 20, 407-416.

[75] Kuna, P. (1998). Longterm effects of steroid therapy. *Wiad Lek*, 51, 12-18.

[76] Kwiatkowska, B., & Filipowicz-Sosnowska, A. (2009). Reactive arthritis. *Pol Arch Med. Wewn*, 119(1-2), 60-66.

[77] Postema, E. J., Remeijer, L., & van der Meijden, W. I. (1996). Epidemiology of genital chlamydial infections in patients with chlamydial conjunctivitis; a retrospective study. *Genitourinary Med*, 72, 203-205.

[78] Haller-Schober, E. M., & El -Shabrawi, Y. (2002). Chlamydial conjunctivitis (in adults), uveitis, and reactive arthritis, including SARA. *Best Practice & research Clinical Obstetrics and Gynaecology*, 16(6), 815-828.

[79] Schumacher, H. R. Jr, Arayssi, T., Crane, M., et al. Chlamydia trachomatis nucleic acids can be found in the synovium of some asymptomatic subject. Arthritis and Rheumatism 199 , 42, 1281-1284.

[80] Lietman, T., Brooks, D., Moncada, J., et al. (1998). Chronic Follicular Conjunctivitis Associated with Chlamydia psitacci or Chlamydia pneumoniae. *Clinical Infectious Diseases*, 26, 1335-1340.

[81] Purcell, J. J., Tsai, C. C., & Baldassare, A. E. (1982). Conjunctival Immunopathologic and Ultrastructural Alterations. *Arch Ophtalmol*, 100, 1618-1621.

[82] Carter, J. D., Valeriano, J., & Vasey, F. J B. (2004). A prospective, randomized 9-monyh comparison of doxycycline and rifampin in undifferentiated spondyloarthritis-with special reference to Chlamydia-induced arthritis. *J Rheumatol*, 31, 973-980.

[83] Lauhio, A., Leirisalo-Repo, M., Lahdevirta, J., et al. (1991). Double-blind, placebo controlled study of free month treatment with limecycline in reactive arthritis, with special reference to Chlamydia Arthritis. *Arthritis Rheum*, 34, 6-14.

[84] Dreses-Werringloer, U., Padubrin, I., Zeidler, H., et al. (2001). Effects of azithromycin and rifampin on Chlamydia trachomatis infection in vitro. *Antimicrob Agents Chemother*, 45, 3001-3008.

[85] Katusic, D., Patricek, I., Mandic, Z., et al. (2003). Azithromycin vs doxycycline in the treatment of inclusion conjunctivitis. *AM J Ophtalmol*, 135(4), 447-51.

[86] West, S. K., Munoz, B., Mkocha, H., Gaydos, CA, & Quinn, T. C. (2011). Number of years of annual mass treatment with azithromycin needed to control trachoma in hyper-endemic communities in Tanzania. J Infect Dis. Jul 15; , 204(2), 268-73.

[87] Williamson, J., Gordon, A. M., Wood, R., et al. (1968). Fungal flora of the conjunctival sac in health and disease. *Brit J. Ophtal*, 52, 127-137.

[88] Mc Cluskey, P. J., Watson, P. G., Lightman, S., et al. (1999). Posterior scleritis: clinical features, systemic associations, and outcome in a large series of patients. *Ophtalmology*, 106, 380-386.

[89] Biswas, J., Aparna, A. C., Annamalai, E., et al. (2012). Tuberculosis scleritis in a patient with rheumatoid arthritis. *Ocul Immunol Inflamm*, 20(1), 49-52.

[90] Fonollosa, A., Segura, A., Giralt, J., & Garcia-Arumi, J. (2007). Tuberculous uveitis after treatment with etanercept. *Graefes Arch Clin Exp Ophthalmol*, 245(9), 1397-9.

[91] Zaher, S. S., Sandinha, T., Roberts, F., et al. (2005). Herpes Simplex Keratitis Misdiagnosed as Rheumatoid Arthritis-Related Peripheral Ulcerative Keratitis. *Cornea*, 24(8), 1015-1017.

[92] Bourcier, T., Thomas, F., Borderie, V., et al. (2003). Bacterial keratitis: predisposing factors, clinical and microbiological review of 300 cases. *Br J Ophtalmol*, 87, 834-838.

[93] Schafer, F., Bruttin, O., Zografos, L., et al. (2001). Bacterial keratitis: a prospective clinical and microbiological study. *Br J Ophtalmol*, 85, 842-847.

[94] Hearter, G., Manfras, B. J., de jong-Hesse, Y., et al. Cytomegalovirus retinitis in patient treated with anti-tumor necrosis factor alpha antibody therapy for rheumatoid arthritis. *Clin. Infect.Dis*, 39(9), 88-94.

Chapter 11

Trachoma and Inclusion Conjunctivitis

Udo Ubani

Additional information is available at the end of the chapter

http://dx.doi.org/10.5772/53861

1. Introduction

Trachoma is the leading infectious cause of preventable blindness in the world today and occurs as mesoendemic, endemic, or hyperendemic disease. The distribution is primarily in tropical developing countries of the world including North and sub-Saharan Africa, the Middle East, and the Northern Indian subcontinent. The disease has also been reported in Southeast Asia and specific regions of Central and South America, Australia, and the South Pacific Islands. Of the more than 600 million people afflicted, approximately 150 million have visual deficits, and 12 million are predicted to be blind by the year 2020.

2. Clinical features

2.1. Symptoms

In the absence of secondary infection, symptoms are minimal and include mild foreign body sensation in the eyes, occasional lacrimation, slight stickiness of the lids and scanty mucoid discharge. In the presence of secondary infection symptoms of acute mucopurulent conjunctivitis develop.

2.2. Signs

2.2.1. Conjunctival

1. Congestion of upper tarsal and forniceal conjunctiva
2. Conjunctival follicles of 0.2 to 2 mm in diameter and are commonly seen on upper tarsal conjunctiva and fornix, but may also be present in the lower fornix, plica semilunaris

and caruncle. Sometimes, follicles may be seen on the bulbar conjunctiva. Follicles are formed due to the scattered aggregation of lymphocytes and other cells in the adenoid layer. Central part of each follicle is made up of mononuclear histiocytes, few lymphocytes and large multinucleated cells called Leber cells. The cortical part is made up of zone of lymphocytes showing active proliferation. Blood vessels are present in the most peripheral part. In later stages signs of necrosis are also seen.

3. Papillary hyperplasia: Papillae are reddish, flat topped raised areas which give red and velvety appearance to the tarsal conjunctiva. Each papilla consists of central core of numerous dilated blood vessels surrounded by lymphocytes and covered by hypertrophic epithelium.

4. Conjunctival scarring may be irregular, star-shaped or linear. Linear scar present in the sulcus subtarsalis is called Arlt's line.

5. Concretions may be formed due to accumulation of dead epithedial cells and inspissated mucus in the depressions called glands of Henle.

2.2.2. Corneal

1. Superficial Keratitis may be present in the upper part.

2. Herbert follicles refer to typical follicles present in the limbal area. These are histologically similar to conjunctival follicles.

3. Pannus which is an infilteration of the cornea associated with vascularization, can develop at any point along the limbal margin but is most pronounced at the superior limbal margin. The vessels are superficial and lie between epithelium and Bowman's membrane; and later on the Bowman's membrane is destroyed.

Pannus may be progressive (infiltration of cornea is ahead of vascularization) or regressive also termed pannus siecus (vessels extend a short distance beyond the area of infiltration).

4. Corneal ulcer may sometimes develop at the advantage of pannus. Such ulcers are usually shallow which may become chronic and indolent.

5. Herbert pits are the oval or circular pitted scars, left after healing of Herbert follicles in the limbal area.

6. Corneal opacity may be present in the upper part. It may even extend down and involve the papillary area. It is the end result of trachomatous corneal lesions.

2.3. Differential diagnosis

1. Presence of large multinucleated Leber cells and signs of necosis differentiate trachoma follicles from Adenovirus follicles conjunctivitis.

The distribution of follicles in trachoma is mainly on upper palpebral conjunctiva and fornix. Sometimes, follicles may be seen on the bulbar conjunctiva.

http://dx.doi.org/10.5772/53861

The corneal involvement of the disease includes lymphoid follicle formation at the limbus. This is a characteristic feature of trachoma and can lead to the development of Herbert's pit.

Associated signs such as papillae and pannus are characteristic of trachoma.

2. Trachoma with predominant papillae is differentiated from palpebral form of spring catarrh as follows:

Papillae are large in size and usually there is typical cobble-stone arrangement in spring catarrh.

The pH of tears is usually alkaline in spring catarrh, while in trachoma it is acidic.

Discharge is ropy in spring catarrh

The corneal involvement of the disease includes lymphoid follicle formation at the limbus. This is a characteristic feature of trachoma and can lead to the development of Herbert's pit. In trachoma, there may be associated follicles and pannus.

3. Sequelae of trachoma

1. Sequelae in the lids may be trichisis, entropion, tylosis (thickening of lid margin), ptosis, madarosis and ankylophearon.
2. Conjunctival sequelae include concretions, pseudocyst, xerosis and symblepharon.
3. Corneal sequelae may be corneal opacity, ectasia, corneal xerosis and total corneal pannus (blinding sequelae).
4. Other sequelae may be chronic daccryocystitis, and chronic dacryoadenitis.

The only complication of trachoma is corneal ulcer and it occurs due to rubbing by concretions, or trichiasis with superimposed bacterial infection.

4. Classification

Trachoma has always been an important blinding disease under consideration of WHO and thus many attempts have been to streamline its clinical profile. The latest classification suggested by WHO in 1987 with the acrimony FISTO is as follows:

1. TF: Trachomatous inflammation-follicular is the stage of active trachoma with predominantly follicular inflammation. To diagnose this stage at least five or more follicles (each 0.5mm or more in diameter) must be present on the upper tarsal conjunctiva. Further, the deep tarsal vessels should be visible through the follicles and papillae.

2. TI: Trachomatous inflammation-intense is diagnosed when pronounced inflammatory thickening of the upper tarsal conjunctiva obscures more than half of the normal deep tarsal vessels.

3. TS: Trachomatous scarring is diagnosed by the presence of scarring in the tarsal conjunctiva. These scars are easily visible as white, bands or sheets (fibrosis) in the tarsal conjunctiva.

4. TT: Trachomatous trichiasis is labeled when at least one eyelash rubs the eyeball. Evidence of recent removal of intured eyelashes should also be graded as trachomatous trichiasis.

5. CO: Corneal opacity is labeled when easily visible corneal opacity is present over the pupil. This sign refers to corneal scarring that is so dense that at least part of pupil margin is blurred when seen through the opacity. The definition is intended to detect corneal opacities that cause significant visual impairment (less than 6/18).

5. The causative organism Chlamydia trachomatis

5.1. Taxanomy

Chlamydial organisms were historically referred to as Bedsonia or Miyagawanella and were initially thought to be protozoa. Because of their small size and the problems encountered with propagation, they were subsequently thought to be viruses. In the 1960s they were classified as bacteria because *Chlamydia* express proteins (e.g., lipopolysaccharides) that are functionally analogous to other bacteria, divide by binary fission, are inhibited by antibacterial drugs, contain ribosomes, and are structurally and morphologically similar to gram-negative bacteria. However, Chlamydia are only distantly related to other eubacterial orders based on phylogenies of ribosomal ribonucleic acid (rRNA) gene sequences. Chlamydiae comprise their own order, Chlamydiales; a single family, Chlamydiaceae; and one genus, *Chlamydia.* The genus *Chlamydia* is comprised of four known species: *C. trachomatis, C. psittaci, C. pneumoniae,* and *Chlamydia pecorum.*

Chlamydia trachomatis is made up of three biologic variants or biovars: trachoma, lymphogranuloma venereum (LGV), and the rodent biovar that includes the mouse pneumonitis (MoPn) and hamster strains. There is 87% to 99% deoxyribonucleic acid (DNA) homology among the human strains and biovars of *C. trachomatis* but only 30% homology for the rodent strains.

With the exception of the rodent strains, C. trachomatis is currently known to infect only humans. The infections in humans include the conjunctiva and lower and upper genital tracts, including the rectum and lymphatics that drain the perineum. These infections are caused by the 19 currently recognized serologic variants or serovars (defined by monoclonal and polyclonal antibodies that react to epitopes on the major outer membrane protein MOMP of C. trachomatis.) of the trachoma and LGV biovars.

http://dx.doi.org/10.5772/53861

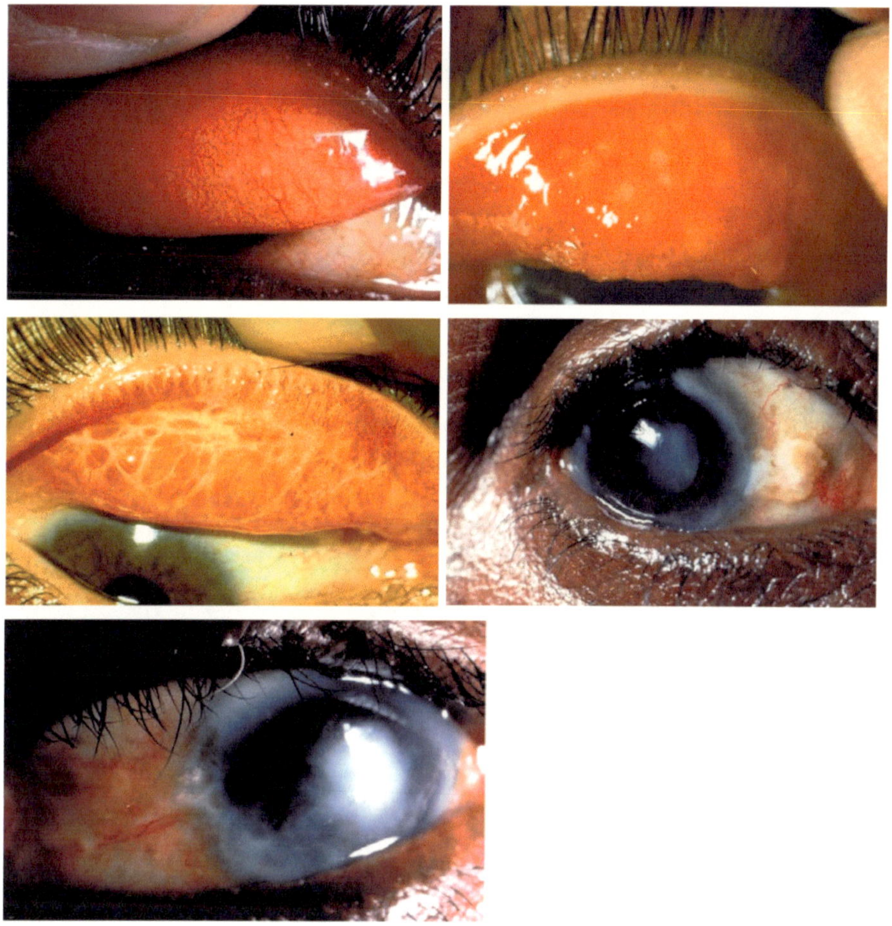

Figure 1. Top left: **Trachomatous Inflammation - Follicular** Presence of follicles on the flat surface of the upper tarsalconjunctiva.Top right: **Trachomatous Inflammation - Intense** With enlarged vascular papillae marked inflammatory thickening of the upper tarsal conjunctiva obscures the deep conjunctival vessels. Middle left: Trachomatous Scarring The scar (white/yellow) lines form a 'network' of fibrous scarring in the tarsal conjunctiva.Middle right: **Trachomatous Trichiasis** There is evidence of one or more eyelashes rubbing on the eyeball.Bbottom: **Corneal Opacity** The patient has significantly reduced vision due to corneal scarring.

Serotyping has distinguished these serovars into different serogroups or classes: B class (serovars B, Ba, D, Da, E, L2, and L2a), intermediate class (serovars F and G), and C class (serovars A, C, H, I, Ia, J, Ja, K, Ka, L1, and L3). Serovars A through K and Ba, Da, Ia, Ja, and Ka were previously referred to as trachoma-inclusion conjunctivitis (TRIC) strains. Trachoma is primarily caused by serovars A, B, Ba, and C, whereas adult and neonatal inclusion conjunctivitis are caused by serovars B or Ba, D through K, Da, Ia, Ja, Ka, L1, L2, L2a, and L3, which are the sexually transmitted strains of the organism. The LGV serovars tend to cause more severe disease and can invade regional lymphatics, whereas the non-LGV serovars are currently known to infect epithelial cells at ocular, respiratory, rectal, and genital mucosal surfaces.

Serotyping has been the most widely accepted technique for classifying C. trachomatis organisms. However, within the last decade, a new technique has been developed based on sequencing of ompA and is referred to as ompA genotyping. (ompA was previously called omp1, but the nomenclature has changed to be consistent with that of other bacteria.) This latter technique has been and continues to be invaluable for evaluating the molecular epidemiology, disease pathogenesis, and transmission dynamics of chlamydiae for STD and trachoma populations.

5.2. Chlamydia trachomatis development cycle

Chlamydia trachomatis are obligate intracellular parasites that are unable to synthesize their own energy (ATP) and are completely dependent on their host for energy. It has a unique biphasic developmental cycle not found in any other bacteria. There is the elementary body (EB) is the infectious form (spore-like particle) that posses a rigid outer membrane that bind to receptors on host cells and initiate infection. and the reticulate body (RB), which is the metabolically active form. Once the EB comes in contact with susceptible epithelial cells, it attaches by divalent cations and polycations, using heparin sulfate as a bridge between receptors on the EB and the cell surface. The EB is taken up into a phagosome by receptor-mediated endocytosis. There is ineffectual lysosomal fusion with the endophagosome because of their rigid outer membrane, and hence intracellular survival is insured.

A vacuole encloses the elementary body and the bacterium is now a reticulate body. Reticulate bodies obtain their energy by sending forth "straw-like" structures into the host cell cytoplasm. It can then replicate itself through binary fission. After division, the reticulate body becomes the elementary body. Anywhere from 100 to 1000 EBs can be produced per infected cell. In many cases, the cell ruptures and dies releasing the infectious progeny, but the cell can also extrude the inclusion body by a process of exocytosis and is released trough reverse endocytosis

6. Diagnosis

6.1. Clinical

A presumptive diagnosis of trachoma can be made based on clinical features, especially in an area where trachoma is considered to be present. The following signs are important indicators for trachoma, and at least two must be present in person diagnosed: follicles in the upper tarsal conjunctiva, limbal follicles or their sequelae, Herbert's pits, typical conjunctival scarring, and pannus. These signs along with conjunctival detection of C. trachomatis in the laboratory confirm the presence of endemic or hyperendemic trachoma in the respective area.

http://dx.doi.org/10.5772/53861

6.2. Laboratory

6.2.1. Cytology

The conjunctiva is swabbed with a Dacron or cotton swab, and the smear is made by rolling the swab over a clean glass slide. Alternatively, the swab can be placed in a special transport media for the respective diagnostic test. Epithelial cells that are clearly separated and the presence of PMNs, lymphocytes, plasma cells, or Leber cells (giant macrophages that contain phagocytosed material) can denote an adequate sampling of the conjunctiva. The degree of inflammation and bacterial superinfection can also be appreciated from these smears. Thus, although not diagnostic for chlamydiae, these findings are suggestive of trachoma. Giemsa stain is inexpensive, and the test is easy to perform, which makes it attractive for developing countries where trachoma is endemic or hyperendemic. However, the sensitivity is only about 60% and, thus, should not be used in areas of low endemicity. With this stain, the inclusion body is visualized as a basophilic, stippled inclusion in contrast to the dark blue to purple color of the cell. However, other entities can also stain similarly: These include goblet cells, bacteria, keratin, nuclear extrusions, and eosinophilic granules. Lugol's iodine stains the glycogen-containing inclusion of C. trachomatis. It imparts a dark yellow-brown color to the inclusion but is infrequently used, because it is insensitive. Commercially available fluorescent [fluorescein isothiocyanate (FITC)] conjugated monoclonal antibodies against the MOMP, which is species-specific for C. trachomatis, or the LPS, which is genus-specific for Chlamydia, are used in this test. The EBs are stained an apple green color and are visualized as extracellular round dots. The sensitivity for this test is approximately 80% to 90%.

6.2.2. Tissue culture

Although the intracellular inclusions of trachoma were first identified by Halberstaedter and von Prowazek4 in 1907, the actual organisms were finally cultured in 1957 by using chick embryos. Today, tissue culture has supplanted the use of eggs, which has made isolation of chlamydiae more widely available, although it is still only performed in specialized reference laboratories. Tissue culture remains the gold standard for C. trachomatis identification but is not 100% sensitive, probably because of the difficulty in maintaining a cold chain (4°C for no longer than 24 hours and then -70°C) from the field site to a specialized reference lab where the culture will actually be performed. Also, because some viability is lost on freezing and some of the trachoma serovars are more difficult to propagate, culture requires technical expertise, can take 3 to 6 days for results, and is very expensive. Many different cell lines are now available for culture, including HeLa and McCoy cells. Additional passages in tissue culture can increase the positive rate but have other drawbacks, including a delay in the reporting time of the results. Fluorescein-conjugated antibodies are used to detect the inclusions in cell culture, which are visualized as intracytoplasmic ovoid, round, or irregularly shaped inclusions. This stain imparts a fluorescing, apple green color to the inclusion body that stands out against the dark red cells that have been counterstained with

Evans blue. Peroxidase-conjugated monoclonal antibodies are also available for the detection of chlamydial inclusion bodies.

6.2.3. Antigen detection

ELISA or enzyme immunoassay (EIA) commercial assays are available to detect chlamydiae, but the sensitivity is only 70% to 85%. However, these assays can be cost effective compared with other commercially available tests such as the DNA detection assays. These tests detect the EB via polyclonal or monoclonal antibodies directed against the genus-specific chlamydial LPS. The antibodies are conjugated with an enzyme that reacts with a substrate to produce a change in color that can be detected by a specific wavelength in a spectrophotometer. One advantage is that a 96-well format can be used to process multiple samples at one time. Less technical expertise is required than for the above-mentioned tests. Another advantage is that the kits contain a confirmatory test.

6.2.4. DNA detection

The commercial LCR and PCR tests are the most recent assays to be developed for detecting Chlamydia. Primers that are specific for the organism anneal to the complementary strand of DNA after denaturation. This target DNA is usually the plasmid, which is only present in C. trachomatis and C. psittaci species. LCR amplifies a signal that occurs when the primers hybridize with the plasmid DNA. In PCR, the actual DNA is amplified after hybridization. Both tests can be used in a 96-well format in which 92 to 94 samples can be assayed at one time. Both products are detected by spectrophotometers that are set at specific wavelengths for the particular assay. An advantage to the commercial PCR test is that an internal control plate can be run in parallel with the chlamydial detection plate to identify which samples have inhibitors. Those samples that contain inhibitors can then be run by in-house PCR assays that employ a DNA purification protocol that removes the inhibitors.

Chlamydial DNA can also be detected by commercially available hybridization probes. These also hybridize with complementary plasmid or ompA DNA. The sample is usually a swab of the conjunctiva that has been applied to a special filter paper immediately after the sample has been obtained from the patient. Occasionally, DNA is extracted from a swab that has been placed in a special collection media and then is applied to a filter. In both cases, the filter is what is probed. The advantage of this technique is that the filter paper that contains the samples can be stored at room temperature under field conditions and transported back to the lab at a convenient time, without the necessity of a cold chain. The sensitivity of the probes is 70% to 90%.

6.2.5. Serology

There are two serologic tests for Chlamydia: the microimmunofluorescent (MIF) test and the complement fixation (CF) test. However, neither is specific for the organism because patient sera can cross react with different serovars and species and may represent current or previous sexually transmitted infection as opposed to conjunctival infection. The highest antibodies detected in the assay, however, are usually found against the initial infecting serovar, even on subsequent infection. This concept is referred to as original antigenic sin. Furthermore, ocular chlamydial infections tend to be chronic and endemic. Thus, these assays cannot be used to diagnose active infection, although occasionally MIF has been used for epidemiologic studies. They are also only available in reference laboratories.

The CF test is the older of the two and detects group-reactive antigen on C. psittaci and C. trachomatis. This test can be used for diagnosing ocular infections resulting from LGV or C. psittaci. The MIF test employs EBs representing C. trachomatis serovars and usually one or two strains of C. pneumoniae and C. psittaci. Sera, tears, and other bodily fluids can be used in this assay. The fluids are serially diluted and reacted against the EBs that have been applied and fixed to a slide in groups of dots. A FITC conjugated antihuman IgM, IgG, IgA or secretory IgA antibody is used as the secondary antibody to detect antigen-antibody binding. The slides are screened under fluorescent microscopy for fluorescing EBs that represents the respective serovar or species. Serum IgM and IgG antibodies appear around 2- to 3-weeks postinfection and persist for 4 to 8 weeks, although the IgG antibodies persist for much longer. Occasionally, IgM titers can rise again with reinfection or relapse of infection. Approximately 80% of children in trachoma endemic areas and 90% of adults with inclusion conjunctivitis will have detectable MIF antibodies. About half of the population in trachoma endemic areas will have both serum and tear antibodies, and the titers are directly proportional to the severity of disease and to the presence of chlamydial organisms in the conjunctiva. In one study in Tunisia, 80% of children with severe disease, 31% with moderate disease, and 17% with mild disease had tear antibodies to chlamydiae. Although the highest titers are usually against the infecting serovar in ocular infections, the MIF test can be used only for a diagnosis of active infection in neonates not in older children or adults. Neonates acquire IgG antibodies from their mothers, and when they develop conjunctivitis, these titers usually do not change during the course of the ocular infection. Most infected neonates do develop a small rise in serum IgM antibodies, usually less than 1:32, which persists for a few weeks.

7. Predisposing factors

Children are considered the primary source of infection because they usually become easily infected from close contacts during frequent play and within small, crowded households. However, female caregivers can also serve as an important reservoir in which the infection is passed to them and then back to their children. Thus, children younger than 10 years are at greatest risk for infection and reinfection.

Young women of childbearing age and other female caregivers are reported to have infection rates that range from 5% to 10%. These infections likely represent transmission within the household from and to children. Adult women develop more severe disease and sequelae than their male counterparts; repeat infection is considered an important factor in disease progression to trichiasis.

Other factors are low socioeconomic status, poor facial hygiene and lack of water. Flies have historically been considered vectors for transmission in Africa. However, data from recent studies do not support the theory. In one study, fluorescein was used to stain the secretions in the eyes of children. Within 15 to 30 minutes, the legs and bodies of the flies were also stained with fluorescein. Eye-seeking flies such as Musca sorbens have been shown to land on the eyes of multiple children as was reported in a study in Africa, but it is not clear how many infectious EBs can be carried on the flies, how long they are viable, and whether the inoculum is sufficient to cause infection. In The Gambia, of 395 flies captured from the eyes of C. trachomatis-infected children, only two were positive by PCR and could not be confirmed. It is certainly possible that flies carry other bacteria from eye to eye, which might promote inflammatory disease and trachoma. Indeed, in many trachoma endemic countries, there are seasonal outbreaks of conjunctivitis resulting from multiple bacterial species including Haemophilus influenzae, Haemophilus aegyptius, Streptococcus pneumoniae, Neisseria meningitidis, N. gonorrhoeae, and Moraxella spp. These infections may actually precede periods of increased trachoma prevalence rates. In a study in Tunisia, moderate to severe trachoma was found significantly more often among children with bacterial coinfections. Furthermore, pathogenic and nonpathogenic bacteria commonly colonize children who reside in trachoma areas. Coinfection of C. trachomatis with these bacteria may be one mechanism that is important for promoting severe inflammation, which results in conjunctival scarring and corneal vascularization years later.

8. Management

Management of trachoma involve curative as well as control measures. The World Health Assembly has resolved to eliminate blinding trachoma by the year 2020. To this, the Global Alliance for the Elimination of Blinding Trachoma (GET2020) was formed in 1998. Control activities focus on the implementation of the SAFE strategy, surgery for trichiasis, antibiotics for infection, facial cleanliness (hygiene promotion) and environmental improvements, to reduce transmission of the organism. Each of these components tackles the pathway to blindness at different stages.

8.1. Active trachoma

Antibiotics for treatment of active trachoma may be given locally or systematically, but topical treatment is preferred because:It is cheaper, there is no risk of systemic side-effects, and Local antibiotics are also effective against bacterial conjunctivitis which may be associated with trachoma.

The following topical and systemic therapy regimes have been recommended:

1. Topical therapy regimes. It is best for individual cases. It consist of 1percent tetracycline or 1 percent erythromycin eye ointment 4times a day for 6 weeks or 20 percent sulfacetamide eye drops three times a day along with 1 percent tetracycline eye ointment at bed time for 6 weeks.

http://dx.doi.org/10.5772/53861

2. Systemic therapy regimes. Tetracycline or erythromycin 250mg orally, four times a day for 3-4 weeks or doxycycline 100mg orally twice daily for 3-4 weeks or single dose of 1gm azithromycin has also been reported to be equally effective in treating trachoma.

3. Combined topical and systemic therapy regime. It is preferred when the ocular infection is severe (TI) or when there is associated genital infection. It includes: (i) 1 percent tetracycline or erythromycin eye ointment 4times a day for 6 weeks, and (ii) tetracycline or erythromycin 250mg orally 4 times a day for 2 weeks.

It is increasingly appreciated that there can be a major mismatch between the signs of active trachoma and the detection of chlamydial infection (Relationship between clinical signs and infection). This is a particular problem for control programmes in determining who should be offered antibiotic treatment; if only those with signs of trachoma are given antibiotic, many infected individuals with significant loads of infection would be left untreated. The WHO currently recommends that mass community-wide treatment should be used.

1. Determine the district-level prevalence of TF in 1–9-year-old children

a. If this is 10% or more, conduct mass treatment with antibiotic throughout the district

b. If this is less than 10%, conduct assessment at the community level in areas of known disease

2. If assessment at the community level is undertaken

a. in communities in which the prevalence of TF in 1–9-year-old children is 10% or more, conduct mass treatment with antibiotic

b. in communities in which the prevalence of TF in 1–9-year-old children is 5% or more, but less than 10%, targeted treatment should be considered

In communities in which the prevalence of TF in 1–9-year-old children is less than 5%, antibiotic distribution is not recommended

8.2. The sequelae

1. Concretions should be removed with a hypodermic needle.
2. Trichiasis may be treated by epilation, electrolysis or cryolysis
3. Entropion should be corrected surgically.
4. Xerosis should be treated by artificial tears.

8.3. Prophylaxis

Since immunity is very poor and short lived, reinfections and recurrences are likely.

Thus following prophylactic measures may be helpful against reinfection of trachoma.

1. Hygienic measures:

Transmission of trachoma is closely associated with personal hygiene and environmental sanitation. Facial cleanliness and environmental improvements the F&E components of the SAFE strategy are primarily targeting the transmission of C. trachomatis between individuals. Numerous epidemiological studies have found an association between dirty faces and active trachoma in children

Eye-seeking flies are a common feature of many trachoma endemic communities and have long been considered a potential vector. Chlamydia trachomatis was found (by PCR) on 15% of flies caught leaving faces of children in a study from Ethiopia.

Many trachoma control programmes actively advocate for general improvements in water supply (for face washing) and sanitation (to suppress fly populations). This drive has fortunately coincided with the setting of the United Nations' Millennium Development Goals (MDG). The target for the seventh MDG is to halve the number of people without safe water and basic sanitation by 2015

2. Early treatment of conjunctivitis:

Every case of conjunctivitis should be treated as early as possible to reduce transmission of disease.

3. Blanket antibiotic therapy (intermittent treatment).

WHO has recommended this regime to be carried out in endemic areas to minimize the intensity and severity of trachoma. The regime is to apply 1 percent tetracycline eye ointment twice daily for 5 days in a month for 6 months.

The future of trachoma control

In previously endemic countries in Europe and elsewhere, trachoma declined in the face of general improvements in living conditions and health. Such changes are beginning to happen in some parts of currently endemic countries. However, for many communities it may take many decades for general improvements in living standards to happen and to have an impact on trachoma. Therefore, it is necessary to pro-actively implement the SAFE strategy as the best validated approach to control this blinding disease. The limited published data on the impact of implementing the SAFE strategy indicate that even in some of the most highly endemic regions, such as South Sudan, significant reductions in the prevalence of active disease can be achieved.

4. The development of an efficacious vaccine:

Vaccine for C. trachomatis that would prevent and resolve infection has been slow largely because of the intracellular nature of Chlamydia and lack of ability to genetically transform the organism. However, recent advances in the field have identified some requirements for vaccine design. It is now generally accepted that MOMP, possibly with other antigens, would be important for a vaccine. However, because of the diversity of MOMP sequences that define different C. trachomatis strains, more than one MOMP would be required. The immune response that must be induced comprises mucosal sIgA antibody and systemic antigen-specific CD 4 TH1 lymphocyte responses. Protection of mice against challenge with

http://dx.doi.org/10.5772/53861

MoPn has been partially successful using vaccine strategies that include conformationally intact MOMP, naked DNA constructs of ompA and intact, nonviable organisms carried by dendritic cells.175 Other attempts at vaccination were less successful and included recombinant poliovirus or Salmonella expressing MOMP, denatured MOMP, or MOMP peptides (summarized in Brunham176). It is likely that a composite vaccine that includes intact MOMP, as well as naked DNA representing ompA from various strains, may be required to stimulate appropriate B- and T-cell responses, respectively. It may also be that only a few MOMP and ompA DNA strain sequences or only specific conserved sequences from MOMP and ompA are required to elicit a protective immune response. The development of the ideal vaccine remains a significant challenge.

9. Adult inclusion conjunctivitis

Chlamydia sexually transmitted diseases account for more than 500 million cases worldwide; but the exact prevalence of adult inclusion conjunctivitis is unknown because infection is usually self-limited and does not always reach medical attention. The primary source of infection is from cervicitis in females and urethritis in males. The spread is from "hand -to genital tract -to eye" (during sexual activity). The incubation period is considered to be approximately 5 to 19 days. Persons between the ages of 15 and 30 years are at highest risk for adult inclusion conjunctivitis.

9.1. Clinical features

Symptoms include:

Foreign body sensation.

Mild photophobia and

Mucopurulent discharges from the eyes.

Signs are:

Conjunctival hyperaemia more marked in the fornices.

Acute follicular hypertrophy predominantly in the lower palpebral conjunctiva

Superficial keratitis in upper hemisphere of the cornea.

Superior micropannus may also occur.

Pre-auricular lymphadenopathy is common finding.

Clinical course: the course of the disease is benign; but often evolves into the chronic follicular conjunctivitis.

9.2. Differential diagnosis

Adults develop a follicular conjunctivitis that can be indistinguishable from that of trachoma. The follicles may be present on both the lower conjunctiva and upper tarsus. The onset is usually acute with preauricular lymphadenopathy on the involved side and a serosanguineous to mucopurulent discharge. After 2 weeks of infection, corneal involvement is more prominent and includes keratitis, subepithelial opacities, and infiltrates that are marginal and/or central. Occasionally there is mild scarring and corneal vascularization referred to as micropannus, but these are late findings, usually among cases that have not been treated.

Otitis media is a common complication of chlamydial conjunctivitis. Although there can be prompt resolution of the disease, In addition there can be a genital tract disease (which failure to treat) resulting in the recurrence of the conjunctivitis.

Inclusion conjunctivitis is caused by serotypes D to K of Chlamydia tachomatis. The LGV strains (L1, L2, and L3) of C. trachomatis are responsible for a much more severe ocular disease referred to as Parinaud's oculoglandular syndrome. This syndrome is comprised of an inflammatory conjunctival response with severe lymphadenopathy involving the preauricular, cervical, and submandibular nodes. The LGV serovars are uncommon in developed countries with few reports in the literature but are very common in tropical and subtropical developing countries. Occasionally keratoconjunctivitis resulting from L2 has been reported as a consequence of laboratory accidents.

9.3. Treatment

The best form of treatment for adult inclusion conjunctivitis is to prevent chlamydial sexually transmitted diseases (STDs). Unfortunately, most chlamydial STDs are asymptomatic for males (approximately 40%) and females (approximately 70%) and usually go undetected because routine diagnostic screening for C. trachomatis is not performed. Thus, it is important to recognize adult inclusion conjunctivitis that is caused by C. trachomatis and treat both the ocular and genital tract disease. Because chlamydial STDs cannot be resolved by topical ocular antibiotics, systemic therapy is recommended. Most cases infected with non-LGV serovars will respond to oral tetracycline250mg four times a day for 3-4 weeks; Doxycycline100mg twice a day for 1-2 weeks or 200mg weekly for 3 weeks, or erythromycin 250mg four times a day for 3-4 weeks; when tetracycline is contraindicated as in pregnant and lactating females.

For LGV, the best treatment regimen for inclusion conjunctivitis caused by C. psittaci and C. pneumoniae is unknown, although 6 weeks of oral antibiotics has been successful in some cases for complete eradication.

9.4. Prophylaxis

Patient's sexual partner should be examined and treated.

Improvement in personal hygiene and regular chlorination of swimming pool decrease the spread of disease.

http://dx.doi.org/10.5772/53861

10. Neonatal inclusion conjunctivitis

Approximately 5% of pregnant women have C. trachomatis infection of the cervix.which if left untreated has 50% chance of the infant developing conjunctivitis. Neonatal inclusion conjunctivitis is more common (about 10 times) than conjunctivitis resulting from N. gonorrhoeae. The incubation period for chlamydial conjunctivitis is 1 to 3 weeks. Earlier infection can occur if there is evidence for rupture of membranes. If left untreated, the conjunctivitis can persist for 3 to 12 months. C. trachomatis is the leading cause of pneumonitis within the first 6 months of life. Rectal shedding of C. trachomatis does occur and is more common among infants with pneumonia. Onset of shedding does not usually occur before 6 to 12 weeks of age and can be as late as 12 months.

10.1. Clinical features

Conjunctivitis in the neonate is characterized by swelling of lids, a purulent discharge, and hyperemia. If without treatment, neonates are at risk for conjunctival scarring, keratitis, and superficial vascularization of the cornea. In addition, these infants if up to 6 months of age are at risk for pneumonitis.

10.2. Treatment

Treating pregnant women is effective in preventing infants from acquiring conjunctival infection, although retreatment may be necessary in high-risk populations. In infants, systemic treatment is recommended for the fact that topical treatment of neonatal inclusion conjunctivitis does not eradicate nasopharyngeal carriage, which can result in pneumonia or recurrent ocular infection. In addition, mothers should be treated for genital tract infection to prevent recurrence of chlamydial conjunctivitis in the neonate.

Author details

Udo Ubani

Dept. of Optometry, Abia State University, Uturu, Nigeria

References

[1] Alemayehu W, Melese M, Bejiga A et al. (2004) Surgery for trichiasis by ophthalmologists versus integrated eye care workers: a randomized trial. Ophthalmology, 111, 578–584.

[2] Batt SL, Charalambous BM, Solomon AW et al. (2003) Impact of azithromycin administration for trachoma control on the carriage of antibiotic-resistant Streptococcus pneumoniae.Antimicrob Agents Chemother, 47, 2765–2769.

[3] Berhane Y, Worku A, Bejiga A (2006) National Survey on Blindness, Low Vision and Trachoma in Ethiopia. Federal Ministry of Health of Ethiopia.

[4] Bowman RJ, Soma OS, Alexander N et al. (2000) Should trichiasis surgery be offered in the village? A community randomised trial of village vs. health centre-based surgery. Trop Med Int Health, 5, 528–533.

[5] Bowman RJ, Sillah A, Dehn C et al. (2000) Operational comparison of single-dose azithromycin and topical tetracycline for trachoma. Invest Ophthalmol Vis Sci, 41, 4074–4079.

[6] Burton MJ, Holland MJ, Faal N et al. (2003) Which members of a community need antibiotics to control trachoma? Conjunctival chlamydia trachomatis infection load in Gambian villages. Invest Ophthalmol Vis Sci, 44, 4215–4222.

[7] Burton MJ, Bailey RL, Jeffries D et al. (2004) Cytokine and fibrogenic gene expression in the conjunctivas of subjects from a Gambian community where trachoma is endemic. Infect Immun, 72, 7352–7356.

[8] Burton MJ, Holland MJ, Makalo P et al. (2005) Re-emergence of Chlamydia trachomatis infection after mass antibiotic treatment of a trachoma-endemic Gambian community: a longitudinal study. Lancet, 365, 1321–1328.

[9] Burton MJ, Kinteh F, Jallow O et al. (2005) A randomised controlled trial of azithromycin following surgery for trachomatous trichiasis in the Gambia. Br J Ophthalmol, 89, 1282–1288

[10] Burton MJ, Holland MJ, Jeffries D et al. (2006) Conjunctival chlamydial 16S ribosomal RNA expression in trachoma: is chlamydial metabolic activity required for disease to develop? Clin Infect Dis, 42, 463–470.

[11] Burton MJ, Bowman RJ, Faal H et al. (2006) The long-term natural history of trachomatous trichiasis in the gambia. Invest Ophthalmol Vis Sci, 47, 847–852.

[12] Centers for Disease Control and Prevention. (2001) Sexually transmitted diseases treatment guidelines,. MMWR Morb Mortal Wkly Rep, 55 (RR-11), 1–94.

[13] Dean D, Suchland R, Stamm W. (2000) Evidence for long-term cervical persistence of Chlamydia trachomatis by omp1 genotyping. J Infect Dis;182:909

[14] Dean D, Powers VC. (2001) Persistent Chlamydia trachomatis infections resist apoptotic stimuli. Infect Immun;69:2442

[15] Emerson PM, Bailey RL, Mahdi OS et al. (2000) Transmission ecology of the fly Musca sorbens, a putative vector of trachoma. Trans R Soc Trop Med Hyg;94:28

[16] Emerson PM, Cairncross S, Bailey RL et al. (2000) Review of the evidence base for the 'F' and 'E' components of the SAFE strategy for trachoma control. Trop Med Int Health, 5,515–527.

[17] Emerson PM, Lindsay SW, Alexander N et al. (2004) Role of flies and provision of latrines in trachoma control: cluster-randomised controlled trial. Lancet, 363, 1093–1098.

[18] Gray RH, Wabwire-Mangen F, Kigozi G et al. (2001) Randomized trial of presumptive sexually transmitted disease therapy during pregnancy in Rakai, Uganda. Am J Obstet Gynecol, 185, 1209–1217.

[19] Hessel T, Dhital SP, Plank R et al. (2001) Immune response to chlamydial 60-kilodalton heat shock protein in tears from Nepali trachoma patients. Infect Immun;69:4996

[20] Holm SO, Jha HC, Bhatta RC et al. (2001)Comparison of two azithromycin distribution strategies for controlling trachoma in Nepal. Bull World Health Organ;79:194

[21] Hsia RC, Ahmed I, Batteiger B et al. (2000) Differential immune response to polymorphic membrane proteins in STD patients. Fourth Meeting of the European Society for Chlamydia Research. Helsinki: Societa Editrice Esculapio.:219

[22] Hsieh YH, Bobo LD, Quinn TC et al. (2001) Determinants of trachoma endemicity using Chlamydia trachomatis ompA DNA sequencing. Microbes Infect;3:447

[23] Jones RB, Batteiger BE (2000). Chlamydia Trachomatis. In Mandell GL, Bennett GE, DolinR (eds): Douglas and Bennett's Principles and Practice of Infectious Diseases, Ed 5. Philadelphia: Churchill Livingstone.:1986-1989

[24] Khandekar R, Mohammed AJ, Courtright P (2001) Recurrence of trichiasis: a long-term follow-up study in the Sultanate of Oman. Ophthalmic Epidemiol, 8, 155–161.

[25] Mabey D, Fraser-Hurt N (2001). Trachoma. BMJ;323:218

[26] Michel CE, Solomon AW, Magbanua JP et al. (2006) Field evaluation of a rapid point-of-care assay for targeting antibiotic treatment for trachoma control: a comparative study. Lancet, 367, 1585–1590.

[27] Miller K, Pakpour N, Yi E et al. (2004) Pesky trachoma suspect finally caught. Br J Ophthalmol, 88, 750–751.

[28] Millman KL, Tavare S, Dean D. (2001) Recombination in the ompA gene but not the omcB gene of Chlamydia contributes to serovar-specific differences in tissue tropism, immune surveillance, and persistence of the organism. J Bacteriol;183:5997

[29] Ngondi J, Onsarigo A, Matthews F et al. (2006) Effect of 3 years of SAFE (surgery, antibiotics, facial cleanliness, and environmental change) strategy for trachoma control in southern Sudan: a cross-sectional study. Lancet, 368, 589–595.

[30] Natividad A, Wilson J, Koch O et al. (2005) Risk of trachomatous scarring and trichiasis in Gambians varies with SNP haplotypes at the interferon-gamma and interleukin-10 loci. Genes Immun, 6, 332–340.

[31] Natividad A, Cooke G, Holland M et al. (2006) A coding polymorphism in Matrix Metalloproteinase 9 reduces risk of scarring sequelae of ocular Chlamydia trachomatis infection. BMC Med Genet, 7, 40.

[32] Natividad A, Hanchard N, Holland MJ et al. (2007) Genetic variation at the TNF locus and the risk of severe sequelae of ocular Chlamydia trachomatis infection in Gambians. Genes Immun, doi:10.1038/sj.gene.6364384.

[33] Polack S, Brooker S, Kuper H et al. (2005) Mapping the global distribution of trachoma. Bull World Health Organ, 83, 913–919.

[34] Rabiu MM, Abiose A. (2001) Magnitude of trachoma and barriers to uptake of lid surgery in a rural community of northern Nigeria. Ophthalmic Epidemiol;8:181

[35] Resnikoff S, Pascolini D, Etya'ale D et al. (2004) Global data on visual impairment in the year 2002. Bull World Health Organ, 82, 844–851.

[36] Rottenberg ME, Gigliotti-Rothfuchs A, Wigzell H (2002) The role of IFN-gamma in the outcome of chlamydial infection. Curr Opin Immunol, 14, 444–451.

[37] Shirai M, Hirakawa H, Kimoto M et al. (2000) Comparison of whole genome sequences of Chlamydia pneumoniae J138 from Japan and CWL029 from USA. Nucleic Acids Res;28:2311

[38] Solomon AW, Holland MJ, Burton MJ et al. (2003) Strategies for control of trachoma: observational study with quantitative PCR. Lancet, 362, 198–204.

[39] Solomon AW, Peeling RW, Foster A et al. (2004) Diagnosis and assessment of trachoma. Clin Microbiol Rev, 17, 982–1011.

[40] Solomon AW, Holland MJ, Alexander ND et al. (2004) Mass treatment with single-dose azithromycin for trachoma. N Engl J Med, 351, 1962–1971.

[41] Suchland RJ, Rockey DD, Bannantine JP et al. (2000) Isolates of Chlamydia trachomatis that occupy nonfusogenic inclusions lack IncA, a protein localized to the inclusion membrane. Infect Immun;68:360

[42] West SK, Munoz B, Mkocha H et al. (2001) Progression of active trachoma to scarring in a cohort of Tanzanian children. Ophthalmic Epidemiol, 8, 137–144.

[43] West SK, Munoz B, Mkocha H et al. (2005) Infection with Chlamydia trachomatis after mass treatment of a trachoma hyperendemic community in Tanzania: a longitudinal study. Lancet, 366, 1296–1300.

[44] West SK, West ES, Alemayehu W et al. (2006) Single-dose azithromycin prevents trichiasis recurrence following surgery: randomized trial in Ethiopia. Arch Ophthalmol, 124, 309–314

[45] West SK, Emerson PM, Mkocha H et al. (2006) Intensive insecticide spraying for fly control after mass antibiotic treatment for trachoma in a hyperendemic setting: a randomised trial.Lancet, 368, 596–600.

[46] Wright HR, Taylor HR (2005) Clinical examination and laboratory tests for estimation of trachoma prevalence in a remote setting: what are they really telling us? Lancet Infect Dis, 5, 313–320.

[47] Wynn TA (2004) Fibrotic disease and the T(H)1/T(H)2 paradigm. Nat Rev Immunol, 4, 583–594.